YO... ...ELL!

D1604496

Dedication

To my children Philip and Victoria, and to all those
who are actively involved in changing our world
into a place of health, love, peace and joy.

YOU DON'T *HAVE* TO FEEL UNWELL!

Nutrition. Life-style. Herbs. Homeopathy.

A Home Guide

ROBIN NEEDES ND, SRN

GATEWAY BOOKS

First published in 1994
by GATEWAY BOOKS,
The Hollies, Wellow,
Bath, BA2 8QJ

Distributed in the U.S.A. by
ATRIUM PUBLISHERS GROUP,
11270 Clayton Creek Road,
Lower Lake, CA 95457

Cover design by Studio B of Kirkbean
Cover printed by Potten, Baber & Murray of Bristol
Set in Plantin by Oak Press of Castleton
Printed and bound by Redwood Books of Trowbridge

British Library Cataloging-in Publication Data:
A catalogue record for this book
is available from the British Library

ISBN: 1-85860-009-X

Appendices

Contents

Introduction

This book was written in response to the many people who have asked me to recommend one which would expand their knowledge of nutrition and allow them to take responsibility for self-healing and the maintenance of health – a tall order!

What I have done is explain most of the different facets of nutrition, albeit in a nutshell, so that they are all available in a single book for easy reference and comparison. Where greater detail is sought in a given area, there are many books written on most subjects outlined in these pages.

In terms of healing, I cover nutrition, herbs and homeopathy in detail, and only touch on the emotional, spiritual and energetic aspects of the self. There is no space for guidelines on consciously harnessing the power within us to direct the physical, energetic and emotional bodies. However, this area is of equal importance to overall well-being, everlasting energy, youth and happiness. A perfect individually-tailored diet will not completely overcome ill-health if thought-processes are negative, the spirit is low and the emotional responses to life are imbalanced.

What I hope to have imparted in these pages is knowledge with which you can restore your own health, and then maintain it in prime condition. To be able to do this really well it is important for you to have an understanding of how disease originates from within the body or mind, and why it is so important to encourage the innate self-healing mechanism, rather than suppress symptoms, wherever possible.

To this end, part one explains the difference between the orthodox and the natural approaches to illness, and therefore the reasons for the vastly different treatment method. This is followed by the evidence which indicates that disease does originate from within, and how simple it is to prevent this from occurring. A brief overview of only two healing arts – naturopathy and homeopathy – is explained, but a great many other very effective ways of stimulating normal life-function are available to us all.

A most important message in these pages is always to look at yourself as a combined physical, emotional and spiritual being, driven by an innate intelligent force – never think of yourself as a bundle of separate components. You have the key within yourself to change the way your body chemistry functions.

All you need is the intention to get on with it: *expect* to be well, program your mind to be fit, young, active and full of the joy of living at all times. Eat the type of food which nourishes the cells and use nature's pharmacy to assist your healing processes.

Never give up hope of a full return to health, as many of the most serious so-called 'terminal cases' have been so restored by natural healing methods. Be happy, positive, and live by the laws of nature, so that well-being can surely follow.

Robin Needes
Singapore, 1994.

Part One

PHILOSOPHY

I: *1. VITALISTS* v *MECHANISTS*

Disease is altered vital function, but its cause is viewed very differently by orthodox and alternative medicine. The modern allopathic doctor has come to believe that disease is the result of a destructive process, be it mechanical or infective. For this reason, he goes about removing symptoms, thereby unwittingly and sometimes deliberately blocking the body's natural healing process, which he views as destructive in many instances. Practitioners of natural healing, because of their different beliefs, call this suppression not cure.

Vitalistic beliefs

These are held by those in alternative medicine but also by a rapidly increasing number of orthodox physicians. Vitalism believes that the body is always trying to maintain the health of all its components and that this function cannot be directed by an inanimate biochemical component. Therefore we are not just a complex mass of chemical and physical reactions, which can be disturbed by outside elements. Instead we are controlled by some force which co-ordinates all the individual reactions that in turn make up a living organism.

Thus ill-health is considered to be a failure of the body's organising force to maintain normal chemical and physical reactions, and is not due to an external agent. Vitalists believe that the controlling force only fails when we deviate from living by the laws of nature, and micro-organisms move in only when the body's defences are weak.

Vitalism further believes that the signs and symptoms of disease are not caused by the external agent or disturbed chemical reactions but are a result of the body's self-healing attempt. To those holding this belief, suppression of symptoms with drugs is harmful, as it inhibits the natural restorative activity. Using inflammation as an example of self-healing, the redness, heat, swelling and pain are termed signs and symptoms but they do not emanate from the microbe – only from the healing effort of the body. The redness and heat results from increased blood supply to the area, the swelling is a result of fluid and white blood cells passing into the tissues for microbe destruction, and the pain is caused by the extra fluid congestion. This process is well documented in medicine.

However, orthodox medicine persists with the belief that the infecting organism caused the reaction, which is therefore destructive. They do not work from the basis that a weakened organising force allows the microbes to multiply for a start, and that the resulting inflammation is a natural response which just needs careful management rather than suppression. In natural healing, it is daily demonstrated that by simply strengthening the health of the patient, the frequency of infections is dramatically reduced. This supports the vitalist belief that disease cannot occur if the organising force is strong, so external microbes are not the cause; they are just opportunists taking advantage of an unhealthy body in which they can readily breed and multiply.

Micro-organisms may determine the type of disease but can only do so after a weakened body has allowed them in to breed on waste matter that it has not been strong enough to eliminate. Chronic disease is slightly different in that the damaged tissue partially causes the symptoms because the healing force is badly weakened and often hardly functioning.

Natural therapists do not object to removing infecting organisms as long as it is done with natural medicine given in conjunction with enhancing the body's resistance. We believe that disease is only possible if the body is susceptible through weakness. As an example of this, it is known that we all have the same germs in the mouth but some develop colds and others don't. It is the strength of the host which determines whether disease will occur or not. Even Louis Pasteur is said to have stated, "the pathogen is nothing, the terrain is everything".

The vital force

This term describes the energy or organising force within all living things, and was so named by the School of Montpelier in the 1700s. It interpenetrates the whole body and is widely believed to be the energy which is captured on Kirlian photography.

Vitalists believe that the vital force is the link between the mind and the body, that it operates the healing power of nature and is responsible for the state of health and vitality. It is what makes living things different from inanimate objects, and is the force which directs all our physical and chemical reactions. Non-adherence to the laws of nature results in a damaged vital force which is then likely to promote faulty body chemistry. This organising force is believed to preserve the function of every cell and protect them from decomposition. Vitalists contend that no living matter can exist without it, as it is the generating force of the organism, and only death terminates it. The introduction of any foreign substance into the body will disturb the normal function of this energy and lead to ill-health.

Mechanistic beliefs

Modern allopathic medical beliefs are called mechanistic, and although they also believe in homeostasis (balance), the orthodox doctor is taught that this is carried out solely by chemical and physical reactions and not by a unifying force. Since the middle of the 20th century, the mechanists have believed that the only difference between the inanimate and the animate is the difference in chemical complexity, and that only an external factor can disturb it. Therefore only an external treatment will cure.

They believe that we function as living organisms entirely as the result of a series of chemical reactions, which could be duplicated if science had all the ingredients necessary to make a human being. Attempts have been made, but so far science has spectacularly failed to prove its ridiculous theory. It has also failed to explain how the living elements came into being in the first place, if not as a result of a controlling force released by a supreme Creator.

The biologists (and therefore the medical schools) hold the belief that a cell's regulating DNA only functions as a direct result of chemical reactions. However, it has been clinically demonstrated that cells appear to have a form of intelligence which directs their function, and therefore their DNA, and that the mind can pass messages to cells and so influence their activity.

Vitalists believe that the DNA in every cell is the mechanical part of its incredibly wide-ranging activity, which is triggered by some kind of unifying force or intelligence. The vitalists have always believed that the animate is different by virtue of a controlling force which is disturbed by the individual's lowered resistance. Therefore the cure is brought about by strengthening the health of the person concerned and not by a suppressive drug. In the past, doctors used to hold the same belief, but the biologists got the upper hand in this century and so modern medicine reversed its theory of disease.

For those who hold mechanistic beliefs, suppressing signs and symptoms makes sense. After all, they are seen as emanating either from the external agent or as a result of the disturbed chemical reactions. Examples of this form of treatment are antibiotics to kill bacteria, antihistamine to block allergic reactions, anti-inflammatory drugs in arthritis, cortisone to suppress eczema and antipyretics to reduce fever. To contend that bacteria and viruses cause disease, and to then proceed to kill them within a living organism, without regard for the danger of this practice, has resulted in a high percentage of hospital beds being filled by people suffering drug damage. This practice is in direct opposition to the physiological functions of the body and is called mechanistic because it interferes with the process of the disease.

Unfortunately this orthodox view has become so widespread that people now routinely suppress the body's disease-eliminating efforts, because they think of them as emanating from the infecting organism and therefore as being destructive. A simple example of this is illustrated by fever, which is the body's method of destroying foreign organisms. The microbe only triggers the body's own healing response of fever, which will then immobilise the invader and destroy it. Any damaged tissue is restored by the body's normal self repair system. Suppressing the fever actually prevents it from destroying the microbe. Eventually a constant barrage of antipyretics and antibiotics weakens the body so that it can no longer throw off infection on its own. We have now reached the stage where even lay-people recognise that these treatments do not cure or halt the incidence of disease; orthodox medicine believes that the suppression isn't strong enough and waits for science to develop more powerful drugs.

The only way to break this vicious circle is to concentrate on building the resistance of the individual. Herbs and minerals can be used if necessary in place of drugs, as they will strengthen the body and cleanse it at the same time as destroying infecting organisms. Several clinical studies have shown that children with fever stay sick longer if given antibiotics. Those treated with just herbal tea and bed-rest recover quicker. When you consider that antibiotics are powerful pesticides, it is easy to understand that although they destroy the infecting organism, the body then has to recover from the effects of the poisonous drug. Any mother who has given her child several courses of antibiotics can testify that the child's health is weakened in the process. All of the orthodox treatments produce seemingly instant cures because the signs and symptoms disappear. However, the failure of these methods to produce a long term cure or to increase the disease-resistance of the individual has resulted in the rapid resurgence of the vitalistic approaches.

The brilliant 20th century biochemist, Roger Williams has described the individual's ability to resist disease as being inter-related with his nutritional health, his external environment and emotions. He further states that we are all biochemically different, and so each person must be examined in this light in order to determine how he can best decrease his susceptibility to disease. This often requires higher levels of particular nutrients in one person than another person would ever need.

By understanding the opposing views of disease, it is easy to see why 20th century doctors use drugs and surgery as their only therapeutic tools. Fortunately, a great many are turning away from this mechanistic belief and learning such things as homeopathy and acupuncture, as well as resolving to find gentle alternatives for drugs.

The disease process according to Vitalists

Acute disease is an acute elimination process which results from the cleansing and healing power of the body. This can only occur when the healing force is strong and the elimination channels working properly. Examples are colds, flu, fever, diarrhoea, boils and other inflammatory reactions. Vitalists assist this process by cleansing the body because it is a natural method for expelling toxins. It is nature's way of bringing disease to the surface of the body for final elimination. Orthodox medicine suppresses these conditions with drugs, because it views them as the destructive result of an infecting agent. Healing efforts and healing cures can only occur if the patient has the power to respond to the natural treatment. This means that the body must be purified and the vital force strengthened.

Sub-acute disease occurs when the vitality of the person is lowered to the extent that he or she is no longer able to manifest a healing reaction. This occurs as a result of deviation from the laws of nature and from suppressing illness with drugs. Sub-acute disease results in such things as mucous and catarrhal discharges, fluid accumulations, fungal infections, low grade fevers, inflammations and general aches and pains.

Chronic disease results if the sub-acute disease is further suppressed with drugs, or if the person's general health deteriorates because of a poor diet and lifestyle. By this stage the body is incapable of expelling anything, and this is when structural and pathological changes occur in tissues in the form of cancer, atherosclerosis, bronchiectasis, emphysema or less severe conditions like glue ear or chronic sinusitis. Symptoms at this stage are caused by the diseased tissue as well as the body's weak effort to eradicate it. Symptoms are also a guide to the fact that morbid disease exists. They act as a trigger to cause a person to look for medical help.

The vitalistic approach to the last two categories is to build the resistance of the patient and remove the cause of disease so that his or her own healing powers are restored. At the same time, we use safe interventionist processes where necessary to help relieve symptoms and restore the self-healing vital force. When the chronic stage is advanced, invasive intervention may be necessary to save life. Those of us who have moved from working within orthodox medicine to alternative medicine often have great difficulty in grasping a totally different approach to disease, but once we see it in practice, all doubts are removed. In fact, observing the healing power of the body can be quite awe-inspiring.

The discovery of all manner of viruses, bacteria, parasites, fungi and drugs to destroy them has done nothing to improve the health of the world and nothing to halt the relentless upward spiral of chronic illness. We were no worse off when we didn't know of their existence because in those days, it was normal to treat people by strengthening their resistance. The result of using antibiotics too frequently, is that we now have to contend with a breed of 'super bugs' which are fast becoming resistant to all drug therapy.

The fundamental truth which has been recognised by vitalists since the beginning of time is that only the health of the individual determines whether he or she will succumb or not. The external micro-organism is not the disease and nor are diarrhoea, fever or inflammation. The latter are the body's self-healing mechanisms actively pushing out foreign invaders. To suppress this is to weaken the healing power inherent in the living organism.

I: 2. NATUROPATHY

This is a healing system using the power of nature, and it is considered an art, science and philosophy. The naturopathic method of healing has existed since the dawn of humanity and its early history is in fact the history of all medicine.

The term *naturopathy* did not exist until being adopted by a German, Benedict Lust in 1902. He travelled to the United States in 1892 at the behest of the famous German physician Father Kneipp with the brief to introduce the Kneipp water cure system to Americans. While in the States, Lust became a qualified osteopathic physician and then practised this along with the broader concept of naturopathy. In the early days, this term indicated healing largely based on fasting, dietary manipulation and hydrotherapy. However, in modern times, naturopathy is not restricted to any particular modalities. It has come to mean natural healing using natural medicine with living by the laws of nature filling centre stage. Diet and fasting are still key modalities in treatment.

After completing all the science subjects, plus anatomy and physiology, diagnosis and pathology, a naturopathic student then spends a few years learning about diet, vitamin/mineral and other supplemental therapy, herbalism, homeopathy, Chinese diagnosis and acupressure, psychotherapy, hydrotherapy, manipulation and massage. The enormous success of naturopathy lies in the fact that it does not rely on just one method but uses whatever is appropriate on an individual basis.

Many of its methods are scientific, as naturopathy is partially founded on the modern sciences of chemistry, physics and biochemistry as applied to human biology and physiology. Its system of diagnosis uses many procedures common to orthodox medicine as well as several which are peculiar to natural healers only. The profession always seeks to keep pace with modern scientific research as well as advances in the natural healing arts.

The foundation of naturopathic medicine is based on the philosophy of *Vis Medicatrix Naturae*, 'the healing power of nature'. This phrase was coined by Hippocrates (460-370 BC) – although natural healing was around long before even that era. This doctor of ancient Greece practised medicine in a naturopathic manner and advocated use of the healing power of nature. He was specific in his opposition to harsh medication, to administration of drugs and to unnecessary meddling by the physician, believing very strongly that the body has a self-healing mechanism that must be aided in every way possible. It is ironic that the modern alternative practice of using drugs is carried out by doctors who swear on the Hippocratic oath. Hippocrates instructed his students to follow nature and do no harm to their patients.

Paracelsus, another famous physician, who practised natural medicine in the 16th century in Switzerland, said that nature is the physician and that the doctor should be her servant, not her enemy, in order to guide the natural healing process. He also emphasised that doctors must give nature what she needs in her battle against disease, and not throw obstacles in the path of recovery by interfering with this power of natural healing – examples of modern interference are panadol to suppress a fever and cortisone to suppress eczema and asthma.

Paracelsus went one step further and said, "In the human being there is present an invisible physician who produces, prescribes, dispenses and administers suitable remedies as occasion demands". Many other visionary doctors from past centuries have also affirmed the principle that the body is a self-regulatory and self-healing organism if the laws of nature are followed.

Philosophy

Naturopathic philosophy has never been static and is forever being formulated. However, it is rooted in the understanding that the curative force is inherent in the body as demonstrated by Hippocrates. It maintains that disease results from a failure to follow the laws of nature, and that a return will ensure that all conditions for proper function and repair of the body will be present. Furthermore, it states that the degree of departure from ideal living conditions determines the degree of ill-health.

The modern concept that physicians must fight disease rather than co-operate with nature to eliminate it, has divided medicine into two fields, *allopathic* and *naturopathic*. The philosophy of the naturopathic physician centres on the study of health and how to promote it, rather than the study of disease and how to suppress it. While the allopathic physician admits that nature does heal, the naturopath treats this fact as a law of nature which must always be obeyed.

Naturopathy arouses, assists and cooperates with the body's healing forces by using natural healing methods and assisting the cleansing and eliminating processes of the body. There is no drug that will restore cell normality when malfunction has arisen from disease; this can only be achieved by establishing normal biochemistry in the body with the help of nature.

When the body is functioning optimally, we are in a state of *homeostasis*. This means that all the internal systems of the body are maintained in equilibrium despite variations in external factors. Homoeostasis is maintained by the body's self-regulating, self-healing and self-repairing ability, but for these to function correctly, the diet must be ideal. If not, it will fail to supply the host of essential nutrients like enzymes and antioxidants, necessary for these functions and for the protection of the body against end products such as free-radicals and waste. When homeostasis is disturbed, disease results, and this begins within individual cells that, in turn, make up specific tissues and organs. When a cell's normal regulating and communication processes are altered, the disease process begins.

Naturopathic therapies

The application of the healing power of nature involves only therapies which support self-healing, and it definitely avoids using anything which interferes with this process. However, naturopathy also recognises that intervention is sometimes necessary but in so doing, it avoids interfering with the self-regulating process. For this reason it uses carefully selected natural treatments like dietary changes, vitamins, minerals, amino acids, herbs, homeopathy, acupuncture, hydrotherapy and tissue manipulation. Even when using these treatments the person is still always considered as a *whole* and not as a *disease*, because ill-health results from the organism as a whole being in a state of disorder. Treatment based on this precept can result in seemingly-unrelated conditions being cured at the same time from a single remedy.

It has been argued that using herbs is akin to drug therapy but in fact although they are an interventionist treatment they have been present in nature since the beginning of the world. Many herbs are in fact used as vegetables or flavourings and form a natural part of normal diets. Nature packages its plant cures with protective ingredients whereas modern medicine extracts a single ingredient or copies it in drug form and administers it with no safe guards and without building the health of the individual.

Naturopathy always aims to remove the cause of disease at the same time as restoring normal body activity. It treats causes, not symptoms, because that is the only way to restore vibrant health. One of the joys of using herbs is that they can be blended to suit the individual case. This means that in an infection, some can be chosen for their antimicrobial properties whilst others can be used concurrently to strengthen the immune system and support detoxifying organs. Because herbs have been present throughout time, the body has developed the means of using them to its benefit without side-effects – as long as the correct dosage is observed and the remedy is appropriate. One of the marvels of living species is their ability to adapt to new agents, but it takes thousands of years to do so completely.

Naturopathy seeks to build a healthy body, mind and spirit, it combats disease by altering the internal and external environment and by natural interventionist methods if necessary. It increases the vitality of the patient so that he or she can throw off disease by means of his or her own self-healing mechanisms. The *whole body* is treated rather than only symptoms. Circulation is improved, toxic waste eliminated from tissues and nutritional deficiencies replaced. Naturopathy uses nothing harmful or dangerous as laid down by Hippocrates and stresses the importance of prevention and education.

Living by the laws of nature

This involves living in such a manner that optimum health of the organism is maintained. The fundamental requirements are:

- a clean environment externally and internally – which means clean air, water and food as well as attention being paid to the function of all the body's elimination channels;
- sunshine and living in a temperature zone for which the body was designed;
- adequate rest, sleep, exercise and attention to personal hygiene;
- whole foods with no additives, eaten in a pleasant environment and to the point of adequacy only;
- a healthy, relaxed state of mind and a correct mental attitude to life – positive, creative, constructive and relaxed.

I: *3. BÉCHAMP* v *PASTEUR*

This chapter is included to highlight a very old theory of disease which has been proven by the work of many eminent scientists over the past 150 years. Most have worked independently but their conclusions have all vindicated the vitalistic approach to healing. In simple terms, these scientists have demonstrated that disease develops from within (when the body becomes toxic) and is not caused by external organisms. Micro-organisms may determine the type of disease but only after a weakened body has provided a fertile breeding-ground of waste on which they can multiply.

The story begins with the birth of Pierre Béchamp in 1816 and Louis Pasteur in 1822. Béchamp became a brilliant but politically uninfluential doctor of medicine, science and pharmacy, whilst Pasteur became a chemist, a brilliant marketing man and a friend of Louis Bonaparte. Béchamp held very responsible posts as professor of several medical universities, and it was he, not Pasteur, who first discovered the air-borne microbe, by finding it in fermentation processes, several years ahead of Pasteur.

Much later in his life, Béchamp found that healthy cells contained living organisms which, under unhealthy circumstances could evolve into bacteria. He called these microzymas, and discovered that they were imperishable and present in all forms of life (plant, up to human) from the beginning and until beyond the end. For this reason he considered these organisms to be a basic constituent of life and that any disturbance of these microzymas was the forerunner of disease in the body.

Béchamp then found that in death the microzymas became bacteria, reduced the body to dust and then reverted to microzymas. After finding these same organisms from past dead animals buried in chalk, Béchamp theorised that the airborne bacteria had evolved from microzymas in dead plant and animal life (human included). He was later to prove this theory and stated, 'The microzyma is at the beginning and at the end of every cell organisation. It is the fundamental anatomical element whereby the cellules, the tissues, the organs, the whole of an organism are constituted living'.

Louis Pasteur stole Béchamp's work in fermentation and then claimed that he discovered airborne germs. However Pasteur, rather than researching further like Béchamp, theorised that all disease was caused by these organisms and therefore that they must be destroyed. Because he was a clever salesman, his view prevailed over Béchamp's and he received funds to develop drugs to kill bacteria. Modern medical belief and its whole treatment-rationale is based on Pasteur's theory that all disease comes from outside. How different the world would be today if Béchamp's view had become established in medicine! Then everyone would have been taught that the airborne organisms are just altered forms of those found in healthy bodies, which only change to a toxic form when a person becomes unhealthy.

After Béchamp came several other scientists, particularly in Germany, who further developed his work. At the beginning of the 20th century, Günther Enderlein (1872-1968) began a life-study of the organisms in healthy blood and their relationship with the healthy human body. He called these micro-organisms *protits*, and found that they could either multiply or disappear. When they did start increasing in number the protits went through a serial evolution before finally becoming pathogenic. Enderlein confirmed Béchamp's belief that illness is always preceded by a change in these micro-organisms, and went on to develop a medicine which would reverse them back to the dormant form. Many illnesses were cured with his treatment and this doctor received world-wide acclaim.

Wilhelm Reich, an orthodox doctor, discovered in the late 1930s that a type of bacteria was present in the blood of most people, but that the numbers of these increased dramatically in anyone with chronic disease. These blood differences could not be seen on standard laboratory tests but only with special magnification. Reich's bacteria only proliferated after toxic conditions had developed in the body. It would seem that Béchamp, Enderlein and Reich were all seeing the same type of organism behaving in the same manner under identical sets of circumstances. That is, the microbes all multiplied and changed into a toxic form only when the body became unhealthy. In health they were few in number and in a form compatible with health.

These were by no means the only scientists who had discovered micro-organisms as a part of human tissue. Other European and American medical researchers also discovered them in inert form within pre-cancerous cells and noted a serial development to a disease-causing type in cancerous tissue. Notable amongst these was William Russell and Otto Schmidt, who were researching during the same period as Enderlein.

Dr Jószef Béres in Hungary, working from a different angle in his research during the 1950s, discovered that identical micro-organisms were present in human cancerous tissue, as in the cells of unhealthy plants and animals. He further discovered that these micro-organisms became obvious only after nutrients were depleted, and that they eventually became indestructible. Dr Béres states that, as a rule, scientists carry out their experiments under conditions where the nutrient supply is still near to normal, and therefore they do not detect these hidden organisms. It would appear that this scientist is also talking about the same type of micro-organisms that the previous researchers had found. That is, a type which only evolves into active form when the body has first been weakened by a failure to live by the laws of nature.

Dr Béres's research found that a lack of micro-minerals in food and therefore in the body, triggered the cancer in which he found the microbes. He believed that dormant pathogenic agents have to be present in all living organisms, but they multiply and are followed by disease symptoms only in case of disturbed metabolism and decreased resistance. He also stated that these microbes utilise the damaged internal conditions of the organism to proliferate and then induce their characteristic symptoms. Dr Béres found, when the micro-organisms were cultured in the laboratory, that by adding micro-minerals, the microbes could be prevented from multiplying and returned to the inactive form compatible with healthy organisms.

Dr Béres' research began with plants where viruses were found to be infecting potatoes, and aphids were spreading these from one to another plant. Some said that these external viruses were causing the destruction of crops, but Dr Béres proved otherwise by planting one half of a seed potato in healthy soil and the other half in mineral-deficient soil. Only those potatoes from the depleted soil were infected and grew deformed and infertile. The potatoes grown in the good soil remained healthy and resistant to surrounding viruses. In further experiments Dr Béres found tiny micro-organisms inside those plants, which had been destroyed by the virus. These organisms could be measured by the millions in diseased plants, but were negligible in healthy plants. Furthermore, the diseased plants, when placed in a suitable soil medium, were able to overcome their disease and begin to propagate again. Reich's findings in human blood parallelled this plant discovery.

During the same period that Jószef Béres was beginning his research, a Frenchman, Dr Gaston Naessens invented an unusual type of microscope (somatoscope) through which he could see a living elementary particle of life that moved and possessed the capability of changing its shape and structure. He found it in all life-forms, and called it *somatide*. Naessens discovered that he could culture the somatide in a laboratory and observe a cycle of development which went through three stages in health, and thirteen more in toxic conditions. Like Dr Béres's micro-organism, he found that the somatide was completely indestructible and returned to the earth after death of the host. Nuclear radiation strong enough to kill any living organism had no effect on it.

Dr Naessen's somatide is probably identical to Béchamp's microzymas and Beres's micro-organism, but the somatoscope shows it more clearly than ever before. All of these organisms develop into disease-causing form only when the body is weakened. Both Naessens and Béres have developed a treatment for returning the micro-organism to the form which is compatible with healthy life, thereby often reversing serious and deadly diseases like cancer.

Furthermore these two brilliant scientists believe that inert micro-organisms are an essential part of life in all things. Béchamp and Reich also held the same belief.

Under the somatoscope, healthy blood is seen to contain three stages of somatide development, as well as a proliferative hormone called trephone, which is necessary for cell division. Life does not exist without trephones, according to Naessens. The somatide development process is halted at the third stage by minerals and organic substances in the blood of healthy people. These minerals act by inhibiting trephone release, which in turn halts somatide change.

However, if a person becomes stressed or otherwise unhealthy, these inhibitors are reduced in concentration, and the somatide cycle continues through thirteen more phases, until the micro-organisms become diverse forms of bacteria and finally yeasts, which are completely indestructible even by massive doses of anti-fungal drugs. Once the somatide has developed to maturity and become extremely active, it bursts and releases an enormous quantity of raw particles capable of restarting the whole cycle. Naessens concludes that a deficiency of the mineral-inhibitors in the diet allows large quantities of trephones to form in the blood which then indirectly lead to diseased cells.

In terms of cancer development, these trephones are thought to cause cells to become more primitive so that they divide rapidly without intervening periods of normal activity pertaining to individual organs. For instance, cancer cells in the liver never function as liver cells. At this early stage the immune system is normally activated to destroy the cancer cells. People whose health is moderately below par may have this process being repeated daily in their bodies. However when we have weakened immune systems (as seen in people developing infections, allergies or auto-immune disease) the malignant cells are eventually not destroyed and so continue to proliferate into a cancerous growth. Once a tumour starts developing, Naessens states that the cells emit a substance which paralyses the immune system and its ability to destroy faulty cells. He calls this substance CXF and says that once CXF is produced, the body's defences are immobilised and the cancer can invade at will.

Dr Naessens has developed a camphor derivative called 714X, which when injected into the lymphatic system neutralises CXF. The immune system then recovers its power to destroy the growth. For anyone interested in being checked out on a somatoscope, the Complimentary Medicine Research Centre in London is presently using one to monitor naturopathic, electro-magnetic and homeopathic treatments. The microscope enables practitioners to determine disease before signs and symptoms develop, and the status of the immune system can also be accurately evaluated.

At this point it should be emphasised that the blood changes precede all forms of chronic and degenerative disease and not just cancer. This is why naturopaths emphasise maintaining the health of all parts of the body through proper nutrition. What this chapter does highlight is the need for food to be grown on organically prepared soil without the use of fertilisers, so that food will contain a wide variety of micro-nutrients.

The evidence that disease evolves from within, and only after we first become unhealthy, has become so overwhelming that it is no longer possible for any thinking person to ignore it. That is, an unhealthy body allows normal internal micro-organisms to evolve into a toxic form, and it also provides external microbes with the toxic conditions that they require in order to breed and multiply.

Researchers have proven their theories by developing means of reversing the process, and yet the knowledge has not become widespread and will not until conventional medical belief-systems are changed. The rigid view that disease comes from without, that the health of the body is irrelevant to the disease-process, and that all parts are separate and not coordinated by a controlling force is the major stumbling block. At least the present strongly-held view that one organism cannot change into another form has irrevocably been disproven by Naessens' microscope.

Since the beginning of the history of medicine it has been accepted that the human body must be treated as a whole, because that is how it functions. Failure to do so does not restore health. In orthodox medicine, that view was changed by biologists, who decided that humans were no more than complex biochemical structures, and therefore each part could be treated separately without taking account of the whole. They gave no credence to the unifying life force in living things, but stated that life derives only from a series of chemical reactions. On this theory is built the 20th century approach to orthodox medicine.

The massive failure of modern medicine to stop the increase of chronic diseases like cancer, arthritis, heart failure, bacterial and viral infections and allergies demands that other areas be explored. At the rate we're going, no-one will be able to afford the incredible spiralling cost of health systems which are clearly not working. In fact to call them health systems is a contradiction in terms.

At a London seminar in 1992, Professor Melvyn Werbach, from the UCLA school of medicine, reported that the rate of cancer in the US had risen from one person in six to one person in three between 1971 and the mid-1980s, and diabetes had increased by a whopping 600% in the same time-scale. Furthermore, when we look at the orthodox medical treatment for disease, statistics from the US and other countries show that approximately one quarter of all hospital beds are full of people put there by drug and surgical damage. In the

UK a government investigation revealed that around 10,000 hospital beds are occupied daily by patients suffering the ill-effects of drugs; 18,000 adverse reactions were reported in one year and 300 of these were in fact deaths caused by drugs. Worse still, the report indicates that the real figures are probably 10 times higher than these because many cases go unreported by doctors.

This is the obvious down side of modern medicine. The less obvious facet is that the suppression of disease by drugs does not cure; it just minimises symptoms and eventually weakens the immune system so that it can no longer heal or prevent cancer. If ill-health were approached by endeavouring to remove causes in the early stages then drugs and surgery would only be needed for life-threatening emergencies. In the old days when doctors had few drugs, they had to rely on knowing the patient and his environment as a whole and therefore used holistic healing methods with success.

The essential message of this chapter is that if we live according to nature we will not self-destruct, but if we follow our present lifestyles we activate micro-organisms within us which cause cellular malfunction and destruction. These organisms were never designed to be activated in a living species. Equally, living species were never designed to be healthy on food grown in devitalised and artificially-fertilised soil.

I: 4. BÉRES DROPS PLUS

This is a mineral supplement composed largely of micro-elements complexed with organic carrier-molecules. The product was developed in Budapest by Dr Jószef Béres.

His original research, thirty years ago, was focused on the humble potato and why it was becoming increasingly unhealthy. Dr Béres proved that the reason for the significant difference between the metabolism of healthy and infected potatoes was largely the excess of macro-minerals (artificial fertiliser) which caused the deficiency of micro-elements in the soil and therefore in the potato itself. These micro-elements play an important role in the biochemistry of plants, ensuring their resistance to disease.

Further down the line, Dr Béres started researching cancer because he discovered that 80% of cases occurred in the areas where the soil and food was extremely rich in lime, phosphorus, potassium and nitrogen (all present in large amounts in commercial fertilisers). In addition to testing the soil, he checked the well-water in the same area and found nitrates and nitrogen derivatives which had not previously been present. This indicated that the water supplies were being poisoned by fertilisers as well. Dr Béres asked himself if this could be the reason for the dramatic upsurge in the incidence of cancer since the 1930s. The death rate from cancer in Hungary was below 3.7% prior to 1930 but it had increased by 15% between 1956 and 1959 and by 20% in 1974. Prior to the Second World War it should be noted that fertiliser consisted largely of compost and animal manure; rich sources of micro-minerals. Only after the war did commercial fertiliser usage become widespread.

Dr Béres first injected mice with surplus levels of the minerals found in fertilisers and many of them grew malignant tumours. In other animal trials, malignancy was induced in those given feed enriched with lime, potassium and phosphorus. Dr Béres then started research on cancer tissue sent in by other hospitals and discovered the same micro-organisms (pathogenic agents) in human cancer tissue that he had found present in unhealthy plants.

The really interesting facet to this is that these organisms only became obvious in tissue (plant and human) after the exhaustion of trace minerals. In plants suffering from viral diseases as well as in cancerous organs in the laboratory, the pathogenic agents then multiplied rampantly leading to (in the case of plants) the eventual destruction of the host. It should be remembered that all soils become deficient in micro-nutrients after a period of using commercial fertilisers, and once the soil is deficient so will be the food grown on it.

When Dr Béres added trace minerals to the laboratory cultures of the micro-organisms isolated from the cancer tissue they actually stopped multiplying. The implication here was that cancer in people could be reversed in the same way. Dr Béres had already discovered that the same pathogens in plants could be inactivated by micro-nutrients to the extent that the host plant became healthy again. Eventually this visionary scientist isolated twelve different minerals needed to inhibit the proliferation of the micro-organisms found in unhealthy tissue. In all, seventeen components became part of the Béres Drops Plus, as Dr Béres felt that the body had to be restored at several levels concomitantly; immune system stimulation being of vital importance.

Dr Béres has treated hundreds of thousands of patients with Béres Drops Plus during the past 22 years and found them to be of enormous benefit in a wide range of diseases. In the early stage of any condition the drops will restore the organism's immune system and its ability to heal itself, and therefore Dr Béres believes that those who have recovered from cancer should take the mineral drops as preventative medicine. Because the product was originally developed to treat cancer, the major part of the research has been done in this area. Among Dr Béres's own patients, the only cancers which didn't respond well were those with poor vascularisation (sarcomas, neuroblastomas *etc*). At the opposite end of the scale, leukaemias responded well and the improvement was lasting.

Between 1975 and 1976 tests were carried out in different hospitals and clinics under the control of several specialists using Béres Drops Plus and dietary improvements. 235 patients with cancer were involved of which 223 already had secondary growths. All were in serious condition and considered to have no chance of recovery or improvement, and none had been cured by surgery, radiation or chemotherapy. At the end of the year 29.8% were 100% cured and 51.1% had tumours regressed to the point that they were almost complaint-free. These results are quite awe-inspiring. A side benefit was that healthy body weights were regained, appetites improved, osteoporosis stopped in some patients, as well as insomnia, fatigue, menstrual problems and visual disturbances. A most astonishing benefit was that of pain relief.

Even in those where morphine was no longer effective, the Béres Drops Plus either completely relieved or notably diminished pain over a period of time. The treatment also stopped hair loss, impotence, allergy and the nausea induced by chemotherapy and radiation, and it assisted the healing of wounds which had been present for years. Those who died in spite of treatment did so either from cardiac failure, pneumonia and other complications, or because their cancer was so advanced and rampant that nothing would arrest it.

Dr Béres summarised his research by saying that the drops are much more effective than the standard chemotherapy offered to patients presently and they are totally devoid of harmful side effects. It is not the minerals themselves which can cure disease; it is their effect of restoring the body's own self-healing ability. Some of Dr Béres' patients opt to combine his treatment with chemotherapy and find to their delight that the side-effects of the drugs are greatly reduced.

On the subject of pain relief, double-blind trials have indicated 40 to 50% greater pain relief with Béres Drops Plus than with placebo, in the case of osteoporosis, periarthritis, spondylosis, arthroses and lumbago. Other doctors have reported success in treating all of the following: poor digestion, fatigue, insomnia, headaches, anaemia, all endocrine (hormonal) disorders, nausea, asthma, bronchitis, cervical lesions, diabetes, allergy, hypertension, epilepsy, ulcers, arthritis, haemorrhoids and multiple sclerosis. Although MS is not cured by the treatment, symptoms are dramatically improved. The product has reached the West only since the fall of communism, but is now in widespread use, and we will see a great many more clinical trials being reported in years to come on a wide variety of diseases.

I have been particularly struck by the effect of Béres Drops Plus on the immune systems of my patients. The T-cell ratios are dramatically restored and even months after stopping treatment, patients remain well. I used to be frustrated by cases of low resistance to infection which responded only 75% to treatment, but most of those who then added Béres Drops Plus to their regime regained 100% health.

A most important lesson to be learnt is that it is disturbance of the organism's mineral balance which alters homeostasis (balance) and by extension, health. Unless we go back to natural ways of living and growing food, the human species will continue to weaken and develop horrible diseases. We are all concentrating on eliminating pesticides from our food and ignoring the more insidious danger of chemical fertilisers.

I: 5. HOMEOPATHY

It is not the purpose of this book to explain the many different healing arts. However, a chapter on homeopathy is included because a great many people are becoming increasingly interested in it and would like to understand the concept behind the type of treatment.

Homeopathy is a natural healing system based on the premise that *like cures like*. This means that a homeopathic remedy cures the same symptoms in a sick person that are produced in a healthy person who has ingested the substance in its natural state. For instance, the symptoms of arsenic poisoning are the same as are seen in a person suffering from food poisoning, and the homeopathic form of arsenic is used successfully to cure this condition. The word *homeopathy* comes form the Greek *omio*, meaning 'same', and *pathos* meaning 'suffering'.

The history of modern homeopathy begins with Samuel Hahnemann, born 1755 in Germany. This brilliant doctor turned away from medicine because it distressed him to see the harm done by blood-letting and the indiscriminate use of drugs. During his research he stumbled upon the knowledge that minuscule doses of Peruvian bark were an effective treatment for malaria. Hippocrates, in 400 BC, had also noted that small doses of herbs were a more effective treatment than large amounts.

Hahnemann started dosing himself (a healthy subject) with Peruvian bark (from which quinine is derived) and noted that he developed the symptoms characteristic of malaria. This was the beginning of what Hahnemann called *provings*, whereby he dosed people who were mentally and physically healthy with minute doses of substances like belladonna and arsenic, and then meticulously noted down all their signs and symptoms. The test subjects had to abstain from all food and behavioural stimulants so that these would not interfere with the symptoms being developed. The resultant provings were then used as symptom-pictures to be matched to those of sick people so that *like would cure like*. The more accurate the matching of the symptom-pictures to the symptoms of the sick person, the more profound the cure. This means that substances which cause specific symptoms in the raw state will cure the same symptoms in a sick person when presented in homeopathic form.

Initially Hahnemann treated people with minute doses of the raw substance but found that they often had severe reactions before getting better. For this reason he developed a system of decimal and centesimal dilutions called *potencies*, whereby the raw substances were successively diluted by a factor of

10 or 100. These were not just diluted but also *succussed* (violently bashed) so that they gained energy with each dilution. Beyond the twelfth potency, no molecule of the original product was present in the solution, and yet Hahnemann found that the higher the dilution the more potent the curative effect. Therefore potentisation removed the drug effect of substances like belladonna but the remedial effect remained.

Other examples of this form of treatment are ipecachuana, which in its raw state causes vomiting; in potency it cures nausea and vomiting. Opium, when potentised, treats coma, and petroleum, where it causes vertigo, nausea and a spaced-out feeling, will cure these symptoms when given in homeopathic form. Therefore, that which causes symptoms of illness in its raw state will cure those same symptoms in an unhealthy person if given in potency.

Today, modern science has an inkling as to why energy remains and works on living organisms. Scan machines point towards a form of memory being imprinted on dilute molecules, whereby they retain a knowledge of the vibratory energy of the raw substance. This memory is then passed onto the patient's energy-field so that it can effect a cure. 200 years ago, Hahnemann popularised the theory of a controlling energy field in living organisms known as the *vital force*. Today the *vitalists* even more firmly believe that it is this force which maintains the health of all living organisms, and it is this area on which homeopathic remedies have their effect.

An area of homeopathy called constitutional prescribing seeks to match a remedy to the person as a whole – that is, to his-her emotional, mental and physical state, since to build health, a person must be treated as a whole and not as a set of isolated components. It is often found that where a remedy matches an individual's personality, the physical symptoms related to that substance also fit many of the health problems to which that person is prone. If this is so, the effect of the remedy will be very great indeed. Where the pertinent constitutional remedy does not cover the present symptoms, it can still be used to strengthen the effect of another remedy chosen for its symptom-match alone.

A fundamental belief within natural healing professions, is that the mind and body are inexorably linked, and if one is affected so will the other. Therefore in chronic diseases the homeopathic remedy chosen should take account of both. In acute conditions where the vital force is relatively strong, it is only necessary to match the symptoms with a remedy for a cure and the personality of the patient can be overlooked.

Some of the most important homeopathic laws of cure are stated as follows:

- cure takes place from the top of the body down – from the head to the feet, from the inside out, and from an important organ to a less important one. An example of this is in asthmatics who as a part of their cure may develop a skin condition at the end of treatment. Suppression of that skin disorder with drugs will drive illness inwards again, back to the lungs in this case, and the asthma will return;

- cure takes place in reverse order of the onset of symptoms. For instance, in rheumatic fever the joints of the extremities are affected before those near the body, and then finally the heart is damaged. A homeopathic cure removes the heart symptoms first and the joints of the legs and arms improve last;
- functional symptoms occur before structural change, and those symptoms are produced by the vital force in exact proportion to the degree of disturbance. Using asthma again as an example, the wheeze will occur before the structure of the lungs becomes damaged;
- small stimuli encourage living organisms, and strong stimuli impede or stop their function altogether. This is expressed by Arndt's law, which we see in action when dosing the body with minerals. The correct dose stimulates the body's enzyme systems whilst a higher dose actually depresses them;
- the quantity of a substance needed to change anything in nature is the smallest amount possible. Why can we not learn from others' experience? Hippocrates discovered this fact 400 years before Christ and still it is ignored by modern science, be it in the area of medicine or agriculture;
- the quality of the action of the remedy is determined by its quantity in inverse ratio;
- action and reaction are equal and opposite.

Hahnemann stated that homeopathy cannot get rid of the cause of disease if it is mechanical or due to poor nutrition. He considered homeopathy to be largely a curative medicine rather than preventative, and stressed the importance of living by the laws of nature for the maintenance of health because a toxic body blocks the flow of the vital force on which homeopathy has its effect.

Part Two

NUTRITION in a NUTSHELL

II: *Introduction*

In this section I have separately introduced many different philosophies and dietary protocols so that you the reader can then make an educated decision concerning your own nutritional requirements. There are many books written on single subjects such as food combining or macrobiotics, but without a concurrent knowledge of other aspects of nutrition, it is difficult to make correct personal choices. For those who are interested in following up on a particular area, good books are listed in the bibliography. The purpose of the chapters in this section is to present each concept completely – and in a nutshell.

The final chapter, *The Naturopathic Lifestyle*, is in part a summation of all the preceding information. More importantly, I have endeavoured to give guidelines on which areas to choose and which to discard, based on a knowledge of your individual biochemical requirements. The laws of nature are highlighted with explanations about why such things as clean water and sunshine are essential to health. Lastly, there is guidance on balancing the diet, how to choose foods with good fats and adequate protein without relying on meat. The menu choices at the end can form the basis for any type of dietary programme, be it the meat-eating, vegetarian, vegan or macrobiotic one that you have settled on.

II: *1. THE ESSENCE OF FOOD-COMBINING*

This is a system of eating which was developed by Dr William H Hay at the turn of the century. It has since been used as the basis of books such as *Food-Combining for Health* by Doris Grant and Jean Joice, as well as *Fit for Life* by the Diamonds.

It all began when Dr Hay himself became very ill with Bright's disease and a dilated heart and was thought to be at death's door. At this stage he decided that medicine, with its obsession for treating only symptoms, was way off track, and he felt he had to treat the cause of his condition instead – a solid naturopathic and Hippocratic principle. Dr Hay started with his diet and decided to eat only natural foods. His calories were reduced to the extent that hunger was assuaged but overeating did not occur. Consequently, his weight fell and he was able to run long distances without experiencing any cardiac distress. Over the next decade, Dr Hay developed his system of food-combining as a means of reducing the acid end-product of digestion, which is still considered to be the major obstacle to a return to health. The main principle of food-combining is that protein and starch should not be eaten within the same meal, as a result of which food is processed better.

Correct food-combining ensures that the digestive system is not over-taxed. Protein requires an acid medium for digestion and carbohydrate an alkaline one, and if the two are eaten together digestion is certainly put under pressure. When meat is eaten with starch the higher acid levels in the stomach will more quickly neutralise the alkaline juices already mixed with the starch food in the mouth. The acidity levels are then reduced in turn by the alkaline in the starch food so that the environment for digestion of meat in the stomach is totally unsuitable. Studies have actually proved that in a mixed meal, stomach acid is one-third lower than when a purely meat meal is eaten.

Where protein and carbohydrate are eaten at the same time a wide range of different types of enzymes must also be produced at the same meal, in addition to both acid and alkaline digestive juices. When this occurs, foods are often only partially broken down and go through the gut fermenting, putrefying and causing gas.

In the early twentieth century it was established that protein in a meal reduces secretion of the starch digestive enzyme, amylase. On the other hand, a protein meal with no starch causes increased secretion of trypsin, an enzyme for protein digestion. This research proved that starch and protein together lead to reduced digestion of food. Incompletely digested protein is a cause of allergic reaction if the bowel is toxic enough to become porous. Combining starch and protein provides the toxicity.

Where digestion is faulty and toxic bowel conditions exist, even alkaline-forming foods are metabolised into an acid end-product. Where digestion works really well, energy levels are markedly improved. Just a few weeks of following this system of separating starch and protein will convince anyone of its value because it reduces fatigue, that heavy feeling (and the desire for a short nap) after a meal. It also ensures a good night's sleep, free of frequent waking and restlessness. For those with any digestive problems whatsoever, food-combining is essential to health.

In addition to correct food-combining, the Hay diet stipulates very high levels of fruit and vegetables because they produce alkaline end-products after being fully metabolised. Most other foods are naturally neutral or acid-forming. For this reason they are recommended in small servings only (as side-dishes to the fruit or vegetables on the plate). Processed and refined foods like white flour products and sugar were not allowed by Dr Hay because their acid-producing potential is even greater than that of natural grain. Acid/ alkaline food values are explained fully in the next chapter.

Dr Hay was decades ahead of his time and was pilloried by his medical peers for his beliefs, but that has always been the tool of the ignorant and is no different today, even amongst intelligent people. Dr Hay cured his own illness by his dietary formula and went on to cure a great many others of serious diseases. Today we are still seeing the enormous advantages of proper food-combining and choice of food.

The essence of food-combining is as follows.

Protein foods

These are dairy products, meat, egg white, fish, low-fat nuts and soya, and they may be eaten with the following:

- all vegetables other than potatoes and artichokes – but you may need to reduce other root vegetables such as carrots, corn, parsnips etc;
- neutral foods;
- acid and sub-acid fruits in small amounts;
- dry wine and cider.

Foods designated as protein are those containing 20% or more protein. Only one protein food should be eaten at a single meal, which means don't eat meat and milk together.

Carbohydrate foods

These include all grains and pulses (except soya) and they may be *individually* eaten with the following:

- all vegetables;
- sweet fruits in moderation;
- neutral foods;
- beer.

Foods designated as carbohydrate must contain at least 20% carbohydrate. Dr Hay did not allow any pulses because many of them have roughly equal proportions of protein and starch. However, their food value is too great to be ignored and small amounts should be in everyone's diet. When beans and lentils are sprouted, they become vegetables, and this is undoubtedly the best way to eat all pulses. Do not eat unsprouted dried beans with grains. Use one or the other with vegetables. A *little* cheese, milk or yoghurt is permissible with a carbohydrate meal.

Neutral foods

These may be eaten with either protein or carbohydrate meals and include the following:

- all vegetables except potatoes and artichokes;
- seeds and nuts;
- herbs and spices;
- wheatgerm;
- fats, oils and egg yolk;
- honey, maple syrup, molasses and raisins, if in very small amounts;
- alcoholic spirits.

Fruit categories

Fruit and vegetables at the same meal are often incompatible – it is better to eat fruit half an hour before a meal or three hours after, unless it forms the major part of the meal. Do not eat sweet and acid fruits together but either can go with the sub-acid category.

- *Sweet fruit* – banana, persimmon, sweet grapes, very ripe papaya and dried fruit.
- *Acid fruit* – citrus, plums, cranberries, strawberries, raspberries, pineapple, pomegranates and mangoes.
- *Sub-acid fruit* – all others such as apples, pears, peaches, cherries, fresh apricots, figs and grapes.

This diet requires combining either animal protein with vegetables or starch with vegetables. It does not combine meat, milk, eggs or fish with bread, pasta, rice, cereal or potatoes. Sandwiches should contain salad, avocado, sprouted alfalfa and a little cheese is permissible. Vegetable and nut/seed spreads are also delicious in sandwiches.

Aside from the food-combining, remember that vegetables and fruit are to form the major part of the diet, and protein, fat, pulses and grains are to be eaten in small amounts. White flour, white rice and sugar have no place in Dr Hay's diet.

II: *2. ACID-ALKALINE BALANCE*

Probably one of the most important factors in health is the correct balance between acid and alkaline in the body. If this is disturbed, disease, allergies and pain ensue.

When food is eaten it is oxidised, and the resultant residual ash is either acid or alkaline. It is the total balance of mineral salts in food which determines this acid/alkalinity, and where sodium, potassium, calcium and magnesium predominate over sulphur, phosphorus and chlorine, the ash is alkaline. Foods recognised by most people as being acid – fruit and vegetables – are actually metabolised into alkaline ash, whereas alkaline foods, like meat and grains, are metabolised to acid ash.

Where acidity predominates, it produces toxic blood, lymph and tissues which means dull skin, malfunctioning organs and cravings for even more harmful foods. Disease occurs, weight problems develop, aches, pains and cramps creep up, digestive disturbance may become a feature, aggression, depression, anxiety and fatigue are likely. Acidity lowers our resistance to infection, and it may also develop where allergic reactions to foods occur, and in people with faulty carbohydrate metabolism. Many factors can upset chemical reactions in the body and the metabolism of carbohydrate is highly vulnerable. When it is disturbed, the glucose from starch foods is only partly oxidised in the energy-producing part of the cells, and organic acids are formed instead of carbon dioxide and water. Sugar, which is neutral in terms of pH (acid-alkaline balance), and dried fruit which is alkaline, will both leave acid residues if carbohydrate metabolism is weak. This accumulation of acids will then cause carbohydrate metabolism to be further disordered. Dr William Hay discovered that incorrect food-combining, whereby protein and starch foods are eaten at the same meal, may also cause alkaline ash foods to become acid, as will eating when unwell or emotionally upset.

Acid-forming foods are important in the diet but they must be balanced by much higher levels of alkaline-forming foods, because the minerals in the fruits and vegetables are used to neutralise the acid ash. Where there is an imbalance, the body will withdraw calcium from bones to neutralise the acid and this is one of the reasons that serious calcium deficiency can often be measured in the bones of people in their thirties. With the increased use of convenience foods, young people are not eating enough fresh fruit and vegetables to balance the very high acid-forming content of their diets. Because a balance is extremely important to the correct function of many systems like the blood circulation, the body will rob other areas like bones to maintain a correct pH level of fluids.

Acid/alkaline-forming foods

The numerical values given to foods denoting their degree of acidity-alkalinity are determined by laboratory analysis, and because mineral content largely determines the values, results can vary according to the soils in which food is grown. This is why figures vary in the case of foods which are borderline acid-forming.

Green vegetable juices and vegetable broth are the strongest alkalisers but nearly all fruit and vegetables have an alkaline ash end-product. However in those with a weaker carbohydrate metabolism citrus fruits are often not properly metabolised to 100% alkaline ash. Cider vinegar can also be a problem in some but by neutralising it with egg shell, the residue becomes alkaline.

Alkaline-forming foods are as follows:-

- all fruit except plums, cranberries, preserved, pickled, canned and sulphured fruits;
- all vegetables except asparagus, broad beans, peas and Brussels sprouts;
- raw milk, yoghurt, whey, egg white, soya beans and tofu, aduki beans and kidney beans, chestnuts, fresh coconut, millet, buckwheat, honey and herbal tea.

Neutral foods are:

- almonds, brewer's yeast and all sprouted nuts and seeds, and pulses which have also been sprouted.

Acid-forming foods are:

- all other foods not in the above categories;
- all meat, fish, gelatine, cheese, egg yolk, butter, cream and any milk which is pasteurised, cooked, dried or canned;
- all nuts except those listed above – however nuts and seeds are close to the neutral range, as are their oils;
- all grains except millet. Refined grains like white flour are more acid-forming than wholegrains;
- all alcoholic drinks, coffee, cocoa, condiments, flavourings, vinegar and Indian black tea;
- all pulses not listed as alkaline.

Freedom from disease and good health requires a diet which is 75-80% alkaline-forming. The naturopathic diet provides this with its emphasis on fruits or vegetables forming the major part of every meal. People who adhere to this rule are not subject to colds and flu or serious chronic disease. Instead their whole chemical balance is correct so that every organ functions optimally.

II: 3. MACROBIOTICS

The term *macrobiotics* was first used by Hippocrates to mean a simple whole-some diet that would promote good health and longevity. The word roughly translates as 'large life' and Hippocrates used it in the broad sense without laying down any rules concerning the type of wholesome food.

Around the turn of the 20th century the concept was redefined by a Japanese, George Ohsawa, and further developed in the latter part of the same century by Michio Kushi. Ohsawa decided that whole grains would form the basis of a modern macrobiotic lifestyle, and proceeded to lay down very firm rules. However the Hippocratic principle of whole natural, un-processed foods is still central to the concept of macrobiotic eating.

The system embodies balance in terms of yin/yang as well as acid/alkaline. It emphasises choosing locally-grown food and eating according to climatic conditions. In terms of fruit, this means that tropical fruits should not be eaten in temperate climates. Ohsawa believes that seasonal health problems like colds and flu in winter are due to eating foods out of season.

The macrobiotic diet

This is largely composed of grains combined with smaller servings of veget-ables. All other foods are taken in very small amounts and everything is supposed to be organically produced.

The basic proportions of each food type are as follows:

- grains 50-60%;
- soup 5-10%;
- vegetables 20-30%;
- beans and seaweeds 5-10%;
- fish, seeds, nuts and fruit 5%, restricted to 3-4 times weekly.

At least two different grains are used every day and served at every meal. A minimum of six different types of vegetables with one serving of pulses are taken daily, and fish and fruit are restricted to three to four times weekly.

The grains in whole form are emphasised, whereas products made from them like pasta and bread are used infrequently. The advantage of this restriction is highlighted by the recent scientific discovery that some whole-grains become glycaemic when tampered with. This means that they may upset blood sugar metabolism. Therefore it is important to eat grains in whole form when such a high percentage of the diet is based on this class of food.

Wheat has been demonstrated to have glycaemic properties from the moment it is crushed, which means that even wholewheat cereal, pasta and bread can be a problem.

The *yin* and *yang* aspect

In terms of this type of balance, cereal grains are largely neutral; beans, buckwheat and millet are more yin and root vegetables slightly yang. Fish is definitely yang, and fruit and non-root green vegetables are very yin.

In this way, the high levels of cereal grains cover the middle ground, beans, buckwheat and millet counterbalance root vegetables and fish is balanced by fruit and other vegetables. Consequently the macrobiotic diet is perfectly balanced in terms of yin and yang.

In the summer more yin foods should be eaten as they are cooling, and this means more light vegetables, salads, light soups and fruit along with the same neutral grains, as in winter. When the season changes to cold, yang foods are increased – beans, seeds, oils, soya and fish.

The acid and alkaline aspect

All food, once it has been fully metabolised in the body, forms an end-product which is either acid, alkaline or neutral in terms of pH values. From this point of view all grains except millet are acid-forming, and so do not fill the neutral area on a pH balance scale.

The diet of a healthy person must contain more alkaline than acid end-products, but the macrobiotic model is only 30-40% alkaline-forming unless millet becomes a significant part of the grain quota. However, a small amount daily of seaweed, with its very high mineral content, would go a long way towards increasing the alkalinity. It is the mineral content of food which determines the degree of acidity or alkalinity. Seaweeds are very high in alkalising minerals so that small amounts would be capable of balancing much higher quantities of grains. Kushi states that his diet does produce a slightly higher alkaline than acid content.

Pros and cons of macrobiotics

The macrobiotic diet is very low in fat and high in fibre, and these features will guard against cardio-vascular disease and cancer. Because everything is organically-grown the food values are very high and the protein is of excellent quality. The proportions of 70-75% carbohydrate, 15% fat and 12-15% protein are in ideal balance. The seaweeds have phenomenal levels of minerals and vitamins, and in fact carotene in the *nori* variety of seaweed equals that of carrots.

Macrobiotics allows no dairy products, animal fats or refined oils – foods are cooked with cold pressed sesame seed oil. Nuts and seeds are encouraged as snacks and they are also made into spreads to replace dairy butter. This ensures that essential polyunsaturated oils are used on a daily basis. Healthy teas such as bancha, dandelion, chrysanthemum and barley replace coffee and fermented black tea.

One disadvantage is that the acid/alkaline balance really has to be watched carefully, which means ensuring adequate levels of seaweed daily and using millet regularly. A less rigid approach would allow more vegetables and fewer grains, and certainly the fruit could be increased. Fruit is very cleansing and should be eaten at least once daily. Kushi restricts it because of insecticides, but if you are buying organic vegetables why not buy organic fruit as well? He also objects to the sugar content, but as all carbohydrates are reduced to glucose by the body, it really doesn't matter whether sugars come from fruit or grain.

Another factor to be aware of is that grains, along with dairy products, cause more health problems than any other food because a high percentage of people are allergic to them. In these people a macrobiotic diet would be unsuitable. Kushi believes that drinking milk in infancy causes grain allergies later, but allergists would not necessarily agree with this statement. However the common grain allergies usually involve wheat, oats, barley and rye, so one could still go macrobiotic using rice, millet, spelt and corn instead.

The question of adequate levels of vitamin B12 also arises in this type of diet. Meat, eggs and dairy products do not form part of a macrobiotic diet, and although fish is allowed, research has shown it to be extremely low in B12. Very small amounts are found in spirulina, brewer's yeast, miso and tempeh, but no other macrobiotic foods. Adequate levels of other vitamins and minerals are also in doubt. For instance, vitamin D is virtually absent, and the very low proportions of dairy products, oily fish and green vegetables would not supply enough calcium for a growing child. Zinc and iron levels may be on the low side unless the bean/lentil content is increased. Seaweeds are not eaten in high enough proportions to supply adequate levels of macro-minerals – trace minerals, however, are well-covered.

Another point to consider when contemplating a macrobiotic diet is bio-chemical individuality. Some people are simply not suited to grain eating and fare better on large amounts of vegetables and fruit, along with small servings of fish, beans, nuts and seeds. It is important to listen to your body in determining your own perfect eating plan. What suits one often causes severe imbalance in another. For instance, some people feel incredibly sluggish, gain weight or retain fluid if grains are eaten every day, whereas others experience a profound sense of wellbeing.

Overall, the concept of macrobiotics is excellent, but from a naturopathic view point, the levels of fruit, vegetables and some nutrients are too low, and the acid-forming content is a little too high. However a slight shift in the percentages will easily change that. A lack of raw food could be altered by taking a percentage of the grains and all of the beans in sprouted form. For natural grain eaters this eating style will bring good health, vitality, balanced emotions and longevity. For those who cannot eat much grain, beans, fish and fruit can be increased a little and vegetables increased a lot, to attain the same percentages of fat, carbohydrate and protein and the same level of health. The root concept of totally natural and seasonal food, balanced protein, carbohydrate and fat and high nutrient levels is 100% compatible with good health, but always listen to your body and adjust the percentages of grains, fruit and vegetables as necessary.

II: 4. WHOLEFOODS

I am often asked about wholegrains, pulses or legumes, so here is a brief chapter on this subject to complement the preceding chapter on macrobiotics.

Grains

Grains are part of the grass family and include rice, wheat, oats, barley, rye, millet and corn. If the grain is whole it means that although it has been flattened, flaked or made into flour – no part of it has been removed.

- *Rice* has seven layers which contain vitamins, minerals, enzymes, protein, carbohydrate, fat and fibre. When rice is processed all of the outer layers, the husk and the germ are discarded leaving only the central white part consisting of carbohydrate and some protein. The final polishing of the white rice with talcum powder or glucose removes any last trace of minerals, B vitamins and most of the protein. Whole grain rice (brown rice) has only the indigestible husk removed; all the nutrients remain. Wild rice is native to North America and belongs to a different botanical family.
- *Wheat* products include bulgur, couscous, semolina, graham flour, bran, flour, gluten and wheatgerm, most of which can be bought as wholegrain products. If wheat is bought and milled at home, it is quite surprising how much bran is present in the resulting flour.
- *Triticale* is a genetic combination of wheat and rye. It is available as flakes or flour and has a higher content of protein than wheat or rye alone.
- *Millet* is a near-perfect food in nutritional terms and is definitely not only for birds! In fact bird millet tastes very different from the grain for human use. It is a common food in northern China, India and Africa and is cooked in the same way as brown rice. The Hunzas in Pakistan consider millet to be a staple food – and these people live to 110 years of age in very good health.
- *Pot barley* is the whole type of barley which contains the bran and the germ, whereas the pearl variety is processed. Barley is a delicious change from rice with a meal and is also often added to winter soups.
- *Cornmeal* is the whole form of corn starch (cornflour) and tastes like the whole corn. Use the finely- ground one as a thickening agent rather than the white nutritionally-dead variety. Allow a little extra time for the thickening to occur as the starch is not released from the wholegrain instantly. Use coarsely-ground cornmeal for Italian polenta and the finely-ground variety for corn bread.

- *Quinoa* is a very old grain about the size of mustard seed, which grows in the Peruvian Andes of South America. Its content of nutrients is very impressive, and is the best of all grains for vegetarians, all the essential amino acids being present. The US National Academy of Sciences describes quinoa as one of the best vegetable sources of protein because it has approximately double the amount found in rice or millet, and 15% more than wheat. It is also a good source of minerals, vitamins, fibre and omega-6 oils. Quinoa is not a grain in the botanical sense: it is classed as a fruit. However, it can be served in the place of rice or millet and is cooked the same way. It is also mixed with other grains and made into pasta.
- *Spelt* is an ancient grain which has again become popular. It is even higher in complete protein than quinoa with a 40% greater content than that found in wheat. This grain is unusual in that all its food value is contained in the kernel, so that even after processing, it contains high levels of nutrients.
- *Amaranth* is another ancient grain – this one was the food of the Aztecs. It too contains all the essential amino acids and can be popped like popcorn, and is sold as flour or as a part of a grain mix in pasta.
- *Buckwheat* is a seed in botanical terms but it is used as a grain. Buy the toasted form as it is easier to cook. Whole toasted buckwheat has a nicer texture than buckwheat groats. Buckwheat is 12% protein and rich in B vitamins and iron as well as the flavonoid rutin, which strengthens capillary walls. Buckwheat pancakes are delicious, though the flavour of the seed is strong and therefore possibly an acquired taste.

When the nutrient layers of grain are removed and turned into vitamin tablets (you pay twice for the one product) the white starch residue is not only of little use to the body, but is actually harmful. If a grain is eaten whole, nature has packaged it with the nutrients necessary for its metabolism, but if it is eaten in a denuded form then vitamins, minerals and enzymes have to be robbed from parts of the body to do the job. Where a person persists in eating white flour and white rice *etc*, they become weakened and less resistant to disease.

Sugar in natural form is either labelled molasses or muscovado, and these contain all the naturally-occurring nutrients. Any other form is processed and even brown sugar or demerara crystals are heavily processed. These are even more harmful than processed grains.

Ten proven effects of processed grains and sugar are as follows:

- the immune system is weakened, in that the ability to resist and fight infection is greatly reduced;
- blood platelets become sticky, and this triggers cardio-vascular disease and cancer;
- B vitamin levels are lowered, particularly vitamin B6;

- triglyceride and cholesterol levels are increased;
- menstrual disorders occur, including P M T;
- hypoglycaemia (low blood sugar);
- constricted blood vessels leads to hypertension;
- suppressed production of digestive enzymes and hydrochloric acid in the stomach;
- an overheated Kreb's cycle (energy production) in every cell, which increases lactic acid in the body. This in turn causes anxiety;
- obesity.

Pulses

These are all dried peas, beans and lentils, as well as fresh French and runner beans, peanuts, bamboo shoots, alfalfa and all soya products like tofu, miso, soya sauce, soya milk, soya oil, soya flour, tempeh and the original bean, cooked or sprouted. The Americans use the term *legumes* for this food family – which is confusing to French speakers, because to them the word means simply 'vegetable'.

Pulses are a very good source of protein, carbohydrate and a wealth of vitamins and minerals. If they are sprouted, the nutritional value increases between 200% and 2000%. Only the soya bean contains all the essential amino acids, but even so it is low on two of them, tryptophan and methionine. For this reason soya should also be combined with nuts, seeds or grains which have moderate levels of these aminos.

Soak beans overnight before cooking and add lemon juice to the cooking water to prevent gas problems occurring during digestion. Rather than buying beans in cans, soak a whole packet overnight and cook them all next morning. Small packets of cooked beans may be frozen and then thawed quickly in a sauce just before serving. Buy a book on sprouting and learn to grow your own beansprouts for salads. Children who have access to sprouts as snacks develop very strong immune systems. Beans may also be bought as flour: chickpea flour is called gram flour and is good as a batter on vegetables. Use lentils in soups and for paté and Indian dahl.

The soya bean has a multitude of uses, and its food value is very high indeed. The sprouted bean is good in salad. Soya milk can replace the cow's variety, and tofu is a low calorie source of quality protein. Only buy soya sauce in the naturally fermented form (*shoyu* or *tamari*) because the commercial ones are synthetically produced with chemical additives. Miso is a wonder-food made from soya, and just two teaspoons put into a soup adds enough protein for the meal. Again be sure of getting a naturally-fermented type as the processed varieties are full of chemicals, salt and sugar and are low in protein and other nutrients.

Nuts and seeds

These are excellent sources of protein, vitamins and minerals, and especially of natural oils. Those highest in the essential polyunsaturated oils are sunflower, sesame seeds and pumpkin seeds, flaxseeds and walnuts. A mixture of other nuts like almonds, Brazil nuts, cashews, hazels and pecans should be used as well. Buy only fresh raw varieties, as the roasted salted ones contain damaged fatty acids which are harmful. If roasted nuts are required, make them yourself in a non-stick pan with no added oil or in a low-heat oven, so that high temperatures do not damage the natural oils inside the seeds. Make only enough to last two or three days, to guard against rancidity.

Toasted pine nuts are delicious sprinkled on a salad, and a mixture of sunflower, sesame and pumpkin seeds makes complete protein. I blend these together with a little soya sauce and put them in a low temperature oven until crunchy. They are mouthwatering as snacks or on salads, but go easy on the soya or they will be too salty. Toasted sesame seeds are useful in many situations, and a paste made from them (*tahini*) is an essential part of many vegetarian recipes. One tablespoon each of tahini and lemon juice, plus one teaspoon of tamari, added to four ounces (115g) of yoghurt, makes a delightful topping for jacket potatoes. Chopped chives on top add colour as well as flavour. This mixture can also be used as a dressing for cooked beans such as chickpeas and served as a salad with vegetables to provide excellent quality protein. If the yoghurt is made from soya milk then the addition of tahini makes complete protein without the need for added beans.

Organic foods

Wholefoods are as nature intended for human consumption, but they should also be organically grown. Some people find that they cannot tolerate whole grain flour, and this is usually because they are reacting to the toxic chemicals sprayed on the wheat by farmers. Fortunately, organic flour is becoming more readily available worldwide. Only public demand will convert farming back to traditional methods, and we all need to play our part in creating this demand by choosing only organic products wherever there is an option. We owe this to our children and grandchildren, because as science is progressing, there will be no nutrients left in food in the next century.

Vitamins and minerals have already been accidentally programmed out of seed stocks in the development of such things as more square tomatoes and perfectly oval shaped potatoes. Many more seed stocks have also been tampered with in similar ways and now science is trying to add pesticides to the seeds so that they will grow with the plant.

The frightening aspect of all this is that, in time, no undamaged seeds will exist in the world. Companies making pesticides are presently buying up seed companies at an alarming rate. If this present situation progresses it will not be long before the only healthy seeds will be found with organic farmers who carefully collect them from their own produce.

II: *5. VEGETARIANISM*

Vegetarians who avoid meat but eat eggs and dairy products are called *lacto-vegetarians*, and those who avoid all animal foods are called *vegans*, although some in this category will eat eggs.

One of the dangers of following the vegetarian route is that meat is replaced by dairy products. Those who discard meat for macaroni or cauliflower cheese are not reducing their fat content, the acid end-product or the chemical load in the body. Cheese, like meat, is an acid-forming food which contains a lot of fat and chemicals. When choosing a vegetarian diet it is important to learn to cook dishes containing pulses, the more unusual grains, nuts and seeds. Buy a few specialist books and start experimenting with recipes, and in time it will become easy to recognise whether you will like a particular dish just by reading the list of ingredients. As with any recipe book there will be a handful of favourite recipes, a few mediocre ones and a lot that are memorably forgettable. Initially, set aside two days a week as meat and dairy-free and experiment. Some good books are listed at the end of this chapter.

The disadvantages of animal protein

Meat is not only very high in fat and cholesterol but contains horrendous levels of chemicals, antibiotics, pesticides and female hormones, all of which get stored in the animal muscle which we eat. People worry about the chemical load in vegetables, when in fact the meat is even more polluted. An anti-candida diet which calls for more protein is difficult to achieve because of the high hormonal and antibiotic levels in animal flesh. Even fish is suspect due to the increasing pollution of the oceans.

Where genuine wild meat is obtainable the situation is greatly improved. However, most venison is now farmed. Wild meat contains extremely low levels of fat and most of that is of the unsaturated variety. Of farmed meats, veal, beef, pork and chicken are the most poisoned. Young calves are taken off mother's milk very early and fed a canned powdered variety to which hormones and antibiotics are routinely added to increase the growth rate and prevent disease. Eventually all manner of processed foods including newspaper and animal testes, gristle, entrails and parts even unfit for putting into hamburgers become part of their diet. Furthermore the animals do not graze freely or exercise and this increases the saturated fat levels in their flesh. Any animal fed in this way often develops cancer very early on and a lot of it does not get removed during butchering.

Food which is considered unfit for human consumption has often been referred to as being fit only for pigs. Well, these days even the pigs get a raw deal as their food is very heavily laden with chemicals and contains wood shavings and newspaper at best. Chickens in battery farms are treated in a disgusting manner: their food also has extremely high levels of chemicals and all the essential polyunsaturated oils are stripped from the feed to give it longer shelf life. This means that eggs lack protective lecithin. They also act as reservoirs for the hormones and antibiotics added to their food. Even the flesh stores these and often contains more pesticides than heavily sprayed vegetables. Conversely, organic eggs are a near-perfect form of protein, and they contain the amino acid methionine, which is a protein vital for proper liver function. It is this amino acid which makes eggs smell of sulphur.

A high level of meat in the diet is known to cause the loss of many nutrients such as calcium, magnesium, iron, zinc, vitamins B3 and B6. It increases free radical activity and acid levels as well as causing cancer. Osteoporosis is more prevalent in those eating meat, mostly because of the raised acid levels in the diet. This indirectly causes the loss of bone calcium. Purines, which cause gout, are very high in meat, and they also cause the destruction of healthy bowel micro-organisms which maintain so many important functions. Eating meat does lead to early rapid growth, but equally it causes early rapid aging due to free radical activity and damaged genes. The high protein content of meat calls for a lot of digestive enzymes, which stresses the pancreas. If large quantities of these enzymes have to be produced for digestion then less may be available for the destruction of cancer cells. Menstrual problems are also often due to excessive fat from animal sources, and this can prevent oestrogen clearance from the blood, with consequent PMT problems.

Meat eaters who are careful to take only small amounts and ensure a high content of fruit and vegetables will not create an imbalance in acid/alkalinity. However all meat should be organically produced, wild or at least freely-grazed throughout life.

Stone Age man was originally a fruit, berry, seed and plant eater and he had big sturdy bones because of the high calcium levels in vegetables. Once the population began to increase, man turned to hunting wild animals and fish to supplement his diet, but this meat was extremely low in fat, the animals grazed freely and contained no chemicals. There are still hunter/gatherer communities in parts of the world and their diets are as much as 25 times higher in nutrients than modern man's diet. These bush people have no dairy products or bread and their meat is wild. However, the rest of us have to buy farmed meat with its toxic load – or become vegetarians.

Pasteurised milk

The cow produces a natural product which is really only meant to feed baby calves. For those humans who wish to drink it, raw milk is better but virtually impossible to find, because governments, under pressure from pasteurisation companies, have made the buying of raw milk largely illegal.

Pasteurisation changes the unsaturated content of milk to a saturated form and damages 42% of the protein, so that it cannot be assimilated. Long life milk is 72% altered, and it is this altered type of protein which causes mucous. Vitamin C is destroyed along with healthy micro-organisms and lactin (a streptococcal antibody). The Wulgen factor, an anti-stiffness ingredient in raw milk which is good for arthritis, is destroyed by pasteurisation, as are all enzymes including those needed for calcium absorption. Americans, with their heavy milk drinking regimes, have the highest incidence of osteoporosis in the Western world. Valuable trace minerals are missing in pasteurised milk, and radioactive iodine used in the process leaves traces in the end-product. Cow's milk given to children under one year is a major cause of allergy, iron deficiency and often leads to gastro-intestinal bleeding. Unpasteurised cheese can often be bought, and a homemade cottage cheese from raw milk is delicious with garlic, herbs or chopped nuts added.

The advantages of a vegan diet

Examination of a great many studies involving those who avoid animal foods indicates that the risk of osteoporosis becomes negligible on a vegan diet, and all manner of other diseases such as arthritis, asthma and psoriasis are improved. The immune system functions better with increased white blood cell activity and increased natural killer T-cells. When meat, eggs and dairy products are avoided a wider spread of foods are eaten, which means that nutrient levels improve dramatically. Saturated fat levels drop and polyunsaturated essential fatty acids are used instead, which protect against all of today's feared diseases. This diet does not contain hormones, antibiotics and disease.

Vitamin B12

Vegans have to concern themselves with this vitamin, as they are at risk of deficiency. The body stores B12 for years and even recycles what is excreted so that what you absorb, you get to keep. Many studies have been carried out on those eating a macrobiotic diet, and although some are B12 deficient, others are not. By examining the results of numerous studies, it is clear that a healthy gastro-intestinal tract ensures that absorption takes place as well as internal synthesis (we make a little B12 in the colon). Factors detrimental to this process are a very low salt diet with too much fruit and soya products and a toxic bowel. It is probable that those who food-combine correctly and therefore avoid fermenting food in the intestines, make all the B12 they need in the colon.

Fermented foods like miso and tempeh as well as brewer's yeast and spirulina all contain natural B12 in small amounts. Those who are concerned should take a supplement occasionally, and pregnant women should definitely do so. In this way the infant will be born with a store of B12. Alternatively, vegans could have a B12 injection every year to maintain stores.

Protein

One of the dangers of a vegetarian, and particularly a vegan diet, is that protein levels become inadequate. We need protein to build muscle, form cells and repair them. All enzymes are made of protein and these are required for every chemical reaction in the body as well as for digestion and the destruction of pre-cancerous cells. Protein is a vital part of haemoglobin to carry oxygen, lipo-proteins to transport cholesterol and the parts of the cell walls which act as transport vehicles for all nutrients going in and out. Antibodies, hormones, adrenalin and insulin are partly made of protein. Two thirds of body protein is found in muscle, other tissue and fluids and almost one third in bones, cartilage and skin.

When insufficient protein is eaten on a long-term basis, muscles become weak and flabby, healing is slow, nails and hair deteriorate, skin looks unhealthy, anaemia develops and fluids are retained. Does this conjure up a picture of a vegetarian you know? Eventually organ malfunction would occur. On the other hand those vegetarians who ensure small amounts of quality plant protein daily are a picture of health and are full of energy.

The daily requirement is much lower than previously thought – remember that berry/root/nut eaters ate sufficient protein. Meat eaters need 50-70g daily depending on weight, and vegetarians who combine their protein sources correctly require 45-50g. Some researchers say that 35-40g daily is enough for a vegetarian woman, as when levels are constantly low the body preserves what it has – it recycles more carefully than usual.

Protein is not hard to come by in a vegetarian diet as long as whole food is eaten rather than convenience meals. As you can see, these three low calorie meals provide nearly 50g of quality protein.

Breakfast
1 cup mixed fruit, 2.2g.
3 tablespoons yoghurt, 4g.
1 tablespoon sunflower seeds, 2g.
1 tablespoon pumpkin seeds, 3.5g.

Lunch
1 sesame pitta bread, 6g.
1 egg, 6.5g.
1 cup mixed alfalfa and mung bean sprouts, 4.5g.
1 tomato and half an avocado, 1.6g.
Strict food-combining would remove the egg and still provide enough protein.

Dinner
½ cup of lentil burgers, 8g.
4 asparagus spears, 2-3g.
½ cup broccoli, 2.3g.
½ cup sweet corn, 2.7g.
1 tomato, 1.6g.

Amino acids

Protein is made up of components called amino acids, and before protein can be absorbed, the digestive system reduces it to the individual aminos. These then travel to the cells where they are reformed into chains of different lengths, and containing a variety of combinations according to the type of protein being made (enzymes, haemoglobin or muscle). Body protein contains up to 23 amino acids, of which the human being can make 15. The remaining 8 are called essential because they must be found in food on a daily basis.

Essential amino acids

Animal protein like meat, fish, eggs and dairy products are called complete protein because they contain all of the essential aminos. Other forms of food protein, like grains, contain incomplete protein because one or more of the essential amino acids are missing, or present only in very small amounts. Some authorities rate soya beans as full protein because they do contain all the essential aminos, but methionine and tryptophan are much lower than the rest. Brewer's yeast and wheatgerm may also be considered complete in that all the essential aminos are present to greater or lesser extent. Combining vegetable sources of protein so that all the essential amino acids are provided in adequate amounts equates to excellent quality complete protein.

Protein pools

It used to be considered that two incomplete proteins had to be eaten at the same meal but it is now known that this is not necessary. Cells contain protein pools and there is a steady stream of them moving from there to the blood and back again, because we continually recycle protein. This means that any amino acid missing at a meal can be found in individual cell pools. However, all essential aminos should be eaten within the same day if possible to maintain balanced protein pools.

Vegetable protein combining

Any food in the left-hand column, if combined with any one food or stipulated group in its opposite right-hand column, will form complete protein.

Nuts, seeds in general	Wheatgerm
Sesame seeds/Brazil nuts	Pulses, wheatgerm, green vegetables or a mix of pumpkin and sunflower seeds.
Sunflower seeds	Pulses, wheatgerm, brewer's yeast or green vegetables. A mix of pumpkin and sesame seeds.
Pumpkin seeds or green vegetables	Grains, wheatgerm, mushrooms or Brazil nuts, or a mix of sesame and sunflower seeds.
Pulses	Grains, Brazil nuts or mushrooms. Sesame or pumpkin seeds.
Brewer's yeast or soya products	Grains, wheatgerm, mushrooms, sesame seeds, sunflower seeds or Brazil nuts.
Grains	Pulses, brewer's yeast, wheatgerm, pumpkin seeds or green vegetables.
Wheatgerm	Grains, all nuts and seeds, soya, brewer's yeast or green vegetables.
Mushrooms	Pulses, brewer's yeast, pumpkin seeds or green vegetables.

Using vegetables as a protein source requires that large amounts be eaten. Added sauce, chopped egg or nuts would increase the protein level.

High calorie nuts are not good sources of protein, as the calories are largely made up of carbohydrate or oil. These include pecans, chestnuts, coconut, filberts, hazelnuts, macadamias, pine nuts and cashews. Sunflower seeds are 30% protein and black walnuts have 40% more than the English variety. Sesame seeds are 25% protein and minerals and are a rich source of the essential amino acid methionine that is limited in pulses.

Protect the protein in your diet

Over-heating destroys protein – pasteurisation, grilling and toasting – so choose cooking methods wisely. Chew food very thoroughly to allow the digestive enzymes to break down protein completely. For those who have poor digestive systems, you will find that the digestibility of beans is increased by sprouting or cooking with a dash of lemon juice and moderate heat releases more protein from beans than the excessive heat of a pressure cooker. Increased levels of protein are needed in convalescence, after surgery, stress, breast-feeding, ill health, jet-lag and loss of sleep.

Net Protein Utilisation (NPU)

This is a method of rating the quality of protein in food according to its digestibility, the amino acid content, its ability to be used by the body and the proportion retained in relation to that which is lost. Where the NPU of a food is high then a great deal less protein is needed in the diet. Vegetarians, by careful combining, can be very healthy on small amounts of protein daily.

NPU is calculated on a scale of 1 to 100 and the numbers have been assigned by scientists. A food rated at 100 would be a perfect protein source and the body would utilise every gram. This means that 1g of body tissue would be developed for every 1g of food protein. Egg is the most perfect food source of protein and has a rating of 94 which means that 94g of body protein is made from every 100g of egg protein.

The following are the ratings of a wide variety of food:

Egg	94
Milk	82
Pasteurised	70
UHT	20
Fish	80
Cheese	70-75
Brown rice	70
Meat and wheatgerm	67
Buckwheat, oats and tofu	65
Soya beans	61
Cashew nuts, sunflower and pumpkin seeds, wheat	60
Mung beans	57
Sesame seeds	55
Walnuts, pistachio nuts and cornmeal	50
Peas, peanuts and chickpeas	45
Pinto beans	35
Lentils	30
Corn and mushrooms	72
Broccoli, cauliflower, Brussels sprouts, okra, potato	60

(*These vegetables have the same amount of protein per calorie as meat but 100 calories of meat is far less in volume than 100 calories of vegetables.*)

The really interesting thing about the NPU rating is that it can be increased by combining two different sources of amino acids; even two different incomplete proteins. This means that a lower volume of protein food will provide more protein units in the body. As an example, three parts of bread to one part egg increases the wheat NPU from 60 to 80, and beans plus wheat results in a 33% increase in NPU. In this way, combinations like brown rice and tofu have the same protein quality as an egg, and sunflower seeds with mushrooms relate in quality to fish. When two proteins are combined the NPU increases by 30 to 50%, and by doing this, smaller amounts are needed. Pulses increase 50% in value when combined with a complementary protein like wholegrain rice.

Menu ideas

Many vegetarian dishes are heavy to digest and high in calories because they combine grains and beans in the same meal. The following menu is for those who prefer lighter food that contains complete protein with very little in the way of dairy products. However, remember that is not necessary to protein-combine at the same meal.

Breakfast choices
- Sugar-free muesli and soya or almond milk.
- Mushrooms and wholegrain toast.
- Fruit with yoghurt, mixed nuts, seeds and wheatgerm.

Lunch/Dinner choices
- Always a large mixed salad at one meal and cooked mixed vegetables at the other. Include a wide variety of vegetables, particularly greens and mush-rooms.

Low calorie protein:
- Sprouted soya, lentils, or mung beans and sunflower seeds to form one third of the salad. All nutrients are increased by a minimum of 500% during sprouting.
- Tofu as burgers with added ingredients like tahini, lemon juice, soya sauce – or grains, grated onion, carrot and celery.
- Tofu with a curried sauce or simply soaked in soya sauce and browned in a pan.
- Soya yoghurt or tofu as a salad dressing base with added tahini, lemon, soya and spring onions or added mint and grated cucumber with garlic.
- A mixture of sesame, pumpkin and sunflower seeds.
- A mushroom dish with added nuts or a little soya or dairy milk as a sauce.
- Low-fat cottage cheese occasionally.
- A vegetable omelette occasionally.

All of these suggestions contain complete protein in the one meal.

Higher calorie protein:
Remember that a little goes a long way. These also contain complete protein.
- Brown rice salad with a yoghurt dressing and herbs or a vinaigrette, chopped vegetables and seed mix.

- Baked potatoes plus soya yoghurt or cheese, spring onions and perhaps mushrooms.
- Nut burgers such as nuts with onions and apple or nuts with mint and grated vegetables. Added wheatgerm makes whole protein.
- Polenta with a spicy tomato sauce and green vegetables. Cheese may be added to the polenta but do be careful not to use dairy products more than two to three times weekly.
- Wholegrain pasta salad with mushrooms and green peppers in the sauce.
- Millet burgers with onion, parsley and grated cheese.
- Buckwheat salad with a soya yoghurt dressing and added natural flavourings such as mint and onion.
- Lentil soup and wholewheat bread.
- Pumpkin stuffed with grain, onion, mushroom and a little seaweed.
- Spinach quiche with a wholewheat base.
- Hummous – this is a complete protein.
- Tabouleh.
- Bean casseroles and green vegetables.
- Lentil koftas, dahl or burgers with mushrooms.

Recipes

Here are some of my favourite recipe books:

> Sarah Brown's *Vegetarian Cookbook*. This is particularly useful as there are many recipes which do not incorporate dairy products.
> *Vegetarian Kitchen* by Sarah Brown.
> *The Cranks Recipe Book.*
> *The Magic of Tofu* by Jane O'Brien.
> Gail Duff's *Country Seasons Cookbook*. This delightful book divides recipes into seasons so that if you cook accordingly all the ingredients are readily available.

All of these books are published in the UK. If you live in another country, you will find vegetarian cookbooks quite easily available, if you look for them.

II: 6. *FATS VERSUS OILS*

In the early part of this century when cancer and cardio-vascular disease (CVD) were almost non-existent we cooked with animal fats and ate butter. Those in the tropics cooked with coconut oil or animal fat. For salad dressings we had access to either extra-virgin olive oil, village sources of genuine cold-pressed flaxseed and sunflower seed oils, or none. Margarines didn't exist, and oils were not commercially extracted with chemicals. Look at what we have today: shelves of giant containers of processed oils, stacks of margarines in the chiller and rows of shortenings for baking. We no longer eat butter or cook with fat but use margarine, shortenings and processed oils instead. At the same time the incidence of CVD, cancer, asthma, chronic ear infections, arthritis and other ailments has gone through the roof. Do you not smell a rat here? No thinking person can possibly ignore the likely connection.

These oil products are totally divorced from anything produced by nature, and are actually highly unsuitable as a food source for any living creature. They are killing us by strangling the life of every cell in the body. Even the expression 'only fit for pigs' is misleading because they too would die of cancer and CVD if fed on the oils we now use every day. It is true that total fats must be lowered. It is true that saturated fat and cholesterol from animal protein must be used in moderation. It is also true that polyunsaturated oils are essential to life; however all of these must be natural and *not chemically processed*. We used to get our polyunsaturates from raw nuts, seeds and any oils made from them were extracted with simple presses. Nowadays we get them from these horrendous oils and margarine on the supermarket shelves. By the time a manufacturer has finished with a sunflower seed, its mother wouldn't recognise it. In fact she'd throw it out, which is what we should do if we want to remain free of cancer and other horrors.

Since the beginning of the 20th century the total fat in our diets has risen by about 35%, and this must be reduced. However a close look at the statistics tells a fascinating tale. Saturated fats from animal products account for only about one third of this increase and of those, milk and butter consumption have gone down by at least half. Meat intake has risen and cheese usage has trebled. The cholesterol intake has not altered in the last one hundred years. The very dramatic increase in fats comes from chemically-extracted oils and margarines, where consumption has gone up ten times! This figure is made up of vegetable shortenings, margarines, salad and cooking oils which are made of unsaturated fats.

The percentage of total fats in the diet has gone up to 40% or more in many cultures. Nutritional researchers are urging a level below 30%, but it should be around 18 to 20% for good health. In countries like Japan, where there is a low level of heart disease, the people consume only 18% of calories as fats, and natural oils form a major part of this. These figures apply only to those following a traditional Japanese diet.

Clearly our health problems are intricately tied up with the processed fats used in commercially prepared oils, shortenings, margarines, salad dressings, mayonnaise, biscuits, cakes, crackers, prepared meals, pastries and a multitude of snack foods like crisps and chips. The rate of heart disease and cancer is certainly climbing with the increase of sales of these products.

Because the oils used in processed foods are polyunsaturated, we are fooled into a false sense of security. The reality is that the oils are extracted by petrochemicals and then heated to excessive temperatures. This leads to a change in the structure of the oil molecule, so that it becomes something not known in nature.

Before explaining the processing of oils and the importance of natural polyunsaturates it may help to first describe the different types of fats.

Fatty acids – what are they?

Just as amino acids are the building blocks for proteins and letters of the alphabet are building blocks for words, so fatty acids form fats and oils. Fatty acids are generally classified according to the degree of saturation or by the number of carbon atoms in a chain.

Saturated fatty acids are so called because all of the carbon atoms are linked to hydrogen. The most common saturates occur in animal fat, dairy products, palm and coconut oil.

Monounsaturated fatty acids contain fewer hydrogen atoms and are therefore softer and disperse more easily. Olive and almond oils are monounsaturates and are also known as omega-9 oils.

Unsaturated (polyunsaturated) fatty acids are the most liquid and are absolutely vital to life, but only as long as they are undamaged. The terms unsaturated and polyunsaturated are interchangeable. It is these oils which this chapter is all about, and an understanding of them is absolutely essential if you are to keep you and your family healthy.

There are two essential polyunsaturates, so called because we cannot make them in the body and must get them from food. In the past we got these oils from raw nuts, seeds, and cold water fish, but now we have a choice. Either we continue to use these and live in good health, or we buy chemically-processed oils and margarines, as well as products made from them, and eventually die from a horrible disease. Statistics indicate that by the end of this century 1 in every 2 people will die of CVD and 1 in every 3 will get cancer. Many will have both. Don't just think of the oils themselves but the crisps, snacks, pastries, biscuits, cakes, dressings, mayonnaises and desserts made from them. Modern medicine is delaying deaths but not preventing serious diseases.

The natural oils are a part of nature, as we are. The polyunsaturates in margarines and other products are not known in nature but are widely available in plastic and vulcanised rubber. Is this what you want to eat? There are literally thousands of polyunsaturates available in industry, and they are all akin to those found in margarine and shortenings. It is the processing of these oils that changes the chemical structure so that they no longer resemble the original natural oil. Feeding these commercial products to the family is no better than a slow drip feed of arsenic. The damage is just as insidious and the outcome as certain.

Triglycerides are the form in which fatty acids are stored in the food chain and in the human body. Fats enter the body as triglycerides which are then broken down into the individual fatty acids before being reformed into the types required by the body, of which one is phospholipids.

Phospholipids are a type of fat which the body forms to use as cell walls. These consist of two fatty acids, one of which is usually a polyunsaturate. Lecithin is the best-known phospholipid and it is used to emulsify fats and cholesterol in the body, dissolve gallstones and supply the B vitamin choline which is essential for liver and brain function.

Cholesterol is a fat-like material found in the food chain but it is also synthesised by the liver in large amounts for making sex and adrenal hormones and for firming up cell walls. Cholesterol is essential for making bile salts, for the vitamin D conversion in the skin and for the making of nerve sheaths. 2000mg may be made by the body in a single day. The main ingredients required for cholesterol manufacture are the acetates which result from the breakdown of all kinds of fats, and also from sugar and white flour. The more of these in the diet the higher the rate of unnecessary cholesterol synthesis. So to lower excessive cholesterol levels in the blood, all of these foods must be reduced. The fatty acids from processed oils and margarine are very readily converted to cholesterol because the human body cannot use these alien products for any important activity, only for energy and fat storage. The incidence of cardio-vascular disease is high because sugar, white flour and total fats in the form of oil and margarine have increased dramatically, whereas our cholesterol intake *per se* has not altered in living memory.

Essential polyunsaturated oils

Another name for these is essential fatty acids (EFAs), and they are some-

Essential Polyunsaturated Oils

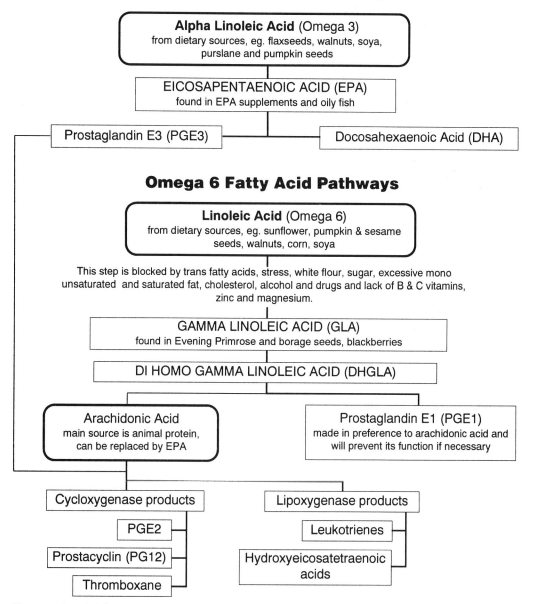

Omega 3 Fatty Acid Pathways

Alpha Linoleic Acid (Omega 3)
from dietary sources, eg. flaxseeds, walnuts, soya,
purslane and pumpkin seeds

EICOSAPENTAENOIC ACID (EPA)
found in EPA supplements and oily fish

Prostaglandin E3 (PGE3)   Docosahexaenoic Acid (DHA)

Omega 6 Fatty Acid Pathways

Linoleic Acid (Omega 6)
from dietary sources, eg. sunflower, pumpkin & sesame
seeds, walnuts, corn, soya

This step is blocked by trans fatty acids, stress, white flour, sugar, excessive mono
unsaturated and saturated fat, cholesterol, alcohol and drugs and lack of B & C vitamins,
zinc and magnesium.

GAMMA LINOLEIC ACID (GLA)
found in Evening Primrose and borage seeds, blackberries

DI HOMO GAMMA LINOLEIC ACID (DHGLA)

Arachidonic Acid
main source is animal protein,
can be replaced by EPA

Prostaglandin E1 (PGE1)
made in preference to arachidonic acid and
will prevent its function if necessary

Cycloxygenase products   Lipoxygenase products

PGE2   Leukotrienes

Prostacyclin (PG12)   Hydroxyeicosatetraenoic
acids

Thromboxane

These are largely inflammatory chemicals but when arachidonic acid is replaced by PGE3,
the effects are greatly reduced. The anti inflammatory prostacyclin is increased by PGE3.
There must be a balance between PGE1, E3 and the cycloxygenase/lipoxygenase
products; our modern diet does not provide this.

times also called vitamin F because they are a form of fatty vitamins. They are called essential partly because we cannot live in health without them, and partly because we cannot make them in our bodies. EFA must be found in the food chain and in their natural state. There are two types:

Linoleic acid (also known as omega-6 oil) is found in sunflower, safflower, sesame and pumpkin seeds, soya beans and walnuts in appreciable amounts. There is some in foods with lower oil content like corn, pulses, kidney, liver and brain. Most nuts also contain linoleic acid, but in combination with much higher percentages of monounsaturated oils as well as some saturates.

Alpha linolenic acid (also known as omega-3 oil) is found in flaxseeds and oily fish like salmon, sardines, mackerel and river trout. It is also found in small amounts in pumpkin seeds, soya beans, walnuts, rapeseeds (toxic) and some green vegetables. Other nuts and seeds contain none.

40% of our fat intake used to come from omega-3 oil but this has now dropped to 3% at best. The omega-6 oils are now much higher in our diets and almost exclusively as dangerous processed oils, margarines and shortenings hidden throughout processed foods.

Throughout this chapter I shall refer to these two types of oils as EFAs, or by their easier individual names of omega-3 and -6, so fix in your mind that omega-6 equates with seeds and omega-3 with oily fish and flaxseeds. Also remember that they are only healthy if they are as nature made them.

Why can't we do without these EFAs? They are as vital as cholesterol for making the walls around every cell in the body, but more importantly they are responsible for the fluidity of the wall, which enables all the nutrients to pass in and out of cells. EFAs also prevent bacteria, viruses and toxic substances from entering and destroying cells. They help prevent cells from becoming cancerous. The health of every white blood cell in the immune system is also dependent on EFA. Our skin, hair and nails require them as well, but one of the major uses of EFA is the formation of little tissue hormones called prostaglandins (PGs). These are made in every cell in the body continuously, as they have very short life spans.

Prostaglandins

These are the really important reason for ensuring omega-3 and -6 oils in the diet. They are made in every cell in the body and control every cell function, every second of our lives. There are three series of PGs, and within each one there are many other types. Fix in your mind that PGE2 is the bad guy, and PGE1 and PGE3 are the good guys. However we do need all of these, but in the correct ratios. Details about prostaglandins are to be found in Appendix Five.

Processed oils and excessive monounsaturates actually block the formation of PGE1 and PGE3. The processed oils are a major reason for the dramatic upsurge in today's killer diseases. None of this information is new; it has been known for about forty years, but wherever big business is involved the knowledge will never be widely disseminated. It should be remembered that in most countries nutrition is not part of a doctor's training, so unless he makes an effort to learn, the same tired, very outdated advice about fats and cholesterol will continue to be given to patients. The only way to put oil manufacturers out of business is to stop buying the products. The solution is in our own hands.

The functions of prostaglandins
PGE1 is made from sunflower, pumpkin and sesame seeds, walnuts, corn and soya:

> anti-inflammatory effect
> lowers cholesterol
> prevents cardio-vascular disease
> essential to nervous system function
> balances hormones
> balances the immune system
> controls PGE2.

PGE3 is made from oily fish, flaxseeds, walnuts, pumpkin seeds and soya:

> anti-inflammatory effect
> lowers triglycerides and cholesterol
> prevents cardio-vascular disease
> essential for the nervous system
> strengthens the immune system
> prevents and shrinks tumours
> controls PGE2

PGE1 and PGE3 are blocked especially by processed oils and margarine as well as white flour, sugar, excessive animal and monounsaturated fats, alcohol, poor nutrition and stress.

PGE2 is made from animal fats:

> inflammatory reactions, *ie* asthma, psoriasis, arthritis, eczema, glue ear, sinusitis, *etc*
> causes high blood pressure, blood clots, atherosclerosis
> stimulates tumours
> depresses immune function
> causes fluid retention
> controlled by PGE1 and PGE3

There has to be a balance between the inflammatory PGE2 and the anti-inflammatory PGE1 and E3. However most people are way out of balance. So the picture is now clearer. If we eat too much animal protein and not enough balancing seeds and oily fish then we get the chronic diseases which are now threatening our lives. Worse still, if we do get the proportions right we can still block the action of the two EFAs with even small amounts of processed oils.

This is exactly what is happening in every so-called civilised country. As these oils find their way onto the shelves of Asian and Mediterranean countries, so too does their rate of CVD climb. Greeks, using only extra-virgin olive oil, have a low rate of CVD even though they're overweight and don't exercise. That is now changing as they shift to the cheap processed stuff. The Hunzas in north Pakistan, who get their EFA from nuts and seeds and use no processed oils whatsoever, live for a 100 years in good health. They do not die of cancer or CVD. They just die of healthy old age. How often do we see that in the rest of the world?

EFA deficiency and disease

This list would go on forever because every cell in the body is controlled by the PGs, and therefore every cell is liable to malfunction.

Anyone consistently deficient, or worse still, blocking the activity with processed oils, will eventually get cancer, CVD or an auto-immune disease like rheumatoid arthritis. However, before that you may suffer from any of the following: poor skin or hair quality, wounds that don't heal properly, poor resistance to infections, inflammatory diseases like eczema, asthma, psoriasis, arthritis, all manner of circulatory disorders, hormone imbalances leading to irregular periods, PMS or even failure to conceive; disorders of the nervous system like multiple sclerosis, hyperactivity, poor learning ability and lack of normal brain development in infants and children, low IQ, depression, anxiety and mood swings.

EFAs form a major part of the brain and are vital to its function. The number of children deficient in EFA is quite appalling, but the reason is obvious – they are routinely allowed all sorts of junk food from supermarkets that are loaded with processed oil. These so called 'treats' are making them sick, and it isn't just the oils. White flour and sugar also block the EFA pathways. It's time to go back to home-baking, using wholegrains and sugar-substitutes like honey and dried fruit and maple syrup.

Cis- and trans-fatty acids in oils

Fatty acids come in the form of molecules. According to their shape they are called either cis- or trans- fatty acids. The cis-fatty acid type are natural to the food chain, and the trans-fatty acid type are made by man during industrial processes and are therefore not meant for eating.

The fatty acids in mono- and polyunsaturated oils like seeds, nuts and oily

Trans-fatty acids, which are formed by exposing mono- and polyunsaturated oil to light, oxygen and overheating, are twisted into a straight molecule not seen in the food chain, and look like this.

fish occur in cis form, but only as long as they are not damaged. The cis molecule looks like this.

Chemical pathways in the body involve a type of lock-and-key action to trigger each reaction, but the key has to be an exact fit. In the case of polyunsaturated oils, a cis-key fits, and reactions progress smoothly to the end-products, prostaglandin tissue hormones. Trans-keys have been twisted out of shape and they not only cannot unlock a reaction, but like any faulty key, once stuck in the lock they cannot be removed, and the whole thing is useless. Because trans-fatty acids are more aggressive than the cis form, they successfully compete for most keyholes and so wreck chemical reactions. In this way, even if cis fatty acids are present in an oil they get elbowed out of line and cannot form prostaglandins. As you have seen this is a very serious scenario indeed and one that is occurring in a phenomenal percentage of people world-wide because of the gross dietary errors concerning fats, sugar and white flour products.

Trans-fatty acids are sticky molecules and so they form fatty deposits in places like blood vessel walls, encourage blood clot formation and constrict blood vessel walls, thus raising blood pressure. They also attack cell walls, making them permeable to invasion by bacteria and viruses. Cis-fatty acids are never used for energy or fat deposits, as they are vital for other functions. However trans-fatty acids can only be used for energy and conversion to storage fat. 15% of these molecules are converted to cholesterol and almost 50% to triglycerides. Cis-fatty acids form the vital PGE1 and E3, which means they control every important life function.

It is also important to know that monounsaturated fats (as in olive oil) compete with EFA for metabolising enzymes, but the EFA are only pushed aside by an excess of monounsaturates. On the other hand, even small amounts of trans-fatty acids overwhelm EFA very quickly.

Saturated fats in meat and dairy products don't have a direct effect, but the body is capable of converting them to monounsaturates. In this way it is easy for meat eaters to indirectly alter their important fatty acid ratios. The problem does not arise in those who always take half of their total fats as natural polyunsaturates.

The processing of oils

This is an area which you need to get a firm grip on so that you do not buy the wrong oils.

Cold-processing of oils involves pressing the oil out of nuts and seeds without the use of heat. Because this is fairly inefficient, and a lower percentage of oil results, very few manufacturers produce oil by this method now. If they do, there is usually a note on the label to the effect that heat over 85°c was not applied and petrochemicals not used. The expiry date will be specified and the product stored in a container in which light cannot damage the oil.

Cold-pressed olive oil is known as 'extra virgin' and is not so easily affected by light and heat, due to its being a 75% monounsaturated oil with very little polyunsaturated content. The only monounsaturated or polyunsaturated oil that should be used for any purpose is a genuine cold-pressed one, and these have a limited life once they have been opened. Heat, light and oxygen all damage oils, but the polyunsaturated ones are destroyed twice as fast as monounsaturates. Light damages an oil 1000 times faster than heat. The oxygen and light trigger rampant free-radical reactions in the oil. So read the label carefully, and if in doubt don't buy. Also don't buy a polyunsaturated oil like sunflower if it is in a bottle, as they are never dark enough to protect the oil from light damage. Bottled extra virgin olive oil is not quite so bad, as this is a monounsaturated oil. Once you've bought it, keep it in a dark cupboard in the kitchen.

Expeller-pressed oils begin with the crushed seeds being cooked for two hours at high temperature to make the oil extraction easier. They are then put into an expeller press which works rather like a meat mincer and forces the oil out of the seeds. The higher the heat the higher the oil yield. This process usually involves heat lower than 100°C. If light and oxygen are excluded during the process then the unsaturated fatty acids are protected. This is the second best type of oil to buy, but only if it comes stored in opaque containers so that light has not caused harm to the fatty acids. Because the heat involved is below 120°C, manufacturers can get away with describing expeller-pressed oils as cold-pressed. I have seldom seen an expeller-pressed oil in anything but a clear glass bottle. In this case, don't buy it.

Solvent-expressed oils covers almost all oils sold in supermarkets and other grocery stores, and it is these oils which are destroying our health. The method is used because it extracts a lot more oil from each food source than by cold or expeller pressing. It doesn't matter what sort of container it's in as the damage has already occurred in the processing stage.

Initially the oil is extracted at low temperature by means of agitating the seeds in chemical solvent, but when the solvent is evaporated off at a high temperature, traces remain in the oil. The refining process in which caustic soda (drano) is stirred into the oil removes fatty acids not required, as well as protective lecithin and lots of minerals. Bleaching follows next, to remove the caustic soda, but all the important colours like beta-carotene and chlorophyll are also destroyed. By this time the oil stinks and tastes bad and so needs deodorising, and this is where the real harm is done to the oil molecules because the temperature used is a phenomenal 250°c. Anything above 120°c and much of the mono- and polyunsaturated molecules get changed from the healthy form to the twisted trans-type. Protective vitamin E in oil is also destroyed by the heat. Incredibly, these oils can also be sold as 'cold pressed' because the heat is applied after the oil is extracted from the seeds.

In the past pages I have frequently mentioned the blocking of EFA by processed oils. It is the trans-fatty acids which do this. A percentage of the cis-type do survive this processing but they are prevented from taking part in the formation of PGs by the physically-stronger trans-fatty acids. Polyunsaturated oils found in nature contain only cis-molecules. Polyunsaturated oils found in processed oils and industry contain trans-fatty acids (plastics *etc*).

The making of margarine and shortening

The clear, refined, bleached unnatural oil is now put through a process of hydrogenation, which effectively thickens the oil so that it is spreadable; the process converts polyunsaturates to saturated fats. Hydrogen gas is pumped into the oil under very high temperatures over a period of at least five hours. If the oil is completely hydrogenated then no polyunsaturates remain in the very hard fat, but the altered fat molecules may well be toxic. Most margarines are only partly-hydrogenated so that they spread easily. It is these which contain known dangers, because more of the cis-fatty acids which survived the oil extraction become changed to the trans-form. So altered is the oil from the original natural form found in seeds that the official description of margarine is 'a plasticised emulsion of edible oils'.

The human body has no use for plastic and can only store it out of harm's way after first converting it to triglycerides and cholesterol. Is it not ironic that the products advertised as cholesterol-free are converted into cholesterol and fat by our bodies, which treat them as foreign invaders? Vegetable shortening and margarine contain 20-60% trans-fatty acids, and often have none in the cis-form. Much of the remainder of the oil has become saturated by the process of hydrogenation. Any essential cis-polyunsaturated molecules are totally elbowed out of the way. Commercial salad dressings are no better, as they also contain high levels of trans-fatty acids. Another point to be aware of is that mixed vegetable oils, commercial salad dressings and margarines often contain higher percentages of cheap toxic oils like cotton seed, peanut and rape seed.

Can anyone really believe that such products as these, are good for the human body? It is madness to even contemplate buying such trash, and again be reminded that these are found inside nearly *all* commercially packaged food. Having said this, there are a few brands of margarine made with cold-pressed oils and thickened with lecithin. This means that the product is safe. The only valid reason for using even a healthy margarine is allergy to dairy products. Everyone else should use butter in moderation.

Butter is better

Because butter is a natural product, it is much more preferable to margarine with its dangerous trans-fatty acids, as long as it is used in moderation. Sensible intakes of animal fats will not block the vital conversion of oils to prostaglandins, whereas even small amounts of trans-fatty acids in oils and margarines will. 1oz (28g) of butter contains 16mg of cholesterol, but the body needs about 2000mg daily. Conversely around 20% of the trans-fatty acids in margarine and processed oils, fried snacks, commercial cakes, crisps, crackers and biscuits are converted to cholesterol by our bodies, which disdain these twisted fatty molecules. A potato crisp may be 40% fat, a third of which is likely to be in trans-form; these snacks are probably more harmful than sweets for children.

Butter contains no cis- or trans-fatty acids, as it is completely saturated and therefore it can be safely heated and used on bread. Vegans can use a little extra virgin olive oil on bread and in baking instead. The internal temperature of a cake is not high enough to damage olive oil, but it will damage EFA in sunflower oil.

In margarine, the essential fatty acids are mostly in trans-form and there are no vitamins, minerals or enzymes left in the product for their metabolism. It contains chemicals from processing and cheap toxic oil like cotton seed. The many dangerous trans-polyunsaturates are not known in nature, and scientists have barely begun to understand their effect on humans. Certainly they are similar to those found in plastic and vulcanised rubber. Labels stating 'high in polyunsaturates' are as misleading as those on processed oil which say 'cholesterol-free'. We need to ask 'what kind of polyunsaturates'?

Nuts, seeds and their oils

Some of you may be interested in the types of oils present in various nuts and seeds, so that you can decide how to use their oils. All nuts and seeds contain blends of saturated, monounsaturated and polyunsaturated oils (EFA); none are wholly composed of one or another. With a knowledge of the proportions of saturates, monounsaturates and polyunsaturates you can decide for yourself whether the oil is safe to heat or not. If the saturated content is very high (coconut) then that oil can be safely heated. If the monounsaturated content is very high (olive and almond) then it can also be heated, but carefully. If the EFA are at 50% or more then they must not be heated or exposed to light and oxygen.

Coconut oil and palm oil are very high in saturated fats (92%) and Brazil, cashew, cotton seed, macadamia, olive, peanut and wheatgerm oils have measurable amounts. Oils containing 45% or more of monounsaturated oil are almond, Brazil, canola, cashew, cob, macadamia, peanut, pecan, pistachio, rice and sesame. Olive oil and almond oil are in the 75% range. In fact all nuts and seeds contain measurable amounts of monounsaturated oil (omega-9). As a source of the polyunsaturates those seeds with both omega-3 and 6 are of the greatest value in health, but don't heat them.

• *Flaxseed oil* tops the list at 58% omega-3, 15% omega-6 and 20% omega-9 (monounsaturate). Don't heat it.
• *Pumpkin seed oil* is 15% omega-3, 40% omega-6 and 35% omega-9. Don't heat it.
• *Soya bean oil* is rarely found in cold-pressed form, but is 10% omega-3,

50% omega-6 and 25% omega-9. Don't heat it.
- *Walnut oil* is 13% omega-3, 56% omega-6 and 20% omega-9. Don't heat it.
- *Safflower/sunflower seed oils* contain no omega-3 fatty acids but are high in omega-6 (65 to 70%), so don't heat them.
- *Canola oil* is 10% omega-3, 30% omega-6 and 55% omega-9, but this oil is one to be avoided because it contains a toxic chemical called erucic acid. Canola is the name given to a new breed of rape seed oil. The latter is very high in erucic acid whereas canola has only about 3 to 5%. However even this is too high, when you consider that this acid causes scarring of the heart and kidneys. Mustard seed oil also contains erucic acid so avoid products containing it.
- *Corn oil* is almost always chemically-refined, because the oil content of corn is very low indeed. However if you can get cold pressed corn oil it has a delicious flavour and contains over 50% omega-6 and 25% omega-9 oils. The corn oil sold in supermarkets is always the dangerous processed type.
- *Sesame seed oil* is roughly half omega-6 and half omega-9 fatty acids. Because this oil is easy to express naturally it is often found in cold pressed form. Look for it in Japanese stores. If you must heat it, keep the temperature very low.
- *Olive oil* is mainly monounsaturated, but it does contain 5 to 10% of omega-6 fatty acids. The cold- pressed form is called 'extra-virgin' olive oil, and words like 'pure' mean petro-chemical extraction. 'Virgin' oil without the prefix 'extra' means 50:50. Olive oil can be gently heated but glass bottles of it should be stored in a dark cupboard.
- *Peanut oil* is another to be avoided as most of the peanut crops in the world are infested with a fungus called aspergillus which produces carcinogenic aflatoxins. It is also high in arachidonic acid like animal fats.
- *Cotton seed oil* is widely used in processed products, but although it contains 50% omega-6 fatty acids, it also contains toxic natural ingredients which affect the liver and gall-bladder, cause fluid retention in the lungs, have a detrimental effect on hormones and may cause cancer. This oil also contains especially high levels of pesticides.

The important thing to remember about all these oils is that they must be genuinely cold-pressed, and if in doubt don't buy. It is better to get a daily supply of the essential polyunsaturates by eating the raw seeds. Commercially roasted and salted ones have had the oils damaged by heat.

- *Coconut oil* is a 90% saturated fat, but it does not act in the body in the same manner as some animal saturates. The caprylic fatty acid content keeps it liquid at room temperature and researchers have discovered that it does not stimulate the production of cholesterol. Neither does palm oil (85% saturated) which is also virtually free of cholesterol and trans fatty acids.

This area concerning the types of fats which increase blood cholesterol is very interesting. The view that saturates do and unsaturates don't is very outdated. Research shows that polyunsaturates in trans-form increase cholesterol as fast, if not faster, than saturated fats. Worse still, the researchers Mensink and Katan have discovered that trans-fatty acids worsen the ratio between HDL and LDL cholesterol, whereas saturated fats do not. Research has even turned up the fact that one of the longest-chain saturated fatty acids found in animal fat (stearic acid) also does not stimulate a blood cholesterol increase. In fact a 1993 report indicated that the stearic acid in palm oil independently decreases total cholesterol and LDL levels. Another clinical study in 1992, where a group of subjects had 70% of their fat intake replaced with palm oil, indicated a significant improvement in the HDL/LDL ratio, and the total cholesterol levels remained the same. It is probable that the stearic acid content of palm and coconut oils prevents the remaining saturated fats from increasing cholesterol counts. Clearly it is nonsense to label all saturated fats as 'bad'.

Evening primrose oil

The seeds of this plant are very important because they contain pre-formed GLA (Gamma-linoleic acid), which is the first conversion from the oil in seeds. For this reason evening primrose oil is used therapeutically in those who are blocking this conversion with trans-fatty acids, white flour, sugar and alcohol excesses or nutritional deficiencies.

GLA also occurs naturally in borage and blackberry seeds, and supplements of these forms can be readily bought. Evening primrose oil contains 72% omega-6, 9% GLA, 19% omega-9 and saturated oils. Glanolin from blackberry seeds contains 17% GLA. A capsule of this oil plus one of vitamin E rubbed into the skin three evenings a week will do more for health and beauty than any expensive skin care product.

EPA and DHA

These occur naturally in oily fish only. Seed sources of omega-3 oils contain only linolenic acid, which must be converted in the body to EPA and DHA. Again this conversion can be blocked by the same conditions affecting the metabolism of omega-6 oils. Although these two essential fatty acids have similar effects in the body, they are not interchangeable. Both must be supplied to maintain health and long life.

Food preparation and oils

All that is needed now is a final reminder about which oils to use for what type of food preparation. Save the cold-pressed flaxseed, pumpkin and sunflower seed oils as well as walnut oil for dressings, or better still get most of your EFA from whole fresh unroasted seeds instead. If you don't eat flaxseeds, be sure to eat sardines, mackerel, salmon or trout three times weekly. Remember that these EFAs are essential to life. Do not buy commercial salad dressings, as they are chemically processed.

Extra virgin olive oil with its high monounsaturated content can be used for dressings and in cooking, as long as only moderate heat is applied.

When stir frying, oil should be put in the pan with a little water, and the vegetables added immediately. The water prevents the oil molecules from overheating. Throughout the cooking process continually splash in small amounts of water, and the resulting steam will cook the food much quicker than when oil alone is used. Just giving the pan an initial wipe with oil should be enough. There is no need for any free-floating oil in most circumstances. The French, who use olive oil almost exclusively have a remarkably low incidence of cardio-vascular disease, in spite of their high saturated fat intake. In 1992 researchers discovered that fats migrate during frying so that part of the saturated fat in meat passes into the olive oil and is replaced by the monounsaturated oil. It is possible that the Mediterranean countries are replacing 50% of their saturated fats with monounsaturated ones simply by cooking food in olive oil.

The best oils to use in high heat cooking are coconut or palm oils, simply because they contain mostly saturated fatty acids which are stable to heat and do not form the toxic products that might interfere with the EFA functions in the body. Coconut and palm oils may be used for frying, baking and roasting. However, remember that too much of a saturated oil adds to that taken in the form of dairy products and meats. Do no more than oil the surface of the pan and use the water technique described above for stir frying.

Avoid all other oils that are not genuinely cold-pressed, and those not correctly stored. Also avoid all commercial food made from these dangerous oils – shortenings and margarines – and this means that you will tend to buy very little in those supermarkets that don't sell natural whole foods. If you eat out regularly, then you need to choose from the menu carefully. Top class restaurants use only extra virgin olive oil, but all the rest cook with processed oils, and worse still they use the same oil over and over. Chinese food is often a lethal source of killer oils so choose steamed dishes only. Fast food outlets are also a danger.

For cooking
● coconut, palm or extra virgin olive oils.

For salads
● genuine cold-pressed sesame, sunflower, safflower, walnut, flax and

pumpkin seed oils, almond or extra virgin olive oil.

Totally avoid
- all chemically processed oils;
- all polyunsaturated oils in clear bottles;
- 'pure' olive oil;
- peanut, cotton-seed, rape seed and mustard oils.

Free radicals and EFA

Anything natural goes off eventually, and this applies to essential fatty acids as well. When oils are destroyed by heat, light, oxygen or rancidity, a chain reaction of free-radical activity is unleashed, which breaks down essential fatty acids into products we don't want.

Nature packages oils in nuts and seeds along with protective antioxidants, and as long as the product is fresh it will do nothing but good. If an oil is genuinely cold-pressed and stored correctly it too contains protective nutrients.

Light, heat and oxygen all cause chain reactions of free-radical activity in polyunsaturated oil, so these need to be excluded at all times. There is no need to ponder over whether a bottle of sunflower oil is genuinely cold-pressed if you are holding a transparent bottle, because the light will cause damage on its own.

Every natural oil can go off once it has been opened for a while, and for this reason it is important to store them in a cool dark place and buy small containers which get used more quickly. Do not avoid something essential to life just because it can go off: rather treat the product like any other fresh food. The major antioxidants are vitamins A, C and E, selenium, sulphur amino acids, and co-factors like zinc, copper, iron, manganese and B vitamins. Vitamins A and E are particularly important in preventing free-radical attacks on the body's fatty acids.

Daily requirements of EFA

In a diet where 20% of calories come from fats, linoleic acids (omega-6) should not be less than 7-10% and linolenic acid (omega-3) intake not below 3% of calories, but a daily minimum has not yet been established for the latter category of fatty acid. The daily amount of EPA in an Eskimo diet is 30ml, which is extremely high. In spite of their excessive total fat intake, these people are protected against heart disease by the EPA levels in fish. It has been established that man is genetically designed to function best on equal levels of omega-3 and -6 in the diet. It is also known that if omega-6 oils are excessive in the diet, they will block the activity of the more delicate omega-3 fatty acids. Those using processed oils are certainly creating this problem for themselves.

When looking at the total fat intake, a minimum of one third should be omega-6 (seeds) and one sixth omega-3 (flaxseed or oily fish). The other half can be a mixture of monounsaturates (in olive oil and nuts/seeds) and saturates (in dairy, meat, coconut or palm kernels). For most people, very few of the dietary fats come from natural essential fatty acids – most are from animal fat or processed oils, margarines and shortenings with their dangerous trans-fatty acids. When you consider the amount of crisps, cake mixes, commercial crackers and biscuits, salad oils and mayonnaise used in western households, the load of trans-fatty acids is high before ever buying any oil, margarine or shortening for home cooking. These days even children have furred up blood vessels because of being allowed these products routinely.

15-20% of total calories from fats is a healthy level to aim for. The Japanese and other Asian countries are well within this range when eating a traditional diet. Those adding greasy dimsum and other oily types of Chinese food, or Western fast foods, consume large amounts of trans-fatty acids. In the West, fats usually form 40-60% of total calories.

Wholegrains and dried peas, beans and lentils all contain natural oils. The wholegrains are in the 2% range but pulses vary widely. Lentils are as low as 1% oil, and soya beans contain 18%, of which more than half is essential fatty acids. This bean is also an almost-perfect source of protein. Nuts and seeds contain fibre, protein and carbohydrate as well as a very high oil content, but again they vary considerably. Chestnuts, which are incredibly high in carbohydrate calories, are only about 1% oil, whereas macadamia, pecan, Brazil and filbert nuts contain 65-70% oil. Pumpkin, sesame and sunflower seeds are 45-50% oil, and coconut and palm kernels are 35% oil, most of which is saturated.

Eggs are 10% fat, milk 3-4%, cheese 20-30% and butter 85%. Eggs from free range chickens contain essential fatty acids, but battery chickens produce none. Oily fish are high in protein and roughly 10% fat, but this varies according to how cold the water was.

Wild game is extremely low in fat (4% or less) and most of this is essential fatty acid. However it is increasingly difficult to find game which is not farmed. The fat content of farmed animals can be as high as 40%, and all of it saturated.

To maintain a level of 15 to 20% of calories from fat is extremely difficult on a western diet, and to ensure that only one third is saturated requires careful planning. However, those who really care for their children's long-term health and freedom from cardio-vascular disease and cancer will take the time to instigate good eating habits from day one.

Remember that junk food is not a treat: it is a slow death.

II: 7. *FREE-RADICALS*

James Bond's controller accused him of having too many of these – the inference being that he was aging. Living cells produce oxygen free-radicals when they consume oxygen for their respiration. When we are young most of these are quenched by a protective system containing co-enzyme Q10. As we get older some leak out into the cells and attack the essential fatty acids which form the cell walls. This leads to the formation of lipid (fatty) free-radicals which damage the life force of the cell. In this way, all the cells of the body are aged. Free-radicals under control are necessary in limited numbers and are even used by the immune system to destroy foreign invaders or hostile cells. Too many is a different story altogether.

A free-radical is a species containing an odd number of electrons so that one has no partner. The lonely electron will do anything to find a mate and destroys other pairs in order to do so. This sets off a chain reaction of cell damage.

Free-radicals not only result from oxygen metabolism but also from processes like chemical processing of oils and hydrogenation of these into margarine, as well as the heating of oils in cooking. When antioxidants in natural oils are used up, rancidity results here as well and is another source of free-radicals. The activity of these reactive molecules is also promoted by radiation, ozone, drugs, pesticides, alcohol, tobacco and even from burnt food such as toast, barbecued meat, smoked and blackened fried food.

Avoidance of free-radicals starts in the kitchen with your shopping list. Remember that all processed oils and margarines are ticking time-bombs. Don't buy or store stale grains, seeds or nuts, as their oils will be damaged. Store butter carefully, because it goes rancid very quickly out of the refrigerator and is often deteriorating while still on the shelves. Almost every convenience food on the supermarket shelf contains or is fried in a processed oil, and these add to cell damage on a daily basis in most people.

Besides damaging cells, free-radicals damage protein, our DNA and cause the deposition of calcium and cholesterol in the artery walls by first damaging the blood vessel linings. The destruction wreaked on the energy production part of each cell (mitochondria) is a direct cause of aging, atherosclerosis and cancer.

When the essential polyunsaturated fats in the body are not protected by vitamin E, free-radicals turn them rancid, and this blocks the formation of prostaglandin hormones – the very things which prevent cardio-vascular disease. The ugly brown markings which are deposited in the backs of the hands and face of older people are also caused by free-radical damage and toxic liver conditions. These pigments are deposited in internal organs as well and in blood clots, which are then particularly resistant to being dissolved. Diseases promoted by free-radicals include cancer, cataracts, rheumatoid arthritis, atherosclerosis, liver and kidney disease, inflammatory bowel conditions, cystic fibrosis and multiple sclerosis as well as premature aging.

To prevent free-radical damage, the diet needs to contain adequate levels of antioxidant vitamins A, C and E, and selenium, with co-factors like B vitamins, zinc, manganese, copper, iron, molybdenum and enzymes such as super-oxide dismutase. The amino acid complex glutathione is also powerfully antioxidant, as are a great many flavonoids in herbs and fruits. A quality multi-vitamin/mineral product covers most of these, although some people need much higher amounts in the short term.

These same vitamins and minerals also restore the immune system, so follow the dosage given in the chapter on the immune system. Always buy natural products rather than those from drug companies, as the body definitely recognises the difference. Until such time as farmers revert to natural methods of fertilisation, which increase soil micro-nutrients, our food will progressively contain fewer vitamins, minerals and enzymes, so seek out organically-grown food wherever possible. In terms of nutrients, the balanced diet is now a myth.

II: *8. METABOLIC FOOD-TYPING*

Who should eat meat and who should be vegetarian is a complex question which has been studied by many. One thing that is clear is that nature has given us a choice, so that the human species can survive in varied and hostile conditions. The meat eating option was built in when populations increased to levels where wild plants were too few to feed humans adequately – in fact hunter-gatherers in Arctic areas found little else to eat during winter, and survival was dependent on a genetic adaptation to metabolising animal protein. This was long before we settled in communities and became farmers of grain and vegetable crops. Years of research has clearly indicated that if we eat according to our individual requirements, the immune system and health will be strengthened. However as Hippocrates stated, 'one man's food is another man's poison'.

Several systems known as *metabolic typing* have been developed to show who is best suited to what feeding pattern. One system uses external signs to categorise biological types. Although this hypothesis is extremely interesting, in practical terms it is difficult to work out, as we seldom seem to fit accurately enough into one area. For instance, a natural meat eater conjures a picture of a short stocky individual with stubby fingers and a short, heavy-jawed face, large muscles and good circulation. His or her digestive system works very well because it is designed to cope with breaking down protein. The vegetarian on the other hand is said to be a lanky, somewhat frail, nervous but creative person. The characteristics of the natural mixed type could be made to fit anyone who isn't strongly inclined to meat-eating or vegetarianism.

Autonomic nervous system typing

Another method of metabolic typing was developed by a Dr William Kelley in the US, and in fact he was the first person to use this expression. Dr Kelley identified the autonomic nervous system as the basis for typing. This part of the nervous system controls all life-processes and is divided into two parts, the sympathetic and parasympathetic, each having opposing functions in the body. In this way we create balance.

Following on from Dr Kelley, W L Wolcott (who had worked for eight years as Dr Kelley's assistant) and his associates at Healthexcel in the US have further developed the system, but based it on oxidative (energy production) and endocrine (hormonal) types, in conjunction with the autonomic nervous system. They believe that if the wrong type of fuel is supplied it will not be metabolised into energy properly, but stored as fat instead. In this manner even low-calorie diets may result in weight increase. Conversely, over-eating of the correct food does not increase weight unless it is done consistently and in excessive amounts.

Another aspect of the wrong fuel being supplied is that foods which naturally form an alkaline ash are processed into acid in the body instead. Take raw milk as an example: this has an alkaline end-product, but if it is unsuitable, a particular individual may metabolise the milk and leave an acid residue. A core premise of this system is that any food can have opposite biochemical influences in two different metabolic types. The researchers have developed a variety of types, and each one has specific biochemic tendencies which require subtle dietary differences. The following illustrates this form of typing in a simplified form, but it goes some way towards increasing understanding.

The *parasympathetic type* tends to be short with broad shoulders and narrow hips. He or she is inclined to be overweight and have a moist skin and poor muscle tone. Bones are small and there tends to be a rounded face and head. On the mental level, the parasympathetic type is emotional, creative, slow to anger and may suffer depression and poor concentration, though tending to be easy-going, friendly and sociable. This type of person is deliberate, needs plenty of sleep and tends toward an alkaline body. When out of balance, the parasympathetic person is poorly motivated, apathetic, procrastinates and is prone to excessive hunger, low blood sugar, allergies, asthma, cold sores, an irregular heart beat and skin problems.

The *sympathetic type* is more lean, with good muscle tone. He or she tends to be tall and slim with narrow shoulders and wider hips. The skin is dry and bones tend to be large. On the mental level the sympathetic person is logical, rational, concentrates well but has difficulty expressing emotions. He or she tends to be anxious, uptight, volatile, highly-motivated and flares up easily. This type runs on adrenalin and other stress hormones. When out of balance, the body is too acid, and therefore craves sweets, has a reduced appetite and is prone to insomnia, digestive upsets, high blood pressure and a rapid heart beat.

The *slow-oxidative type* is too alkaline and so energy levels are low. There is a tendency to depression and lethargy, digestive problems and a slow metabolism, with weight-gain. Appetite is poor and protein is rejected in favour of carbohydrate. This is similar to the parasympathetic person. However, a slow-oxidiser can also be a sympathetic metabolic type, even though that seems a contradiction in terms. Mentally, emotionally and energy-wise, they are opposites, and yet it is amazing to note that their biochemical requirements are similar. This illustrates the complexity of this method of typing and the reason for the various combinations containing subtle important differences.

The *fast-oxidative type* is similar to the sympathetic personality, but more extroverted. Concentration is poor because of fast thought patterns – getting hyped up but exhausted by the effort. These people burn carbohydrate too quickly, crave fat and protein and become acid. Appetite is good, and because of the fast metabolism, basal body temperature is high. Clearly it is not enough to only know whether one is a sympathetic or a parasympathetic type; the oxidative rate has also to be evaluated (the rate at which nutrients are burned for energy production). Only by carefully determining which types predominate in each person can the diet and supplements be decided.

Diets for different types

The *sympathetic diet* requires high-complex carbohydrate, moderate protein and low fat levels. The protein needs to be from pulses, fish, eggs, poultry and low-fat dairy products. In fact an extreme sympathetic type would be calmed by a vegetarian diet. Vegetables and fruit should be eaten in abundance and all types are suitable. These can form the bulk of the carbohydrate content of the diet.

The *slow-oxidative diet* is the same as the sympathetic except that the fat needs to be very low (10% of calories) and the protein a little higher. These people should avoid dairy products, salmon and red meat because of the fat levels and the high calcium in the milk products. Calcium slows the metabolism in a slow oxidiser and the fat binds magnesium so that it is not available to balance calcium. Very often a sympathetic person is also a slow oxidiser, which means that the acid/alkaline balance will not be too far out of balance. The proportion of fat and protein will depend on which type is dominant.

The *parasympathetic diet* requires a higher protein and fat content (20-30% of calories) and a lower level of carbohydrate. This means that all meat and the oily fish like salmon are suitable as well as dairy products. The parasympathetic person does better on root vegetables and should restrict simple carbohydrate in the form of fruit. He or she does well on grains of all types but needs less than the sympathetic person.

The *fast-oxidative diet* is similar to the parasympathetic one but the carbohydrate must be lowered further. Grains contain *phytates*, that bind calcium so that it cannot be absorbed, and fast oxidisers need extra calcium to slow the rate. If grains are sprouted, soaked or fermented, the phytates are neutralised.

A look at this type is extremely interesting, for here we find that the mental, emotional and energy-related characteristics closely mimic the sympathetic, but their dietary requirements are virtually opposite. Whereas the high-carbohydrate diet works well for the sympathetic, it causes fast-oxidisers almost to jump out of their skin with nervous hyper-irritability. The fast-oxidiser does better on a diet more suitable for the parasympathetic, yet in terms of personality, fast oxidisers are as different from parasympathetics as slow-oxidisers are from sympathetics.

This type of person tends to have blood sugar fluctuations and hypo-glycaemic tendencies due to the rapid combustion of carbohydrate. For this reason it is best to avoid foods that aggravate the situation – glycaemic foods. The worst of these are wheat of any kind, processed rice, corn, potatoes, yams, beetroot, bananas and fruit juice. Eskimos are a good example of fast-oxidisers, and they do very well on a high meat and fat diet and would not survive on a high carbohydrate one. They do not develop CVD if they follow their traditional diet.

Where a parasympathetic type is also a fast-oxidiser, the acid/alkaline levels will be fairly even. However, the dominant facet needs to be ascertained professionally in order to ensure the correct type of carbohydrate. The Healthexcel address is given in the bibliography for those who would like to be evaluated.

According to Dr Kelley, early signs of eating incorrectly are low energy and slow mental faculties, followed by headaches, mood swings, poor digestion, food craving after a meal, weight problems and allergies. For instance, if you notice that carbohydrate saps your energy, and meat and fat give you a feeling of wellbeing, then you are a parasympathetic type. If you are also mentally calmed by meat and fat then you may be a fast oxidiser as well and should eat accordingly, although I would still restrict fat to 30% of calories.

Bill Wolcott has highlighted a case which demonstrates the value of a higher fat and protein intake for the parasympathetic/fast-oxidative type. A 48 year old man with the early stages of CVD was put on a low-protein, low-fat and high-complex carbohydrate diet by his doctor. However, his symp-toms worsened. When this man reversed his eating pattern to fit in with his autonomic and oxidative type, he lost 80 pounds, his cholesterol normalised and his tachycaria disappeared – all this on a higher fat/protein intake com-bined with low carbohydrate. This sort of situation keeps us humble in the face of the forces of nature and reminds us that we are indeed all bio-chemically individual.

ABO blood groups and diet

Most people think of blood groupings in terms of transfusion, but in fact a great deal of research has linked ABO groups with disease-susceptibility and diet. The naturopathic doctor, Peter D'Adamo in the US has for many years routinely used blood-typing profiles of his patients to determine their ability to deal with the different classes of food. In combination with previous researchers' conclusions he has evolved the following patterns.

Group O was the first known blood group and still predominates in several areas: most notably in isolated communities and island people who have not been infiltrated by other races. Group O people produce high levels of protein-digestive enzymes, and the palaeolithic diet was a high protein one. This group is best suited to small amounts of food, and the diet should be largely vegetables and fish with low fat levels. Dairy products and grains are not suitable fare for group O individuals according to this system of typing.

Group A2 is thought to be the second blood group to appear in man and developed primarily in two areas initially. In Africa the blood group is thought to have evolved as protection against parasites (blood groups also determine disease-susceptibility) and in the far northern latitudes as a protection against severe cold. 45% of all Laplanders belong in this group, which was first seen 30,000 to 100,000 years ago. The incidence of group A2 is now highest in Europe, and it is speculated that this gene has some disadvantages to Asians, and so the group was eliminated there. A2 people do very well on meat, seafood, grains, nuts, seeds and vegetables.

Group A1 is a much newer blood group which evolved as man had to adapt to warmer climates after the ice age. It is dominant in the temperate climates of Europe and in Asia above 30° latitude. Around 40% of these people are fully adapted to dairy products, but all are unsuited to meat and pulses. They do very well on seafood, eggs, grains, vegetables, nuts, seeds and fruit. This group is the first to become well-suited to a vegetarian diet.

Group B appeared only 10,000 years ago after the glacial melting which followed the ice age. This group is dominant in Egyptian mummies! It is also common in Mongolians, Indians, East Europeans and in the Middle East. Group B individuals are completely adapted to dairy products and have always used fermented milk, which has no relationship in terms of food value with our present day pasteurised and long-life varieties. Abundant diets high in carbohydrate are suitable for group B. About the same time as this group developed, humans settled in communities and began farming grains. Like group A1 these people could also successfully follow a macrobiotic diet.

Group AB is the newest group which appeared well after the fourth century and probably not until the seventh century. These people are the result of parents with A and B groups and they are well adapted to all modern foods. This includes farmed meat as opposed to an O group preference for fish and low-fat wild meat. Dairy foods are well tolerated as are new vegetables such as the nightshade family: potatoes, tomatoes, peppers and aubergines, which are very common allergens in other blood groups.

In addition to food-typing it is particularly interesting to be able to link ABO groups with disease-susceptibility, and by extension instigate prevention appropriately.

Eating according to climate

It is widely recognised that in the tropics, food requirements are very different from those in the frozen lands of the far north. Much has to do with storing sunshine because the body needs daily amounts in health.

The Frozen North

Where little light is seen for months on end, the diet is very high in saturated fat for its insulation qualities, but equally it is very high in highly-polyunsaturated fats. The latter have two important protective functions: one is to guard against heart disease, and the other is to store the sunshine needed during the winter months. Sunlight is stored in cis-chemical bonds found in unprocessed polyunsaturated fats occurring in oily fish. Essential fatty acids are also part of the photosynthesis process by which plants absorb sunshine.

Eskimos fit into this category, and it is interesting to note that they do not suffer from winter depression (SADS) because the fish they eat has successfully stored UV rays. SADS has been recognised as an illness brought on by a lack of broad-spectrum light and northern Europeans, with their modern diet high in saturated fat and very low in essential fatty acids, suffer a high incidence of this condition. Nature has provided them with oily fish, nuts and seeds that are high in essential fatty acids, but these foods have fallen out of favour.

Indigenous races from very cold climates thrive on diets higher in fat and protein and low in carbohydrate. Root vegetables are stored for winter, and greens are available only in summer. The parasympathetic or fast-oxidiser types originated in this same climatic area, and the diets are similarly structured.

The Tropics

Where sunshine is available all year round, the diet is very low in fat and high in fruit and vegetables. Even fish and meat have a low fat content in comparison to that found in the north. The fats which occur naturally in the food chain are the moderately unsaturated and monounsaturated ones, as well as saturated coconut oil used in cooking. Avocados are an example of a unsaturated/monounsaturated food source.

Saturated and monounsaturated oils are not particularly sensitive to sunshine, which means that they are not harmed in the skin by the tropical sun. The polyunsaturated content of this diet is just enough to maintain essential fatty acid function, but there is no excess to be stored. Remember that polyunsaturated oils are damaged by heat, light and oxygen and this occurs in the skin as well as in the bottle. Dr Robert Buist, a researcher in Australia, believes that the rapid rise in the incidence of skin cancer in his country is not only due to the damaged ozone layer, but also due to the large amounts of processed polyunsaturated oils stored just below the skin.

The use of saturated fat has been reduced in western countries in favour of processed oils and margarines. This has occurred in the home as well as in all food processing, and the result is the phenomenal rise in the amount of oil stored in the body. Even tropical Asia has abandoned its natural saturated oils for cooking in favour of the poisonous processed polyunsaturated varieties. Only *cold-processed* polyunsaturated oils are used within the body – the rest have to be stored, which means under the skin as well as in other areas. Excessive sunshine not only destroys these stored polyunsaturated fats but there is a knock-on effect of free-radical formation causing skin spots and cancer.

Tropical diets should be low in fat, high in carbohydrate (fruit, vegetables and whole grains) and contain moderate levels of protein from fish and poultry rather than fatty red meats and dairy products. The sympathetic/ slow-oxidiser originated in warm climates, and the diet dovetails well with the tropical one.

The Mediterranean

Where the climate falls between extremes, the indigenous oils are monoun-saturated as in that expressed from olives. Here there is no need to store sunshine. However, like the tropics, temperatures are still great enough to harm an excess of polyunsaturates, and so they occur naturally in the diet only in the amounts required.

It is very clear that nature packages food according to climatic requirement, and to deviate radically is to court ill-health. For instance a person reared in the tropics who accidentally found himself marooned in reindeer territory would very soon become weak, sickly and a potential wolf target if he tried to exist on a Laplander's diet. Modern people, loving processed food, are ignoring the need to incorporate climatic guidelines into their dietary pattern.

II: 9. CONTRASTING THE CHINESE AND JAPANESE DIETS

Because we live in a very cosmopolitan world and enjoy foods from many different cultures, it is interesting to have a knowledge of their nutritive values. I have chosen to highlight two Asian diets because they have subtle differences that are important in determining whether health or disease will prevail. Many believe that the Chinese diet is very healthy, but in fact this is not usually so. Chronic degenerative diseases are as common as in the West; cancer is the foremost cause of death, cardio-vascular disease a close second, and there are all the usual health problems arising from stress, pollution, lack of exercise and poor nutrition.

Traditional Chinese diets vary according to the regions. For instance, in the north, grains form the staple food, to which cooked vegetables, soya and a little meat is added. Wheat, rice and some millet are the most commonly used grains. In the south the diet is more varied, with rice forming the staple grain, to which more meat, fish, beans and vegetables are added. Unfortunately, white rice with its low nutrient level has long superseded the wholegrain variety, which is considered fit only for peasants. In the 1950s, Norman Joliffe conducted a nutritional survey in Taiwan, which indicated an alarming deficiency in B vitamins, iron, vitamin A and protein in the Chinese diet. The vitamins and iron are found in whole grains, fruit and vegetables, and these are not eaten in adequate amounts, even in affluent communities.

Chinese meat-eating habits have varied according to agricultural need. Until 400 BC they were heavy meat eaters, and only changed because the rapidly expanding population needed a cheaper food source. Grains then became the staple, but in the south, because rice had a lower food value than millet and wheat, pulses like soya were added. As communities became more affluent meat consumption again increased.

Today the traditional diet is still deficient in nutrients because grains consist of only white rice, white flour and noodles, and vegetables are treated as side dishes. The calcium content is also very low because oily fish and green vegetables are not eaten in adequate amounts. Asians are largely lacking in the enzyme which digests milk and should not use this as a calcium source as adults.

Research indicates that right up until the 1950s many Chinese in China lived on inadequate diets and this resulted in their stunted growth and poor resistance to disease; life-span was also relatively short. These days the situation has improved somewhat as dietary patterns have changed to more protein, vegetables and fruit, but resistance to whole grains has remained widespread.

A survey reported by Dr F M Baber on child-rearing in Hong Kong in the 1970s illustrated how customs and feeding habits affected growth and development. Breast-feeding was stopped very early indeed, but only 52% of infants were given good quality milk formulas; the rest were fed evaporated or sweetened condensed milk. White rice congee was introduced at just four months, at which time milk consumption was sharply reduced. At this stage upper respiratory tract infections and diarrhoea became very prevalent. By six months of age most infants were being given fish and liver, but only in minute amounts and often only the water in which they were cooked. Vegetables were added at eight months, but again in insufficient amounts or as soup broth.

As a result of Western education, fruit was introduced at six to eight weeks, but the variety was very restricted. The rice staple food was always the processed white variety. Dr Baber's survey indicated that this diet, so deficient in vitamins, minerals and protein, resulted in slow growth, weak flabby muscles and frequent infections. At eighteen months to two years, when they started eating an adult diet, the situation improved, but although the growth rate accelerated the children never caught up that which they had lost.

The Chinese adult, following traditional eating patterns, will eat processed noodles or white rice congee for breakfast and tea or perhaps coffee with condensed milk, none of which builds health. Many others start the day with a sweet white roll and soft drinks, or go to a Western fast food restaurant and eat fried sausages, bacon and eggs, thus setting themselves up for cardiovascular disease. Lunches during the week often consist of noodles in broth with a few vegetables on top, or white rice topped only with meat and two to three sprigs of greens.

Western fast food restaurants are packed all day long with Chinese eating poor-quality high-fat foods and white rolls. Dimsum restaurants and hawker stalls serve very tasty food, but much of it is soaked with oil and fat, or made of white flour and white rice. The same oil is used over and over, which is extremely harmful to the body. The evening meal at home is possibly the only nutritious one of the day, as more vegetables are eaten, home made soup served as well as fish, in addition to the ubiquitous white rice or noodles.

In Chinese cultures, holidays and feast days are associated with using a lot more oil in the cooking pan. Unfortunately only petro-chemically expressed oils are utilised, and extreme heat is applied in the stir fry technique. It doesn't matter whether it is corn, mixed vegetable or peanut oil; what matters is whether it was cold-pressed or not. Even if it were, which is rare, the heating would damage the molecular structure of the oil. Only coconut oil or palm oil is safe to over-heat. This is widely used in South East Asia, but not in the Far East. Woks should have no more than the surface greased with oil, and then water splashed in during the cooking process to prevent burning. Olive oil can be used safely if excessive heat is avoided.

Salt fish with its powerful cancer-causing nitrosamines is a part of the southern Chinese diet, and is being given to very young children. Research has not only linked the eating of salt fish to naso-pharyngeal cancer (NPC), but also indicates that it is more prevalent in those who were given salt fish as children. Studies in both Malaysia and Hong Kong indicated a significant association between NPC and the consumption of salt fish in early childhood. In Hong Kong, 80% of those with NPC were given salt fish before two years of age, and where the food was introduced at weaning, the incidence was even higher. China's most prevalent cancer, gastric cancer, is also linked to diet, and again it is salt fish as well as pickled vegetables and infected fungi which are associated. However, other dietary faults like eating processed grain, the use of fertilisers and pesticides, and the presence of nitrates in the water supply must also be causative agents.

On the plus side there is an increasing number of young Chinese eating from salad bars in restaurants at lunch time. This may be a reaction to the fact that as a race they are rapidly gaining weight, because of turning to fast foods, sweet bread, biscuits and soft drinks, but whatever the reason, it is a healthy trend. Another plus sign is that those following the traditional diet do tend towards a good balance between carbohydrate, protein and fat. The carbohydrate, however, needs to change to a wholegrain variety, and vegetables should be increased. The habit of adding sugar during the cooking of most dishes also needs to stop.

The traditional Japanese diet is much healthier. It is also based on grain, fish, meat and vegetables, but there the similarity with a Chinese diet ends. Although white rice is a staple food, other wholegrains are frequently eaten, such as 100% buckwheat noodles. The use of fat and oil is much reduced and the little food which is fried seldom oozes grease. Meat is not eaten as often, because fish is the main source of protein and this is just as likely to be eaten raw as cooked.

Seaweeds form a small but daily part of the diet and this food source is extremely rich in nutrition. Cardio-vascular disease is rare in those eating seaweeds, as they contain 10-20 times the minerals of land vegetables. They also contain alginic acid which binds the toxins in the body for elimination. Where minerals are very high in a diet, there is a strong alkalising affect in the body, which purifies all systems and prevents disease. Seaweeds contain appreciable levels of protein, carbohydrate, calcium, potassium, sodium, iron, iodine and trace minerals as well as all vitamins, chlorophyll and antioxidant enzymes.

Another factor in the Japanese diet is the obsession with quality: deadly chemical sprays are not permitted and vegetables reach the markets really crisp and fresh. A wide variety of vegetables is common, and soya products are an important staple food. Miso soup, tofu and naturally brewed soya sauce (*shoyu* and *tamari*) are in daily use. Miso is a rich brown puree of soya beans fermented with sea-salt and a cereal grain. It is one of the world's wonder foods in terms of nutritional value.

Breakfast in Japan is also a healthy meal, and includes cooked cereal, nuts, seeds and a raw salad. Teas tend to be herbal, such as chrysanthemum or unfermented green tea. In common with all Asians, the Japanese cannot digest milk, but the high fish, seaweed, tofu and sesame seed content ensures adequate calcium.

Although the incidence of cardio-vascular disease, arthritis and cancer have been much lower in Japan than in the West, they do match mainland China for having the world's highest rate of stomach cancer. This is possibly due to the fiery pickles like wasabi which must abrade the stomach like a scouring pad in a frying pan. There is also a high incidence of cerebro-vascular accidents, which is thought to be due to persistent stress combined with a high sodium intake – albeit in natural form. Unfortunately Western fast food has also hit Japan and those who are changing from the traditional diet are gaining weight and developing typical Western chronic diseases.

The serious consequences of fast food have been widely publicised and yet Asia is turning a blind eye and welcoming junk food with open arms. It is really important that they learn from the mistakes of the West in this area and quickly turn back to a traditional diet.

II: *10. JUICE FASTING*

Fasting is described as the complete abstinence from food – which actually means water only. However most authorities on the subject now agree that juice fasting is of greater value than only water as a therapeutic tool. By abstaining from food, the digestive system can be rested and the body can concentrate on cleansing and rejuvenating the entire system.

We are only as healthy as each individual cell in the body. If they are suffocated by waste products, then oxygen supplies drop, cell function diminishes and by extension, organ function also. Extended periods of stress, lack of exercise, over-eating and toxic bowel conditions decreases liver, kidney and digestive function. Cells then suffer from nutrient depletion and toxic accumulations, which prevent proper oxygenation. Juice fasting reverses all of this.

How it works

Once digestion has stopped, the body can spend all day working on spring cleaning every cell. The juices are largely absorbed directly from the stomach, so that little activity is called for by the pancreas and intestines. The vitamins, minerals and enzymes in juices assist the cleansing process. At one time it was thought that enzymes in food were not absorbed and used, but this theory has been proven wrong. What is not yet known is whether the enzymes are absorbed intact or whether they undergo some transformation in the walls of the stomach before reaching the blood stream. Certainly raw juices add enzymes to our storehouse and they are used to regenerate and rejuvenate all parts of the body.

During a fast, the body lives off glucose stored in the liver for the first day, and then breaks down non-essential body protein and fats thereafter. These are converted to glucose for energy. Protein breakdown is reduced fairly quickly as the body recognises the need to recycle amino acids for vital repair. Triglycerides become the main source of fuel after the glucose in juices is used up.

When the body starts living off itself, preservation is very strong and so damaged and decomposing cells are destroyed first, while vital organs are never digested or damaged. Fasting is a wonderful garbage-disposal system, and is the first line of defence against diseases like cancer and arthritis. The fast stimulates the process of new cell growth and regenerates cells of the brain and all the vital organs first. Cellular oxygen levels are raised so that energy production is enhanced along with the making of protein, fat breakdown, bacterial destruction and DNA synthesis. In this way every cell can again function perfectly. Enzymes are involved in every phase of this cleanup, and with none being needed for digestion, metabolic enzymes are spared for all the essential body functions.

The digestive process itself is rested and its function greatly enhanced after the fast. Metabolism is markedly altered for the better by a juice fast, as is shown by a proper weight maintenance once food intake is returned to normal. All the elimination organs get a spring clean and function so much better after a fast. When mega-nutrients are supplied in juices, the skin, liver, kidneys and lungs can more readily expel accumulated toxic waste.

Other benefits of fasting

Almost all chronic conditions are improved by juice fasting, simply because it enables the body to self-heal. Throughout time, fasts have been used to cure arthritis, heart conditions, diabetes, toxic poisoning, psoriasis, eczema, depression, schizophrenia, and a study indicated that fasting is more beneficial in treating acute pancreatitis than any drugs. The list of conditions improved by fasting is endless, and includes serious illnesses like cancer, kidney and liver abscesses, nephritis and congestive heart failure. The immune system is markedly affected by a fast, to the extent that all bacterial and viral destruction is greatly enhanced. The phagocytes which engulf them increase their activity, and killer T-cells also work faster. Allergic complexes are less likely to form, and there is even an increased resistance to infection after the fast is over.

Juice fasting has been used for six months on end in complete safety and there is always the added benefit of disease and age regression. It is well known that communities consuming restricted calories live longer, look younger and suffer less disease. Regular fasting keeps the metabolic rate tuned up and prevents cellular degeneration and aging. Even one week at a time is of great value.

Juice versus water fasting

Those who follow water fasts for more than a few days should be admitted to a hospital or fasting clinic where they can be monitored on a daily basis by qualified personnel. They must also severely restrict activity, and rest during the day to conserve energy. Conversely, on a juice fast, life continues as normal and daily moderate exercise is important. It is usual to have a great feeling of wellbeing.

It is said that hunger disappears sooner on a water fast, and certainly fat is broken down more quickly, as no nutrients are being provided. However energy levels may be lower, muscles feel weak, and heart problems are emphasised, because of the initial heavy loss of sodium, potassium, magnesium and calcium. People with slight heartbeat irregularities often find that water fasts worsen the problem dramatically and a shift on to juices immediately produces a marked improvement. In some cases this becomes a complete cure after a few weeks of juices.

A great many physicians in Europe have vast experience in fasting patients, and almost universally now follow the juice regime. The process is widely used as a cancer therapy and this is where the advantage of juices over water becomes really obvious. Cancer often regresses well on water only, but the results of the many documented studies clearly show quicker regression, and the cancer is more likely to disappear entirely on juice fasts. The alkaline juices speed the process of disease recovery, acid excretion is hastened, and the minerals prevent the loss of cellular oxygen.

Supporters of water fasts point to the Swedish tests where people walked for days on no food. However these were fit people, not sick ones. The very interesting feature of these studies is that even after ten days of marching about thirty miles a day, the fasting individuals maintained normal blood levels of sugar and protein, which just demonstrates the body's extraordinary ability to maintain balance even during a total absence of nutrients. Additionally the walkers suffered no energy depletion and had an increased feeling of wellbeing throughout the route march.

Side effects
Where a person has high levels of toxins in the body, their rapid release can cause some initial ill effects like headaches, dizziness, dark urine, body odour, bad breath, skin irritations and catarrhal excesses. In water fasting, aching limbs, palpitations, nausea and even disturbances of hearing and vision may occur; some also experience unpleasant complications such as a pounding heartbeat or a sudden drop in blood pressure, severe weakness, gout or kidney stones.

However these conditions are rare if fasting is done with juices. Where toxic headaches occur, it is important not to reach for pain-killers; rather increase the fluid intake and rest more often. In some cases, fasts have to be preceded by an extended period of fruits and vegetables so that the cleansing process is more gradual. Those trained in iridology can determine the degree of toxicity within each person and adjust the diet accordingly.

Hunger may be a problem initially, but this wears off within two to three days and does not return until the body is cleansed. Another factor is that we are conditioned to eating at certain times, and the so-called hunger pangs in the first few days are often just habit. Drinking a glass of water and getting on with some other activity will stop the feeling. The most common problem in fasting is that you miss chewing on food in the first few days.

Contra-indications

It is generally recognised that children, pregnant and breast-feeding women should not fast, although in an infection, it is of benefit even for these people. Anyone with a serious illness, diabetes, heart disease or T B should only fast under qualified supervision.

Juices

These must be freshly made from raw fruit or vegetables – preferably organically grown. Never used canned, frozen or packaged juices. Where pesticides have been used, fruit and vegetables must be washed very thoroughly with a brush and water, to which cider vinegar has been added. A final rinse in plain water follows. Though fruit and vegetable juices are rich in vitamins, minerals, enzymes and sugars, they must be consumed soon after extraction, as within ten minutes the enzymes begin to disappear from the juice. Additionally, fruit and vegetable juices are rich in colours (which increase red blood cells, digestion and assimilation), natural antibiotic-type substances, natural hormones and many active healing elements.

Some people confuse juicers with food-processors. The latter just breaks up food to a pulp, whereas a juicer extracts the liquid part of the plant and leaves all the solids in a hopper. When buying a juicer be sure to get one with a metal grater inside, as the plastic ones are useless for vegetables.

A juice fast literally means liquid only, so all the solid part is discarded. If squeezing citrus fruits, strain them into a glass so that none of the pulp is drunk.

When making juices, never mix fruit and vegetables together – except that apples are permissible with vegetables. Fruit is very cleansing and vegetables are regenerating. Purists use only one fruit at a time in a juice, and the most powerful cleansers are apples and grapes. Both of these fruits have an amazing number of nutrients, which not only cleanse and rejuvenate cells, but also attach to toxic metals like lead and mercury and eliminate them from the body.

When deciding on fruits it is useful to include any specific to your condition. For instance, in arthritis, the berry fruits are especially beneficial and the best vegetable juices are carrot, celery and beetroot. When mixing vegetable juices, use a very wide variety, but always include carrots and celery. Carrot juice is a 'cure all', and celery cleanses all the tissues of waste. Greens make juice a little tart, but extra carrot and green beans add sweetness. The oxalic acid in raw spinach cleans and heals the digestive tract, but when it is cooked, this acid accumulates in tissues if eaten in excess. Cabbage juice is another green which acts on the digestive tract. It heals the linings and will eradicate a gum infection or a stomach ulcer. Parsley strengthens the kidneys and adrenal glands, but a little goes a long way. Go lightly on beetroot and radishes as they are quite strong juices, although of great benefit. Beetroot improves the red blood cell count in anaemia and cleanses the joints, liver, gall-bladder and kidneys. Always add either wheatgrass or barley green powder to vegetable juice, for their powerful antioxidant properties. Leafy greens like parsley, cress and spinach need to be packed into the juicer with the plunger in place before switching on, or they tend to miss the grater and not be juiced. Fruit juices must be diluted 50:50 with mineral water but vegetable juices may be drunk neat, but slowly.

Potassium broth

This is a vegetable broth very rich in potassium, but it also contains many other minerals and vitamins. The soup should be simmered very, very slowly for one hour with the lid on, until all the nutrients have left the vegetables and are in the liquid. Strain out the liquid so that no fibre remains, and drink it at whatever time of day you prefer to have a hot soup rather than a cold juice. Do not use stock cubes, which may be from animal sources or loaded with chemicals. A little added Vecon or some other natural vegetable stock is permissible to enhance the flavour, but added salt is not allowed.

Recipe:
1 potato, unpeeled and chopped.
1 cup each of finely sliced carrots, celery and onions.
1 cup of green vegetables – and vary the types used.

Add garlic and herbs for flavour, cover with mineral water and simmer.

Beginning a juice fast

Initially it is a good idea to wind down food intake by eating only fruit and vegetables for two days before beginning the fast. No vitamins, minerals or other supplements should be taken, and all non-essential drugs avoided. Those on cardiac drugs, insulin or long-term cortisone should not stop taking them. Those who are very ill may need extra vitamin C and even some organic honey each day.

During the two days before, and on the morning of the first day, epsom salts or castor oil may be taken in orange juice to cleanse the bowel. Alternatively, take one to two tablespoons of flaxseeds swallowed whole with a glass of warm water. Usually normal bowel function continues during the first two days of a fast, because waste from previous meals is being eliminated.

Daily enemas are important if a fast is to last more than four to five days.

This is because the cleansing process expels a lot of waste into the bowel, and without solid food stimulation, it may not be expelled. Stagnant toxins will then be reabsorbed into the bloodstream and defeat the object of the fast. For an enema, one pint of body-heat water is prepared with a little added lemon juice. The water flow needs controlling so that it does not enter the bowel too quickly, and this can be done partly by ensuring that the canister is not held up too high. Enemas are taken while lying down on one side with the knees pulled up, and the water held for five to ten minutes if possible. Put some KY jelly on the end of the tubing for easier insertion.

Fasting programme

7am	A cup of warm mineral water with lemon juice added.
8am	A glass of fruit juice, diluted 50:50.
11am	One glass of vegetable juice or herbal tea.
1pm	One large mug of potassium broth or vegetable juice.
4pm	One cup of herbal tea.
7pm	One glass fruit juice, diluted 50:50.
9pm	One mug of potassium broth.

Mineral water may be drunk in between if required, and it is particularly beneficial if it is hot, with added lemon juice. Do not use tap or distilled water during a fast, as the pH is usually too acid. When drinking juices, small amounts should be sipped and held in the mouth for a period as though chewing. This is because carbohydrate digestion begins there, before continuing in the upper part of the stomach.

During the fast and after the early morning lemon tea, dry-brush massage the skin for five minutes before taking a hot shower, which should be followed by thirty seconds of cold water. This ensures that the skin works well as an elimination organ. At some time every day, go for a short walk in the sunshine, and if possible a rest after lunch is recommended. Exercise is to be limited during a fast otherwise tissue repair and the elimination process is inhibited. Daily deep breathing exercises in fresh air improves lung function.

Breaking the fast

Day 1	Add half an apple twice daily and chew it thoroughly and slowly.
Day 2	Add the soup vegetables to the potassium broth and start varying the whole fruit.
Day 3	Add a salad dressed with lemon juice and a little olive oil to one meal.
Day 4	Steamed vegetables are added to the diet.

Day 5   Add some fresh raw nuts and seeds and live plain yoghurt to the fruit.

Day 6   Add an egg, a small serving of fish or pulses at one meal.

Day 7   Add whole grains to one meal such as brown rice, millet, cornmeal, oatmeal, barley or rye bread.

Day 8   A normal wholesome diet. However reduce the food intake to only what is necessary and continue the habit of a daily vegetable juice.

Golden rules

- Eat slowly.
- Chew thoroughly.
- Do not eat when tired, upset or stressed.
- Do not over-eat.
- Follow correct food-combining.
- Do not drink water with a meal.
- Keep all elimination channels open:
  bowels – fibre and exercise;
  skin – dry skin brushing, hot and cold alternating showers;
  lungs – deep breathing exercises;
  kidneys – 6-8 glasses of fluid daily.

Food elimination programmes can be varied to suit individual needs, but they should always begin with a period of liquids only. A useful variation is as follows:

Days 1-7   juice fasting.

Day 8   add half an apple twice daily.

Days 9 & 10 eat a full serving of fruit twice daily at 8am and 7pm.

Days 11 & 12 add vegetables to the soup once daily and steam a plate of mixed vegetables in place of the lunch or dinnertime broth.

Days 13 & 14 eat a raw salad once daily to replace one vegetable juice.

By this time the day's menu will be as follows.

7am   Warm water and lemon juice.

8am   A bowl of fresh fruit.

11am   A glass of vegetable juice.

1pm   Cooked vegetables or soup.

4pm   Fresh fruit.

7pm   A raw salad.

9pm   Herbal tea or clear broth.

After a total of 2-3 weeks, re-introduce other food, as for days 5-8, listed under 'Breaking the Fast'.

II: *11. DRY SKIN BRUSHING*

It is important to realise that the skin is a major elimination organ and if it is not functioning properly then the kidneys, lungs and liver have to work much harder. Roughly one third of body waste is eliminated through the skin, and if the pores are clogged and the circulation to the upper layers is poor, then toxins accumulate in the tissues. Skin is also capable of absorbing oxygen, vitamins, oils and water through its surface and transporting them to the blood stream. Again, if the cells are clogged this will happen very inefficiently. The first hormonal conversion of vitamin D from the sun occurs in the skin, and if this function is disrupted the next two vital conversions in the liver and kidneys will be prevented.

Dry skin brushing removes any dead surface cells and keeps the pores open. It stimulates small capillaries to open up and improve the circulation, as well as stimulating circulation to muscles and fat cells. In this way they too function better. Tired, sluggish fat cells are less responsive to insulin and less likely to release fat stores for fuel. Medical science has proven quite conclusively that a mixture of skin brushing and hot/cold showering improves resistance to infection quite dramatically. The routine also has a marked anti-aging and rejuvenating effect.

Use a natural fibre brush, as synthetic bristles will damage the skin. Use the brush dry, and on dry skin, as the shower comes after the brushing process. Start at the soles of the feet and work up the legs brushing in a circular motion, always in the direction of the heart. Work on each leg until a warm glow develops in the skin. Then dry brush the arms starting from the palms and working towards the shoulders in the same circular motion. The pressure used will depend on the degree of skin-sensitivity, but in time, more will be tolerated. After the arms, brush the back, abdomen and finally the chest. The whole process takes about five minutes and is best done twice daily to improve circulation and all skin functions.

II: *12. ROTATION DIETS AND FOOD FAMILIES*

All foods are divided into families, which are determined by their chemical constituents, and the rotation diet is designed to prevent repetitive eating of any single food group. The most widely-used variety is the four-day rotation programme, whereby the system remains clear of any given food for three days on end. Very sick people need to work on a seven-day rotation.

With the preponderance of packaged food in today's diet, a single product may be unknowingly eaten every day. Dairy products, wheat, corn, sugar, eggs, soya and yeast tend to be hidden everywhere, and some chemical additives are used very repetitively. This is quite aside from the deliberate eating of the same foods over and over, simply because it is easier. When we ate according to seasons the diet was naturally diversified to a certain extent, and although some foods would be eaten daily for weeks on end, at least afterwards they disappeared from the table for a period of months.

The main reason for following a rotation diet is to reduce the chance of developing food allergies. It will help in discovering any offending food, and the procedure will increase a person's tolerance of an allergen following an initial period of avoidance. A side-benefit is that rotation ensures a wide range of food intake.

The following is a four-day rotation plan, and although grains are present on three of the days, the gluten ones are all restricted to day one only.

The four-day rotation diet

Day 1	Day 2	Day 3	Day 4
PROTEIN:			
Chicken, turkey, duck, quail, pigeon, pheasant, eggs, sesame/pumpkin and sunflower seeds, brewer's yeast	Beef, venison, fresh-water fish, pine, cashew and pistachio nuts, cow's milk products, crustacean shellfish.	Lamb or pork, almonds, walnuts, pecans, hickory, peanuts, sheep's & goat's milk products. Soya products.	Saltwater fish, mollusc, shellfish, rabbit.
STARCH:			
Barley, malt, rye and products, oats and oat cakes, wheat, wheat germ, wheat bran, bulgur, semolina, cous-cous.	Rice products, arrow-root, buckwheat.	Dried beans, peas, lentils, sago, coconut, tapioca, millet.	Corn products.
VEGETABLES:			
Chives, shallots, garlic, onions, leeks, truffles, mushrooms, artichokes, marrow, pumpkin, butternut, courgettes, asparagus, lettuce, cucumber, chicory, endive, dandelion, mint, basil, oregano, thyme, sage, rosemary, bamboo shoots, marjoram, savory, lemon grass.	Carrots, parsnips, celery, parsley, celeriac, fennel, sorrel, chervil, plantain, avocado, turmeric, bay leaves, cardamom, cinnamon, ginger, coriander, cumin, dill.	Peas, beans, potato, tomato, egg-plant, spinach, chard, mung bean sprouts, peppers of all kinds, beetroot, alfalfa sprouts, fenu-greek, tamarind.	Sweetcorn, rutabago, swede, turnip, radish, cabbage, cauliflower, collards, kale, Brussel sprouts, mustard/watercress, broccoli, kohlrabi, chinese cabbage, mustard seed, horseradish.
FRUIT:			
Any melon, lemon, lime, orange, tangerine, grapefruit, pomelo, blueberry, huckleberry, cranberry.	Rhubarb, banana, mango, gooseberry, figs, mulberry/juniper berries.	Dates, prunes, cherries, plums, apricots, sloes, peaches, nectarines, crabapples, pears, apples, rosehips, quinces, loquat, boysenberries, loganberries, strawberries, raspberries, blackberries, tamarillos.	Grapes, raisins, currants.
DRINKS			
Lime, peppermint tea, mint, lemon verbena, thyme/sage and camomile teas, dandelion & chicory coffees, Barley-cup. Melon and citrus juice.	Ginger tea, fennel tea, cow's milk yoghurt, juices from fruit and veg above.	Fenugreek tea, apple and pear juice, rosehip tea, goat's milk, soya milk, carob, tomato juice, apple cider	Wine, coffee, rooibosch tea, grape juice.
OTHERS			
Gherkins, sesame/safflower/sunflower oils & seeds, cane sugar, molasses.	Hops, gelatin, suet, rice syrup, maple syrup.	Walnut oil, soya sauce, lecithin, fructose, sugar beet, honey, date sugar, carob.	Corn oil, wine vinegar, corn sugar.

The following foods may be used on any day but none should be repeated within 4 days: Poppy seeds, macadamia nuts, filberts (hazelnuts), chestnuts, Brazil nuts, water chestnuts, yams, okra, olives, nutmeg and mace, capers, allspice, cloves, sweet potato, papaya, passion fruit, kiwi fruit, pineapple, pomegranate, vanilla, lychee, lotus root, taro, Chinese spinach (een choi), Ceylon spinach (saan choi).

The following is a list of food families. If you wish to move a food from one day to another on the rotation plan, be sure to shift every part of that food family at the same time, or the rotation will be no more.

Banana – banana, plantain, arrowroot.

Beef – beef, veal, all milk products, rennet, gelatin, suet.

Beet – sugar beet, spinach, chard.

Bird – all fowl and game birds: chicken, turkey, duck, goose, pigeon, quail, pheasant, eggs.

Blueberry – blueberry, cranberry, huckleberry.

Buckwheat – buckwheat, rhubarb, sorrel.

Cashew – cashew, pistachio, mango.

Citrus – lemon, orange, grapefruit, lime, tangerine, citron, pomelo.

Composite – lettuce, chicory, artichoke, dandelion, sunflower, tarragon, chamomile, endive, safflower, white wormwood, garland chrysanthemum (*tong ho*).

Conifer – juniper, pine nut.

Crustacean – crab, crayfish, lobster, prawn, shrimp.

Freshwater fish – salmon, trout, pike, perch, bass.

Fungus – mushrooms, brewer's yeast, truffles.

Ginger – arrowroot (East Indian), ginger, cardamom, turmeric.

Gooseberry – currants, gooseberry.

Grape – grapes, raisin, wine, brandy, currants, muscadine, cream of tartar.

Grass – wheat, semolina, corn, oats, barley, rye, maltose, rice, malt, millet, bamboo shoots, sugar cane, lemon grass, molasses, sweet corn, bulgur, hominy grits, popcorn, sorghum, wild rice shoots.

Laurel – avocado, cinnamon, bay leaf.

Lily – onion, garlic, asparagus, chives, leeks, shallots, aloe vera.

Melon – water melon, cucumber, cantaloupe, pumpkin, zuccini, acorn, marrow, gherkin, butternut, all types of vegetable melons and the fruit varieties.

Mint – mint, basil, hyssop, marjoram, oregano, peppermint, rosemary, sage, thyme, savory, lemon balm.

Mollusc – abalone, snail, squid, clam, mussel, oyster, scallop.

Morning Glory – sweet potato, water spinach (*ong choi*).

Mulberry – figs, mulberry, hops.

Mustard – turnip, radish, watercress, cabbage including Chinese varieties, cauliflower, sprouts, kohlrabi, kale, broccoli, collards, cresses, horseradish, swede, rutabaga, Chinese kale (*gaai laan*). Other Chinese vegetables are: *baak choi, choi sum, taai goo choi, chuk gaai choi, daai gaai choi, jiu la choi, wong nga baak.*

Myrtle – allspice, cloves, guava.

Palm – coconut, date, date sugar, sago.

Parsley – carrot, parsnip, celery, anise, parsley, caraway, chervil, coriander, cumin, dill, fennel.

Pea – peas, dry beans, green beans, soya beans, lentils, licorice, dill, fennel, peanuts, carob, alfalfa sprouts, fenugreek, tamarind, senna.

Pepper – black and white pepper, peppercorn.

Pineapple – pineapple.

Plum (Rose family) – plum, cherry, peach, apricot, nectarine, prune, almond.

Potato – potato, tomato, eggplant, peppers, paprika, cayenne, tobacco, tamarillo, chili, Chinese boxthorn.

Rose:

   a) *Pomes* – apple, pear, quince, pectin, cider, loquat, rosehip.

   b) *Stone fruit* – almond, apricot, cherry, peach, plum, sloe.

   c) *Berries* – strawberry, raspberry, blackberry, loganberry, youngberry, boysenberry.

Salt water fish – cod, tuna, mackerel, eel, halibut, plaice, anchovy, sole, sardine, hake, haddock.

Spurge – tapioca, cassava.

Swine – all pork products.

Tapioca – Tapioca (Brazilian arrowroot), castor oil.

Walnut – walnut, hickory, butternut, pecan.

II: *13. THE NATUROPATHIC LIFESTYLE*

This has been unchanged throughout time and involves living according to the laws of nature, as follows.

Clean air

This can be difficult to find, but it helps if you avoid living in industrial zones and downtown areas where pollution levels are highest. Ionisers clean the air and increase negative ions. All sorts of air-filtering systems are now on the market which will improve the quality of the air inside your home.

Clean water

It is not only toxic micro-organisms that need avoiding in water supplies, but all the added chemicals as well. Some of these are put in at the instigation of governments, but none will build health and most serve to unbalance mineral levels in the body. At worst some, like fluoride, can actually cause insidious damage, because it is uncontrolled in water supplies. Fluoride in toothpaste is all that is needed to protect your teeth. Swallowing it is harmful longterm. Several European countries have banned water fluoridation and produce toothpaste free of this mineral for children under 4 years, because they often swallow the paste after tooth cleaning. Researchers believe that water-fluoridation is implicated in Alzheimer's, cancer, mongoloid births and the fragility of bone in osteoporosis.

Many sources of well water are badly polluted with chemicals because anything added to the soil eventually finds its way through to the water table. Heavy levels of nitrogen, phosphates and potash are found in well water in areas where these fertilisers are added to crops. Researchers believe that a mineral imbalance in human beings and plants caused by fertiliser is what leads to chronic disease.

Factories pollute the air and cause acid rain which enters our water supplies. Governments empty effluent and factories flush toxic chemical waste into our rivers, lakes and the sea. We are destroying all sources of clean water and already have to filter everything. There are many good water filters on the market but it is wise to check your local consumer research council to find which ones are the best. They must remove all chemicals and leave the minerals and be particularly effective in removing fluoride. If you choose not to use a filter, drink distilled water and take kelp tablets for the minerals or use mineral water and vary the brands.

Sunshine

Everyone feels well after a day out in the sun and the quality of sleep that night is first class. Sun through the eyes goes from the retina to the pineal gland, which secretes the hormone melatonin. The effect brightens the spirit and causes a feeling of good cheer and happiness. However, to be effective, UV light needs to reach the eyes without the barrier of eye glasses or contact lenses. Just half an hour daily is enough even on cloudy days, for the UV rays to have their effect.

When sunshine is lacking, emotional and mental health suffer, and because the brain communicates with the physical body, that too becomes sick. If the mind is unhappy, the cells become unhappy and then cease to function properly. So try to spend a part of every day outside and remember to remove your specs. If you also take heed of the advice to include omega-3 oils in your diet (oily fish or flaxseeds) you will store extra sunshine in your cells for the winter months.

Sun is absolutely essential to life, but to be most effective a small amount should be absorbed and stored every day. Aside from maintaining the happiness of all your cells, UV light has the following specific effects: it causes the skin to form vitamin D, it increases the function of the immune system and all our hormones. Blood cholesterol and triglyceride levels are reduced, cholesterol plaque shrinks back and high blood pressure is lowered. A little daily UV even protects against skin cancer, whereas those who use sunscreens at all times are more prone to malignant melanomas. In 1982 the *Lancet* reported that skin cancer was considerably more prevalent in office workers than those working outdoors without sunscreen creams. This highlights the need for moderation in all things including sunshine exposure.

Rest and sleep

Those who require only five hours sleep at night are extremely lucky, as they can do so much more with their days. However most need six to eight hours of restful sleep. Adequate rest is essential to mental and physical health, and a healthy person will fall asleep readily and wake refreshed. Those who have disturbed sleep are stressed and must deal with this in order to improve sleep quality. Those who wake tired even after enough hours sleep may be suffering from hypoglycaemia, mineral deficiencies, stress or illness. If a brief nap in the middle of the day increases the afternoon's energy levels then don't ignore what your body requires.

Recreation

Doing things that bring pleasure and relaxation are not only healing but essential to health. Time should be set aside on a daily basis for something relaxing like reading, watching a film, painting, dancing, playing sport, enjoying scenery and fresh air in the country, or whatever equates with pleasure in your mind.

Regular social contact with friends is of utmost importance. This can be through classes, sports groups, bridge, mother-and-toddler groups, coffee mornings or dinners. Loneliness, a feeling of isolation or having no time for yourself also leads to ill-health because you are not then mentally strong. If you are unhappy and have no time to recharge your batteries you cannot give to others successfully. So be a little selfish for a part of every day and don't feel guilty about it!

Love, laughter and joy

If the mind is happy the immune system functions well, and in fact the whole physical body functions well. Emotions enter cells just as easily as they are transferred to those around us, and this means all cells. For instance unhappiness in the immune system means that it cannot fight infection or that it starts attacking its own tissue, and if the liver cells cry they cannot detoxify adequately.

It used to be thought that a happy emotion had to originate in the mind in order to transfer to the cells. However researchers have discovered that just moving the mouth into the smile position causes increased happiness. The smile triggers the release of chemical messages which travel to the brain. Conversely, moving the face into pouting, crying, angry or fearful expressions causes chemical changes that make the brain unhappy. It then sends identical messages to cells of the body. At the same time the heart rate, breathing and skin-conductivity change with the different emotions.

Love involves touch, be it between lovers, friends or parents and children, and touch definitely increases happiness. One of the major benefits of massage is simply touch. It brings relaxation, peace of mind, freedom from pain, a sense of security and a feeling of general wellbeing. Repressed and unhappy emotions may be released through touch. Everyone knows that the love of a pet towards its owner is healing and certainly increases happiness.

To be well as a whole, love, laughter and joy are as essential as a good diet. Go and see an amusing film whenever possible, read funny books, seek out people who make you smile or laugh. Enjoy!

Spiritual development

This is an oft-ignored facet of human growth. We cannot be healthy unless we are physically, mentally and spiritually strong. Time for prayer and meditation should be set aside on a daily basis or at least four times weekly. Meditation is a way of getting in touch with your inner self and finding peace and clarity of mind.

A great many people with busy lives, allowing no time for spiritual growth, have been brought to a grinding halt by serious illness. Those who then reassess their lifestyles and instigate a daily meditation period will often express gratitude for the illness. This is because they discover their essential inner being, learn to listen to it and discover a whole new dimension to existence. A combination of adequate rest, recreation and spiritual growth leads directly to peace of mind, a positive mental attitude and freedom from stress.

Hygiene and elimination

The skin is an elimination organ, and to function correctly it needs the stimulation of regular dry-brush treatment, followed by washing in hot water. A final cold shower stimulates the circulation and nervous system and serves to contain the body's core heat. Aerobic exercise which causes perspiration also increases skin elimination.

The lungs eliminate carbon dioxide from the body. Deep breathing exercises increase oxygenation of the tissues, which is central to proper function. Most people shallow-breathe all day long, never fully expanding the lungs and using the full oxygen/carbon dioxide transfer potential. Carbon dioxide, which is an end-product of energy production in the cells, is released from the venous capillaries into the lungs for removal from the body. Inhaled oxygen is transferred to the haemoglobin molecules in the arterial capillaries of the lungs for transport to all cells in the body.

Daily deep breathing increases the health of all the tissues. Inhale by first pushing out the abdomen and then expanding the lower ribs before filling the upper part of the lungs. Exhale slowly.

The bowel and kidney elimination channels are largely controlled by diet. However exercise and freedom from stress also play an important role.

Exercise

This is important for firm muscle tone, to increase metabolism, improve circulation, skin function, lymph movement and the cleansing of tissues. Muscle tone, flexibility, strength and endurance are improved by power-lifting techniques or floor and stretching exercises. For the health of the cardio-vascular and respiratory systems, exercise needs to be of the aerobic variety. T'ai ch'i has been shown to increase the immune system function, and in fact all moderate forms of exercise do this. However, athletes, with their very heavy training programmes, have a lowered immune function because over exercising stresses the body.

Aerobics. This type of exercise must be continuous, rhythmical and at a rate which significantly increases cardiac output. Thirty minutes four times a week is the minimum considered necessary for health. An additional cooling-off period of five to ten minutes at the end, when exercise is done at a slower rate, is important to prevent the pooling of blood in peripheral areas. Aerobic exercise improves breathing and oxygen use, lowers blood pressure and strengthens the heart and circulation. It also creates a feeling of wellbeing. Those who don't exercise develop cancer, cardio-vascular disease, obesity, diabetes, pulmonary disease or aches and pains due to poor oxygenation.

When exercising, avoid becoming dehydrated, by drinking fluids beforehand. Use electrolyte drinks that are free of glucose, and don't take salt tablets as they draw water from the tissues to the gastro-intestinal tract. Always exercise in clean air areas as carbon monoxide combines readily with haemoglobin in the blood, and this prevents oxygen being transported to the tissues. To work out your safe aerobic pulse rate, subtract your age from 220 and multiply this by 0.8. Do not exercise above this rate.

A balanced diet

That which is balanced for one is a disaster for another, and it is important to find your own food pattern which brings permanent health and vitality. Health is not just freedom from disease but a deep sense of wellbeing with boundless energy, freedom from stress, perfect emotional balance, physical fitness and a strong immune system. All of this is attainable through proper nutrition because the mind and the body are interlinked. If one is healthy so will be the other.

Most people who think that they are well, are in fact muddling along with a body and mind which is no more than barely free from obvious disease. A profound sense of wellbeing is unknown to the majority. Science tells us that we should live to 120 years in good health, but most of us are lucky if we make it to 70 or 80 years old, and very few are in excellent health at this stage.

Fanaticism has no place in nutrition, but those who avoid all processed food are not fanatics. They are just seeking to eat in the way that has been considered natural throughout time. The fanatics could be said to be those who eat nothing but junk. What you do occasionally will do you no harm – it is the routine which is most important, and there is no need for good quality food to be lacking in flavour. There are hundreds of good vegetarian books around now and even meat-eaters should learn to make dishes with grains, beans, nuts and seeds, as they may eventually be necessary for survival. Unless we prevent farmers from polluting our meat sources, and factories and governments from polluting our waters, all animal protein will become unfit for human consumption in the very near future. Then man will have to make yet another adaptation to total veganism in order to survive.

A balanced diet means a balance between carbohydrate, fats, protein and fibre, and if the food supplying these factors is organic and unprocessed, there is a good chance that all the vitamins, minerals and enzymes will also be present. However, this is where rigid patterns end, because we are all bio-chemically different. It was the brilliant biochemist Dr Roger Williams who first proposed what he called the *genetotrophic theory of disease*. In simple terms it means that people become ill if their unique genetic need for certain nutrients is not met. Dr Williams demonstrated that although we all need the same nutrients, some require much higher doses of particular ones than others in order to remain healthy. Dr Williams discovered B vitamins like folic acid and pantothenic acid and contributed a wealth of nutritional know-ledge through his books and teachings. He lived in good health until 91 years old.

As an example of Dr Williams' theory, the natural grain eater will be healthy on a much higher percentage of cereals in his diet than the natural meat-eater. Grains contain a lot of fibre, and yet where cereal is a genetically unsuitable food, severe constipation may and often does occur. Frequently a person is strongly attracted to an unsuitable food, even without allergy being present, so desires are poor guidelines for choosing an eating pattern. It is important to listen to your body's reactions when experimenting with food patterns to find your optimum energy levels.

Soil depletion

If all food were organically produced then vitamin and mineral supplements would probably not be necessary. However, after decades of artificial fertilisa-tion and overcropping most farmers are raising food on dead soil. Dr Béres discovered that cancer was rampant in areas where chemical fertilisers were used, and this is because micro-nutrients are leached from soil and food by these. Even a major mineral like magnesium is widely deficient in the food chain now, as is the vitamin C in an orange. Farmers no longer leave fields fallow or rotate crops, so that each food can add different ingredients to the soil; worst of all they use chemical fertiliser instead of animal manure and compost.

A US department of agriculture report looked at the mineral content of foods from eleven farms using modern agricultural methods. Over just one four year period, the following depletions had occurred: sodium 55%, po-tassium 28%, calcium 41%, magnesium 22%, iron 26%, copper 68%, zinc 10%, manganese 34%, phosphorus 8%. Considering that this depletion increased year by year, the implication is quite frightening in terms of health ten years down the line. Everyone is looking at pesticides and very few are aware of the dangers of fertilisers. It is interesting to note that the phosphorus levels dropped very little. This is one of the big three used in chemical fertiliser, and it is antagonistic to calcium and magnesium.

In an ideal situation, everything is organically-grown. Again, think back to how your parents or grandparents grew vegetables. Remember the days of compost heaps, animal manure and rotating the vegetables in the garden. It wasn't difficult, and the food tasted real because of the high levels of natural minerals and vitamins. It is important to return to this method of growing food, and it will only happen on a larger scale if we all demand organically-grown produce from the shops.

Finding your bio-type

For those who are not able to use any of the bio-typing offered by nutritional computer and hair analysis, use your blood group as a basis for starting the treasure hunt. Next you could relate this to your autonomic/oxidative type to find your optimum eating pattern.

Group O – avoid all grains and most dairy products. Eat fruit, nuts and live yoghurt for breakfast or vegetable juices. For lunch and dinner eat lots of vegetables with fish or meat as a side dish once daily. At the other meal use beans, nuts, seeds, egg and occasionally cottage cheese with the vegetables. Fruit should be taken between meals. If your wellbeing improves, stay with this pattern for a few weeks and then try grains in full servings on a daily basis. If it is an unsuitable food, changes will occur in your body or mind. It may be no more than a subtle shift in energy levels or moods.

Group A – avoid all meats and restrict dairy products. For breakfast eat cereal, fruit, nuts and yoghurt, toast or porridge. Vegetable juices may be used in place of the fruit. For lunch and dinner eat a plateful of vegetables with a vegetarian grain dish at one meal. Use eggs, pulses occasionally, seafood or nuts and seeds at the other meal and ensure complete protein is eaten on a daily basis. See the chapter on vegetarianism for how to do this. Grains should be part of two meals every day and fruit eaten between meals. If the energy levels are good and no ill effects occur such as weight gain in spite of the low calorie intake, stick with the diet for long enough to feel the benefits. Then experiment with meat if you wish.

Group B – follow a vegetarian diet and include dairy products which are unpasteurised, or fermented if possible. This means natural cheeses, quark and yoghurt or kefir. You could start by following a macrobiotic diet and use yoghurt in place of fish. If this eating pattern leads to a feeling of wellbeing then don't change something which is working well, although meat may be quite suitable in small amounts.

Group AB – all foods are said to suit this relatively new blood group so start with a diet containing meat, fish, eggs, dairy, grains, beans, nuts and seeds, and eliminate one thing at a time for two weeks on end. In this way you will discover if any type of food is harmful. Fruit or vegetables should still be the major foods eaten at every meal. This is the only group fully adapted to the potato family.

Whatever group you are, remember to food-combine correctly.

Important food considerations

Acid-alkaline

Whatever type of food is eaten, there are certain basic requirements which are necessary to all. The acid-alkaline end-product must be correct, and this requires 75% of the diet to be alkaline-forming. If two meals a day contain vegetables as the main dish and other foods are treated as a side dish, this will automatically occur as long as fruit is eaten at breakfast or between every meal. Macrobiotic devotees must be careful to include alkaline grain (millet) as a major part of the grain portion, or take some in sprouted form. They must also routinely use seaweed in their cooking.

Raw *versus* cooked food

Two thirds of the diet should be raw for optimum health. Ideally breakfast is totally or at least half-raw, and lunch consists of salad with raw or cooked food as a side dish. In winter a hot soup could be added. For those who can't cope with a big plate of raw food, turn the vegetables and sprouts into juice. Again, find your own optimum balance but work towards the ideal over a period of time.

There are some who opt for nothing but raw food, but this is usually neither necessary nor particularly desirable. Cooked vegetables release some nutrients more readily than do raw ones, and for this reason a little is beneficial. One of the most important reasons for eating raw food is that it is living food and contains enzymes, vitamins and minerals as nature intended us to use. A scientific crystallisation technique which measures the living energy of substances shows that raw food leaves strong patterns, sick plants form weak patterns and cooked ones, none. Natural vitamins also form very different patterns from the chemical ones, and anyone experimenting will soon discover the difference between the natural types and those made by drug companies.

Plants radiate measurable energy, which starts to diminish as soon as they are picked. Even fresh milk straight from the cow contains energy which also is slowly reduced to nil over twenty four hours. Juices made from fruits and vegetables lose 60% of their living enzymes within half an hour of being made. It is known that we do absorb these enzymes, as they have been isolated in the bloodstream.

It is known that we are born with a limited enzyme potential and as we get older the enzymes grow increasingly weak. Much research has proven this. We begin to die only as our enzyme potential runs down and therefore all body function is jeopardised. To maintain youth through a bank account rich in enzymes we must subsidise our own stock from live raw food. This is why the major part of our diet must be raw as nature intended. Higher calorie foods contain the highest stock of enzymes, so sprouted seeds, beans and grains, as well as avocados and bananas have more than lower-calorie fruits and vegetables. Those who eat too much cooked food would be well advised to take enzymes with their meals, as the digestive ones are robbed from the metabolic store needed to maintain every living body function. Longevity absolutely depends on maintaining our 'enzyme potential' storehouse with plenty of raw food.

Basic food volumes

The following broad percentages are generally recognised by all health authorities as being optimum for human nutrition. The figures are in terms of total calories.

Carbohydrate	70-75%
Protein	10-15%
Fat	10-20%

If the food is whole and natural, the fibre content will be high when these ratios are followed. However, the concept of biochemic individuality means that for some people, these ratios require altering in order to maintain optimum health.

Fats

Fat content needs breaking down into categories. Only half may be saturated or monounsaturated, with the ceiling on the saturated portion at one third. Omega-6 oils (linoleic) must form at least one third of the fat content, and omega-3 oils (linolenic) at least one sixth. It would be better if each of these EFAs formed a third each of the total fats. Vegetarians often consume 20% of their total calories as polyunsaturated oil, with virtually no other fats in the diet. Omega-6 is found in sunflower and pumpkin seeds, walnuts and soya. Omega-3 is found in flaxseeds and oily fish with small amounts of pumpkin seeds and walnuts.

On a 2000 calorie diet, 10-20% of calories as fats are very quickly achieved:

1 quarter avocado   (8g)

1 tablespoon nut butter	(7g)
Half a tablespoon oil	(7g)
1oz pine nuts or half cup grated coconut	(14g)
1oz of cream cheese	(10g)
Half cup cooked soya beans	(5g)

This is a little over 20% of calories (44g). Any meat, milk, eggs or butter would be extra, as would be any cakes, biscuits, pancakes or crisps.

Considering that only one third of the allowance (14g) should be saturated this would be covered very quickly with animal fat alone:

1 egg	(2g)
1oz cheese	(4-6g)
4oz lamb leg	(9g)
4oz chicken thigh	(2.5g)
5oz fresh salmon	(7g)
1 tablespoon butter	(7g)
Half cup ice cream	(4g)

In addition to these food sources, all those which contain unsaturated fat also have a varying amount of saturated fat. Peanut butter, low-fat yoghurt, fish, nuts, grains and pulses are examples of this. In fact, many processed peanut butters are 50% saturated palm oil.

The unsaturated half (22g) could be made up from some of the following:

5oz of mackerel	(9g)
5oz fresh salmon	(7g)
Half avocado	(8g)
1 tablespoon linseed (flaxseed) oil	(12g)
1 tablespoon sunflower oil	(12g)
2.5 tablespoons mixed sesame, sunflower and pumpkin seeds	(8g)
3 tablespoons flaxseeds	(8g)
2 walnuts	(8g)
Half cup cooked soya beans	(2.5g)
Quarter cup wheatgerm	(2g)

Remember that some of these also contain saturated or monounsaturated fat. 5oz fresh salmon contains 7g saturated and 7g unsaturated fat. Avocados and seeds have monounsaturated oils as well as the unsaturates. The only good sources of omega-3 oils are flaxseeds and oily fish, so in a 2000 calorie diet one of those servings above is necessary for health on a daily basis. Even though this amount represents only 3% of calories, very few people manage to achieve it.

In today's diet the saturated fats and 'plastic' polyunsaturates are really difficult to control, whereas the essential polyunsaturates are frequently deficient. Care needs to be taken with the latter to ensure adequate amounts of the two essential types, omega-3 and -6 oils, from the only good sources – oily fish, flaxseeds, pumpkin seeds, sunflower seeds, walnuts and soya. To reach a level of 10% of calories from fat, which is usually necessary for reversal of cardio-vascular disease, you would need to be a vegan with a little oily fish added or a vegan taking flaxseeds daily.

Carbohydrates

The carbohydrate percentage is made up of grains, fruit, vegetables, pulses and some nuts. Of the 70-75%, only 10% should be found in white flour, or sugar products. The rest must be from whole grains, fruit and vegetables etc. if good health is to be a reality. Each person must find his own balance of these foods, all the time keeping acid/alkaline balances in mind. Again, the easiest way to do this is to eat full plates of vegetables or fruit at every meal and treat whatever goes with them as a side dish.

When comparing the food levels of carbohydrates, protein, fibre and fat we find the following rough estimates in percentage terms.

	Carbohydrate	Protein	Fibre	Fat
Grains	80-85	8-15	1-3	1-3
Nuts	10-15	10-15	2-4	50-80
Soya beans	37	38	52	20
Tofu	16	54	0	29
Lentils	67	27	4	1.7
Mung sprouts	38	22	38	1
Soya sprouts	35	41	145	9
Other beans	69	25	5	1-5

Vegetables are largely water, but contain quality carbohydrate, protein, fibre and fat. With the water content removed from the equation we have the following approximate estimates in percentages remaining.

	Carbohydrate	Protein	Fibre	Fat
Cauliflower	58	30	11	2
Carrots	81	9	8	1.5
Broccoli	53	31	13	3
Swiss chard	58	29	10	4
Potato	89	10	3	0.5
Onion	78	18	3	1
Lettuce	52	10	36	2
Spinach	51	38	6	4

Protein

On a 2000 calorie diet 50g is 10% of calories. Protein requirements can also be worked out by weight, i.e. 0.8g per kilo of ideal body weight. This figure has a healthy margin of safety built in and the minimum requirement is lower. When the quality and quantity of protein is very high as in vegetarian combinations, less is required. The quality of protein in vegetables and sprouted food is extremely high in relationship to calories.

As an example, here are the protein values for 100g of some vegetables and sprouts.

Broccoli	3.5g	Kale	4.5g
Swiss chard	2.4g	Leeks	2.2g
Cauliflower	2.7g	Mushrooms	2.8g
Potato	2g	Mung sprouts	4g
Spinach	3.5g	Soya sprouts	6.5g
Peas	5.7g	Lentil sprouts	8.4g
Brussels sprouts	4.9g	Alfalfa sprouts	5.1g
Beans	2g	Collards	3.6g
Sweetcorn	3.5g	Avocado	2.3g
Onions	2.5g	Bamboo shoots	3.0g

The major danger of excessive protein is the death of cells. Dr P Schwartz, an expert on the subject, states that amyloid (a by-product of protein metabolism) damages the cell in the same manner as free radicals, and it is a major cause of aging and disease. Meat also causes acidity, a release of inflammatory chemicals, mineral and vitamin imbalances, osteoporosis, cancer and has no fibre. A protein level of 10% is very quickly achieved with a balance between vegetables, seeds, pulses, grains and a little fish or egg. For instance, if beans are eaten for lunch, fruit, nuts and yoghurt at breakfast, and vegetables at two meals, then just 4oz of fish takes the percentage over 10% in a 2000 calorie diet.

Wonder foods

These are foods which supply an incredibly wide range of nutrients, which are fully absorbed and utilised so that small amounts are sufficient.

Spirulina is a fresh water plant (bought as powdered supplement) which contains all the essential amino acids, plus nine others in an alkaline-forming state. The beta-carotene content is 25 times higher than in carrots and the B_{12} content is at least twice that of raw liver. There is also a very wide range of minerals and vitamins and a high percentage of pigments like chlorophyll. Both omega-3 and -6 oils are present. This product is capable of independently sustaining life and will chelate and remove heavy metals from the body, cleanse the blood and tissues, protect against free radicals and alkalise the body.

Wheat grass or *barley grass* juices also contain a similar but reduced amount of proteins, vitamins, minerals and pigments along with many useful enzymes, and therefore have similar properties to spirulina. The enzymes include super-oxide dismutase (the anti-aging free radical scavenger). Wheat grass juice has been used to shrink tumours, heal wounds, other skin conditions and increase haemoglobin levels. The chlorophyll in wheat grass and spirulina has remarkable healing properties. Grasses can be grown at home cheaply for juicing or they can be bought in powdered form.

Aloe vera juice has anti-inflammatory properties. It heals skin, sprained ligaments, the linings of the digestive and the genito-urinary tracts as well as keeping the bowel functioning well. It also has anti- bacterial properties. This product must be cold-processed and unpasteurised, or it is of no value.

Brewer's yeast contains all the B vitamins except B_{12}, as many amino acids as spirulina and a wide range of minerals including GTF chromium for blood sugar control.

Sprouted foods are an excellent way to eat seeds, nuts, grains and beans as all the nutrients are increased by the sprouting process. Some vitamins and minerals increase by as much as 2000%, and the protein content is improved in quality so that the body uses it better. Some grains and pulses come very close to being complete protein after they have been sprouted. The grains or beans become a highly digestible food even for those normally unable to eat unsprouted produce, and soya beans in sprouted form are considered to be an almost perfect food. A major advantage of these foods is that they are grown on unfertilised soil or in water and have no pesticides on them. The Hunzas who live in complete health until a great age use sprouts and the Chinese have used them throughout time. Sprouts contain very high levels of enzymes which prevent cancer by their antioxidant activity. The process of sprouting causes protein levels to rise, B vitamins to increase by 200% to 1500%, and vitamin C goes up by 500%. The sprouting of wheat increases its vitamin content by 600 to 1000%. The minerals in grains and beans which are bound to phytates are released by the sprouting process and available for use in the body. Buy a good book on sprouting and start doing it at home so that these foods are available for daily use. The commercial varieties are often forced with chemicals and grown in dirty water. The quality of the seeds and grains need to be very high or they won't sprout well. Old or diseased stocks cannot grow into healthy vibrant plants.

The naturopathic diet

• Everything should be organically grown and fresh.

- 80% alkaline-forming (largely fruit and vegetables, with grains, seeds and pulses if in sprouted form).
- Two-thirds raw.
- 80-85% fruit, vegetables and grains. Those unsuited to grains can use fruit, vegetables and buckwheat (a seed), and perhaps a little of the non-gluten grains (corn, millet, rice).
- 5-10% pulses, fish, eggs, meat, dairy.
- 10% seeds, nuts and oils. All oils to be genuinely cold pressed.
- High fibre from wholegrains (not wheat bran), fruit and vegetables.

Beverages
- 6-8 glasses of water or juice daily.
- Herbal teas, miso (a Japanese soya drink), fruit and vegetable juices, soya and nut milk with carob or blended banana added.
- Cereal or dandelion coffee.

Do not drink less than half an hour before a meal or until one hour afterwards.

Fruit and vegetables
- Fruit three times daily, preferably 30 minutes before or 3 hours after any other food except a little live yoghurt or nuts and seeds.
- A vegetable juice at least 3 times weekly.
- Two platesful of vegetables daily, and at least one to be raw. Eat a wide range and include garlic every day.
- Cooked vegetables may be lightly steamed, stir-fried, baked or made into a soup.
- Include a small amount of seaweed daily.
- Sprouted grains, seeds and pulses should be eaten every day as a part of a salad or added to the juice.

Wholegrains
- Preferably millet, corn, spelt, quinoa, rice and buckwheat.
- Barley, rye, oats and wheat in smaller amounts.
- Feeding brown rice to your dog and eating the white variety yourself, ensures that your respective life- spans will come closer together!

Pulses
- Soya beans, black-eye peas, chickpeas, kidney beans, pinto and lima beans, lentils, tofu and tempeh etc. Put these into sauces to serve as a main course in the same way as meat is presented.
- Pulses can be sprouted; lentils and mung beans are particularly easy to do.

Seeds and nuts
- Buy these unroasted and unsalted. You may gently roast them yourself but

only make three day's supply at a time.

- Eat at least two tablespoons of seeds daily (flaxseed, sunflower, sesame, pumpkin). Remember that half the fat content of your diet must be found in omega-3 and -6 oils (see 'Fats', earlier in this chapter).
- Use sprouted seeds in salad and between meals (alfalfa, cress, sunflower, buckwheat).
- Nuts can be cooked as loaves or patés but keep the heat low to avoid damaging the oil contents.
- Store fresh nuts in the fridge or freezer – although long freezing destroys the protective vitamin E.
- Make nut milk for cereals and salad dressings.

Fish, meat and dairy
- Use these in small quantities only.
- Follow a rule of *either/or*.
- Restrict animal protein to once daily only, other than cow's milk yoghurt or eggs occasionally.
- Fresh cold water fish three times weekly, or flaxseeds daily for vegetarians. Poach, steam or bake the fish.
- Meat should be organically raised. Lamb is probably the least polluted of all farmed meat, but it needs to be casseroled so that the fat can be skimmed off the surface.
- Lamb's liver or kidneys or organic beef and chicken liver have very high nutrient levels.
- Free range chicken and eggs. If the skin is removed, organic chicken is low in fat and most of it is unsaturated.
- Live low-fat yoghurt, home-made cottage cheese from fresh milk, or a little hard cheese occasionally. The goat's variety is best.
- Shellfish from clean water sources.

Natural sweeteners
- Organic or wild honey – others contain sugar fed to bees in winter.
- Molasses is what is left after sugar has been refined, and it is full of vitamins and minerals.
- Muscovado sugar is the unprocessed form.
- Dried fruit will sweeten a porridge if added during the cooking process.
- Maple syrup or rice syrup.
- Carob. This is a chocolate substitute loaded with nutrients and without any caffeine.

Natural flavourings
- Vegetable stocks, such as *Vecon*.
- Herbs, garlic, ginger, parsley, lemon grass, french mustard, yeast extract,

tahini (crushed sesame seeds), tamari (naturally brewed wheat-free soya sauce), lemon, cider vinegar or wine vinegar and vanilla.
- Do not use malt or distilled vinegar, as they destroy red blood cells and interfere with digestion.

Dressings
- Extra virgin olive oil or cold-pressed seed oil with lemon juice or cider vinegar, mustard, herbs and garlic.
- Nut milk (blend one quarter cup of nuts and one and a quarter cup of water) with added lemon juice, honey and a little sea-salt.
- Yoghurt with added tahini, lemon juice, a little soya sauce and garlic, or with horseradish, garlic and parsley.
- Yoghurt with added mint, garlic and grated cucumber.
- Yoghurt with added mayonnaise, garlic and fresh herbs.
- Do not always use cow's milk yoghurt. Make soya milk yoghurt instead, and silken tofu can be used as a base for dressings.
- Mayonnaise, homemade with extra virgin olive oil or a seed oil and egg yolk, mustard, vinegar and lots of garlic.
- Italian *Pesto*. Make your own with fresh basil, olive oil and real parmesan cheese.
- Tomatoes puréed with added nuts, garlic and herbs.
- Vegetable stock and puréed tomatoes in equal amounts with added cider vinegar, garlic and oregano or basil.

These can all be used on salads or poured over cold cooked beans, pasta or grains. Lots of other very tasty dressing and dips can be found in health food books.

Spreads
- Nut cheeses, where ground-up nuts are blended with *Rejuvelac* (a wheat ferment), tahini, spring onions and herbs, or with cooked finely-chopped vegetables and stock.
- Houmous (hummus): a Greek/Lebanese dip made of chickpeas, lemon, garlic, parsley and tahini.
- Babar ganoush: a Lebanese dip which is made the same way as houmous, except that cooked aubergines replace the chickpeas.
- Lentil spread: cooked lentils mixed with cooked vegetables and spices.
- Olive paté: a blend of olives, olive oil, capers, garlic, parsley and wine vinegar.
- Avocado-based spreads like *Guacamole*.
- Cottage cheese, homemade with added flavourings such as garlic or ground-up nuts.

Most of these recipes can be found in the books recommended in the chapter on vegetarianism.

Living dangerously

Because a good diet involves whole natural foods, it is obvious that at least 75% of food in supermarkets is on the *avoid* list. It is easy to forget that our present lifestyle based on convenience food is fairly new, and only present in westernised societies. Those who have forgotten how to eat in a healthy manner will look at this list and feel that there is nothing left to eat! To them I can only say *work into it slowly*. Think back to the type of food prepared by your mother or grandmother in the 1930s to 40s, when everything was made at home from whole natural food. Although sugar and white flour was used, many other processed foods were not. Fruit and vegetables were not artificially fertilised or sprayed, and animals were not fed huge doses of hormones, antibiotics and garbage food. Chickens and eggs were free-range and eggs were only available at certain times of the year when the hens were laying. Food was eaten according to season and not frozen. Processed oils and margarine were virtually non-existent, and in northern Europe cold-pressed flaxseed oil could be ordered weekly for home delivery with the milk.

For us, at the end of the twentieth century, it now requires real effort to find what our immediate forebears took for granted, but if we are to feel alive and well at all times we must search out unadulterated food and water. We must also accept that more time needs to be spent in the kitchen, so that home baking using natural ingredients again becomes a norm. Biscuits, cakes, waffles, ice cream, pasta and bread can all be made from whole natural ingredients. Some supermarkets are bowing to pressure and stocking whole organic food, and we can encourage this by buying these products in preference to the food grown with artificial fertilisers.

Avoid

- Processed and refined food, and everything made from them – white flour, white rice, pearl barley, corn starch, sugar and so on. This includes commercial cakes. biscuits, pastry, bread, crumpets, waffles, packaged cereals, doughnuts, sweets, chocolate, ice cream and jams. Besides the obvious, remember the following: sweetened yoghurts, flavoured milk, processed cheese, orange coloured cheese, canned soups, vegetables and fruit. A maximum of 10% of the carbohydrate content of the diet can come from processed grains if necessary.
- All additives, like so-called natural flavourings, colourings, preservatives, artificial sweeteners and dyes.
- All chemically-extracted oils. Margarine and whipped-up cooking fats.
- All rancid food; old butter and grains, old seeds, nuts and oil.

- Chemicals in food and water – and this includes fertiliser as well as pesticides.
- Excessive salt and fast foods. If all processed foods are avoided a little sea salt added to protein is alright.
- Canned drinks, squashes, and sweetened juices. Use unsweetened fruit juice, preferably freshly made in a juice extractor.
- All processed meats like bacon and salami, sausages and ham because of nitrites in them, which are carcinogenic.
- Tap water. White and malt vinegar.
- Peanuts, and all deep-frying.
- All enriched food, as added synthetic vitamins are harmful.
- All household toxic chemicals – air fresheners, sprays, *Chlorox*, etc.

Restrict

- Alcohol to wine, and only with a meal. Buy a good quality chemical-free type, and don't drink every day.
- Tea and coffee to once daily at most.
- Grains that have not been soaked overnight, sprouted, fermented or subjected to long slow cooking. Europeans have always served soaked muesli. It is a norm in Switzerland, Germany and Austria.
- Dairy products to low-fat yoghurt and natural cottage cheese, or a little hard cheese sometimes.
- Strong spices to very occasional use.
- Any natural food which doesn't suit your bio-type.
- Meat to small servings of low-fat types, preferably organically raised.

Menu choices

Early morning

- Hot water and lemon juice or a vegetable juice with added powdered spirulina, wheat or barley grass and aloe vera juice.

Breakfast

- Fresh fruit, a little plain live yoghurt, chopped fresh nuts and seeds.
- Unsweetened soaked muesli with sweet fruit, nut milk or soya milk.
- Fresh, sweet fruit and buckwheat pancakes.
- Fresh acid fruit and poached eggs with tomatoes.
- Wholewheat toast or black rye bread with cooked mushrooms and tomatoes, a vegetarian spread or a little butter, honey or vegetable extract. Sweet fruit may be served with this meal.
- A large glass of mixed vegetable juice with blended sprouted produce

instead of fruit on some days. An apple may be added to the vegetable juice.

- Fruit at breakfast is a good habit for everyone, and to eat fruit only is cleansing and detoxifying. However, this should not become a routine for most people, as many bio-types require grains or other substantial food at breakfast. Just remember that any fruit can be eaten as long as it is taken 30 minutes before other food, and it can also be eaten at the same time as a little live yoghurt, nuts and seeds. Otherwise, food-combine carefully, or your breakfast will ferment and you may experience a bloated sluggish feeling.

Mid-morning

- Fruit and herbal tea, cereal coffee, or miso. A few nuts if hungry.

Lunch

- A large plate of salad vegetables; lettuce, cucumber, tomato, cauliflower, broccoli, radish, spring onion, avocado, grated carrot, sweet turnip, courgette, green beans, watercress, mushrooms, onion, fresh herbs etc. Use spinach, cabbage or chicory as a base instead of lettuce sometimes. A very large handful of sprouted produce should be added daily and a little seaweed as sources of mega-nutrients.
- Make a tasty dressing or dip from the dressings list.

Side dishes:

- brown rice salad or Italian polenta;
- buckwheat salad;
- wholegrain pasta (wheat, corn, millet, quinoa, spelt);
- potato salad or a jacket potato with live flavoured yoghurt and spring onions;
- chickpeas or tofu concoctions;
- mixed home roasted seeds and nuts;
- wholegrain bread and a vegetarian spread;
- low-fat cottage cheese;
- home-made hot vegetable soup, containing barley, beans or lentils;
- peppers stuffed with a grain mix or pumpkin stuffed with a grain and seaweed mix;
- nut loaf or patés;
- home-made pizza with a wholewheat crust;
- home-made spinach quiche with wholewheat crust – no crust if food-combining.

Mid afternoon

- Herbal tea and fruit.

Dinner

- Fruit may be served as a starter half an hour before the main course.
- A large plate of mixed vegetables preferably half as salad and the rest stir-fried, steamed or baked in a soupy sauce.
- Vegetarians will eat in the same manner as lunch but carefully combine vegetable protein. Even meat-eaters should have some days without animal protein. They may also reverse the lunch and dinner menus if desired.

Side dishes:

- fresh oily or white fish with lemon juice or a light low-fat wine sauce;
- an omelette or a cheesy vegetarian dish;
- lamb fillet and mint dressing;
- free-range chicken breast or wild game in a non-dairy sauce;
- shellfish from clean water sources.

Remember that meat servings must be small.

1½ hours after dinner, herbal tea, miso or grain coffee.

Notes

- If allergies are present, rotate all other foods so that the same things are not eaten on consecutive days.
- Don't eat if your are upset, tired, in pain or ill.
- Do not overeat and do not eat too close to bedtime.
- Chew food very thoroughly.
- Never go hungry.
- Do not drink water with meals as it dilutes the digestive juices.
- Eat slowly and in a relaxed manner.
- Don't cook in aluminium pans.
- Follow food-combining.
- Juice fast from time to time to cleanse your tissues.

If you eat good quality food at least 90% of the time, not only will your physical health be vastly improved but your mental wellbeing also. Many negative personality trends will disappear without effort so that you become easier to live with and more able to cope with other people's mood swings. You will find yourself looking at every day optimistically. smiling a lot and having a deep sense of inner peace and joy. If the whole family eats correctly, then the effect will be really noticeable in terms of family life, relationships and problem solving as well as physical wellbeing.

'Our food should be our medicine – our medicine should be our food'.
Hippocrates 400 BC.

Part Three

DISEASE CONTROL

INTRODUCTION

The following chapters are presented in such a manner that readers can readily treat themselves. However, naturopaths never look at a person as a *'disease' per se*. We always follow the holistic approach of treating the individual as a whole. Only in this way can we pinpoint the causes of symptoms and instigate the correct treatment. Sometimes only the diet or its nutrient content is at fault, but at other times environmental, emotional or spiritual problems need to be addressed before health is restored. Many people need a lengthy period of detoxification to cleanse the tissues, bowel, liver and kidneys before any other treatment can be started. In the following diseases, I have highlighted all these features and it rests with you, the reader, to do your best at viewing yourself in a holistic sense and making changes in the appropriate areas.

The first two parts of the book have taught you how disease arises and how to prevent it with a healthy lifestyle. Part three highlights the power of the mind over health and the role of toxicity and allergy in disease, in addition to dietary specifics relevant to each condition.

The purpose of including herbs and homoeopathy alongside supplements is to give you a choice of treatments to complement the diet. Additionally, with knowledge of the function of each supplement, you can more readily choose those which are relevant to yourself. Unfortunately there is no space in this book for itemising deficiency symptoms of all vitamins and minerals, but everyone should own a book on this subject.

In most of the following 'diseases', it is certainly not necessary to take everything suggested, but sometimes herbs and homoeopathy are required in conjunction with supplements to effect a cure. Homoeopathy alone will often eradicate many symptoms, but remember that if your diet and its nutrient content is inadequate, good health will not be maintained. *'We are what we eat'* can also be expressed as, *'What we eat turns into us'*. It is our routine which is so important; if that is wholesome then no harm is done by occasionally eating or drinking a food which does not build health. Re-read part two from time to time as a reminder of the path you should be routinely following.

In nearly every chapter I have only given adult doses of supplements. Space permits nothing more, but a good book about vitamins and minerals will indicate the correct dosage for all ages of children. However, these are usually designed for disease prevention and treatment doses may be considerably higher. If in doubt, seek the guidance of a naturopath or nutritionist, as they are the only people highly qualified in this field. The appendix contains a chapter about herbs which details the method for determining children's doses of plant remedies.

I wish you health, happiness and good fortune, for such should be our expectation throughout life!

III: *1. THE IMMUNE SYSTEM*

The immune system is like a huge army with many ranks, all designed to protect the human body against foreign invasion. It acts as a barrier, recognises invaders, traps them, destroys them and holds their fingerprints for swift retribution should invaders of the same family return.

Stem Cell in Bone Marrow

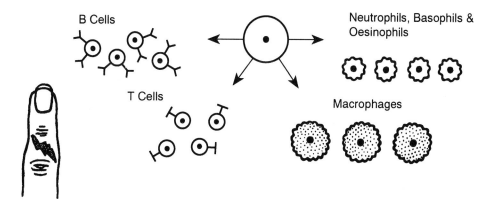

B Cells

Neutrophils, Basophils & Oesinophils

T Cells

Macrophages

The *barrier* part of the system consists of the acid pH and sebum in the skin, the mucous membrane in the mouth and nose with its cilia to move organisms out again, tears for flushing the invader and acid gastric juice to destroy anything making it as far as the stomach. Lysozyme is an enzyme which breaks down bacterial cell walls and it is found in perspiration, saliva, tears, nasal secretions, urine and tissues.

The *moving and active* part of the immune system begins in the red bone marrow. Here a stem cell forms all the major blood cells, both red and white, but only the latter are part of the immune system. See the diagram for a quick memory-trigger of the unfamiliar names to follow. The stem cells make white cells called *lymphocytes* of two types, T-cells and B-cells. In addition they make *phagocytes*, which come in the form of large *macrophages* and tiny *neutrophils, basophils* and *eosinophils.* All these cells leave the marrow and travel to the blood stream, where they have specific duties within the immune system army.

The eosinophils are seconded to deal with things like allergies, but the basophils are the look-outs, and as soon as an invader is sighted, they call up the tiny neutrophils. These can squeeze through blood vessel walls and are the first line of defence against invaders in the tissues. The macrophages are divided into two groups: the fixed type make their homes in lymphatic tissue, and from there they reach out to trap and imprison any microbes going by in the lymph flow; the wandering macrophages also live in the lymph nodes and spleen, but they will be mobilised to move out into the blood stream and travel to the site of foreign invasion whenever the little neutrophils call for assistance.

Phagocytes (neutrophils and macrophages) act by engulfing foreign invaders, stunning them from inside with lysozyme and then presenting them to the T- and B-cells for specific action.

Neutrophils live only a few hours, so we can make billions of them in a day. The wandering macrophages which come speedily, when the neutrophils call, have the job of assisting in trapping microbes as well as mopping up all the debris from the battlefield. This includes dead neutrophils. Additionally they ensure that the body makes extra neutrophils when necessary, so that this rank of the army is kept up in numbers.

The host cells that become infected will often secrete a substance called *interferon*, which passes from an infected cell to neighbouring uninfected ones, to leave the message that they must protect themselves. They do this by producing antimicrobial protein to stop the invader from breeding inside healthy cells. Macrophages also produce interferon, and the combined effect inhibits the spread of infection. The other major antimicrobial protein circulates in the blood and is called *complement*. The army mobilises this in response to antibody activities and coats a microbe to attract phagocytes to the area, like bees to honey. The microbe is then destroyed.

Now for a look at our specific resistance mechanism, the powerful T- and B-cells which form the higher ranks. These are made by the stem cells in the bone marrow, and the T-cells then travel to the thymus gland in the chest to be programmed. The B-cells are processed elsewhere, before both types make their home in lymphoid tissue like the spleen and lymph nodes.

T-cells are activated by foreign invaders and then divide into killer, helper, suppressor and memory T-cells. The killers destroy microbes which are served up as stunned prisoners by the macrophages. The helpers stimulate the formation of antibodies and the suppressors inhibit them so that a balance is maintained. The suppressors also inhibit the killers once the war is over, or else the killers would run amok and destroy healthy tissue. Memory T-cells remember the fingerprints of invaders and cause an immediate response should they dare show their faces again. When the ratios between the various T-cells are unbalanced, all kinds of problems can arise.

People with allergies or auto-immune diseases have too many helpers and therefore too many antibodies, whereas AIDS victims have greatly reduced killer T-cells and all the ratios are unbalanced. In allergy, the immune system is making antibodies against food. This occurs because it is weakened by such things as stress, pollution and a poor diet. An auto-immune disease is one in which the immune system is making antibodies against its own tissue. This triggers a destructive attack because the body tissue is being recognised as an invader. Again this can only happen if we are weakened by poor lifestyles. Rheumatoid arthritis, lupus erythematosus, rheumatic fever and multiple sclerosis are all auto-immune diseases.

T-cells and macrophages secrete chemical messengers called *lymphokines*, and these trigger the production of helpers and suppressors. Indirectly they are responsible for the rejection of transplants by increasing the helpers, but they also send messages which lead to the destruction of tumours, fungus and many bacteria. The T-cell function is to see to the actual annihilation of foreign invaders, to attract antibodies and macrophages and to increase their effect. They are like the generals in the army.

B-cells are responsible for our antibody system. There are thousands of different types of B-cells and each responds only to a specific foreigner (antigen). B-cells stay put in lymphoid tissue and first become plasma cells which in turn make antibodies. They do this at the rate of 2000 per second each, whenever they are activated by a specific invader. The antibodies die of overwork in four to five days. Each B-cell secretes only one type of antibody, and this action is stimulated by the entrance of a foreigner whose markings are recognised by the memory B-cells. They are also mobilised by a totally new invader being presented in a straitjacket by a phagocyte.

Antibodies belong to a group of proteins called *globulins*, and for this reason they are also known as *immunoglobulins* (**Ig**s), of which there are many different types: **IgG** enhances the phagocytosis process and neutralises toxins. It also protects the foetus and new-born. **IgA** protects the mucous membrane barrier against invasion, and **IgM** is specific in action against microbes that kill. **IgE** is involved in allergic reactions and **IgD** stimulates antibody production. Every part of our immune system is inter-related and they all constantly support each other.

The immune response to microbial invasion

- The microbe (antigen) enters the tissues having got past the barriers.
- The basophils (in the blood) and mast cells (basophils residing in the tissues) immediately release chemicals called *kinnins* to attract the neutrophils to the area. At the same time they release histamine to dilate blood vessels and make the walls more porous, so that phagocytes can move into the tissues to begin the war. This happens in allergy as well.
- The neutrophils set about immobilising the microbes by engulfing them. The latter are also coated with complement to attract more neutrophils, and interferon is produced to prevent microbial invasion of healthy areas.
- Neutrophils call up the heavies – macrophages which remove the dead neu-

The Immune System Fighting Infection

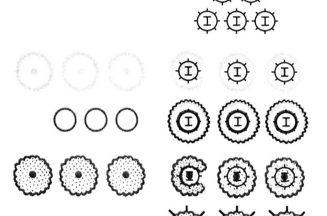

The invader enters and multiplies rapidly. This attracts the immune system.

Enter the Neutrophils to engulf the microbes.

Complement stick to the free microbes and attracts more immune components.

Enter the macrophages to assist the Neutrophils and clear the debris. The microphages contain the microbes and dead Neutrophils.

The macrophages develop the invader's marking which attracts the T and B cells.

The macrophages present the microbe to the T and B cells

B Cells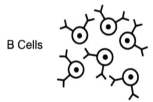

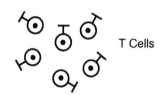 T Cells

The specific B cells divide into 4 types

The specific T cells divide into 4 types

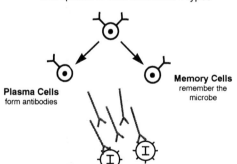

Plasma Cells
form antibodies

Memory Cells
remember the microbe

Antibodies attach to the microbe and activate the complement system which is fixed to the microbe. Destruction of the invader begins

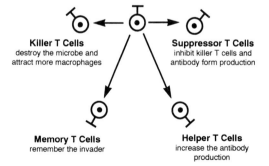

Killer T Cells
destroy the microbe and attract more macrophages

Suppressor T Cells
inhibit killer T cells and antibody form production

Memory T Cells
remember the invader

Helper T Cells
increase the antibody production

trophils with their enclosed microbes, as well as clearing any other debris. Additionally they ensure that a constant supply of neutrophils is being made, and secrete a chemical messenger for communicating with T-cells.
• Macrophages then develop surface-markers relating to the particular microbes inside them and present their bundles to T-cells, which then enlarge and divide into the four types. The killers destroy the stunned microbe. The helpers stimulate the formation of antibodies against that specific organism once it has been presented to the B-cells for recognition. The suppressors ensure that antibody production and killer T-cells are controlled and stopped once the infection is over.
• Once the specific antibodies have been mobilised, they travel to the site of the invasion, combine with foreign invaders and activate complement to coat microbes. This attracts more phagocytes and killers to the area. The co-operation between the different ranks is awe- inspiring.
• The next time the same family of microbes enters the body, memory-cells act fast and trigger the specific antibodies to be made immediately and in enormous amounts. These travel at the speed of light to the site of invasion, get chummy with the microbes by forming antigen/antibody complexes, secrete complement to coat them – and then the whole process of destruction begins and is over before any symptoms occur. This is known as the *secondary response*. The first time a microbe enters the body, the antibody response takes a few days to begin and then slowly increases. This is called the *primary response*. When you recover from an infection over a period of days, it is caused by the primary response, but when you recover without ever getting any signs and symptoms, the secondary response has been at work.

Damage to the immune system

If this whole amazing army is to function properly, it must be protected from breakdown. A good diet is the first line of defence. If the immune system does not receive a wide variety of vitamins and minerals it starts knocking like an old car and missing beats. Equally damaging are processed foods like white flour, sugar, oils and margarine because they block immune system functions very dramatically. Studies have shown that just one teaspoon of sugar in an infection will reduce neutrophil phagocytosis by 50% within half an hour, and the effect lasts five hours. Conversely, fasting increases phagocytosis by 50%. An interesting hypothesis is that insulin and vitamin C compete, and therefore the sugar which raises insulin levels in the blood prevents vitamin C from strengthening immune function. Studies also indicate that where fat and cholesterol levels are raised, antibody response is slow and phagocytosis inhibited.

Vaccinations stress the immune system by causing it to over-react. Receiving microbes in concentrated form is not what the immune system is designed to cope with! Stress, anxiety and depression also have potent inhibiting effects on immunity. Experiencing relief of allergic reactions and minor infections when on holiday clearly demonstrates this aspect. Antibiotics and other drugs, the contraceptive pill, alcohol and smoking also impede the immune system, and those using antibiotics several times a year will be well aware of becoming weaker in the long run. Eating food to which you are allergic means that the antibody system is forever being activated and so it becomes impossible to correct the important ratio between helper and suppressor T-cells. Illnesses including candida, operations and burns keep the immune system under constant stress, as does pollution. By this term I mean not only the air we breathe, but the chemicals in water and food. Free radicals and lack of antioxidants, excessive sex, marathon running and the removal of tonsils or the spleen will also reduce immune activity. Toxicity in the body as a result of poor bowel function means that there is no rest for many parts of the immune system, and this often results in the development of an auto-immune disease like rheumatoid arthritis or lupus erythematosus.

To maintain a healthy immune function we need good quality organic food, filtered water, filtered air in the house, exercise, relaxation and happiness. Stress-release techniques alone powerfully strengthen immune function.

Psychoneuro-immunology

This literally means the mind/brain influence over immunity. The brain, the immune system and our hormones are known to communicate with each other, and every cell can receive brain and hormonal messages. Not only can the mind influence the activity of the immune system, but our emotions can also enter white blood cells. In other words stress, unhappiness or joy can be received in the cells. If the immune system is unhappy it cannot function properly, and in cancer, it eventually becomes paralysed and completely unable to destroy foreign cells.

Once we realise that we are responsible for our own lives and can influence that and every part of our bodies with our minds, a sense of inner strength is born; fear, victim attitudes, despair and self-pity disappear. These negative emotions are replaced with enthusiasm, positive thoughts, excitement and an inner drive. The immune system and hormones also respond in a positive manner and happiness prevails all round – in the cells as well as in the mind. ***Happy cells do not malfunction.***

The reason that some people experience 'spontaneous' recovery from terminal cancer is normally due to a shift in attitude from a helpless to a positive area. Once these people consciously take charge, everything changes for the better, whereas helpless people, with their unhappy immune systems, continue to grow lumps.

T-cells have receptors for sex and stress hormones as well as endorphin messengers from the brain. In this way immunity can be influenced by the mind. For instance, when we are stressed, the release of cortisole hormones depresses the immune system, and when we are happy, immune function increases. T-cells also produce their own types of hormones and endorphins for talking back to the brain. This means that when the immune system is depressed it can complain to the mind in an effort to rectify the situation. Additionally, T-cells produce special messengers called *lymphokines* for communicating with each other. The brain too has receptors for lymphokines in order to listen in on T-cells talking to each other and to receive status reports from the immune system. So when the latter is fighting an invader, lymphokines act like messengers to all parts of the army as well as to the brain. Equally, when immune function is depressed because of receiving unhappy hormonal messages it can shout at the mind to rectify the situation. T-cell hormones are also received by the endocrine glands (thyroid, thymus, adrenals, ovaries etc.) and so influence their activity as well.

These discoveries have given us a scientific explanation for the long-known fact that *the immune system can be activated by the mind*. It has been proven over and over (with blood tests) that cancer and AIDS patients can increase their killer T-cells and phagocytes by visualisation techniques – by thought. A positive mind is the only pre-requisite for a successful outcome. A stab of fear, despondency about the chances of a cure, or resignation to eventual death profoundly inhibits immune system function, whereas a fighting spirit galvanises it into action. Happiness and health are inexorably linked.

All types of visualisation involve messages passing from the brain to relative parts of the body – and even stress-release techniques – encourage the immune system to increase activity. Everyone has seen that extra sleep, relaxation and holidays will often clear all manner of infections, whereas stresses predispose us to colds and flu. Stress in moderation is the spice of life, but what is stressful to one is not so to another. The aim of relaxation techniques and meditation is to increase the body's resistance to stress so that higher levels are tolerated without harming the immune or glandular systems.

Repair of the immune system

This involves taking steps to avoid all that damages the immune function, in addition to restorative measures. Follow the naturopathic diet and lifestyle, as all those aspects are important to immune function. Dry skin brushing followed by hot and cold showering has alone been shown to increase resistance to infection, and regular walking raises natural killer T-cell levels. For those who also need nutrients to rebuild their immunity or protect it against doses of toxic drugs or radiation, supplements are discussed below. Remember that stress is particularly harmful to immune competence, and failure to deal with it may result in an auto-immune disease or cancer in the long term.

Hormonal effects on immunity

The *thymus gland* is the field marshal of the immune system and as such is responsible for priming the T-cells to ensure proper forma-

tion and function. Thymic hormones also tell lymph nodes that their function in life is to fight bacteria and reject foreign cells. As we age, the thymus shrinks, and so our T-cell function is reduced. This process can be delayed by reducing stress and taking antioxidant vitamins and minerals to prevent free radical damage to the gland. We can also stimulate its activity with other nutrients such as thymus glandular supplements. However, because of the difficulty in finding unpolluted animal sources of thymus gland ingredients, many manufacturers have stopped making them. Nutrients which stimulate the thymus and prevent damage are: the amino acid arginine, vitamins A, C, E and B6, the minerals selenium, zinc and magnesium.

The *thyroid gland* stimulates the primed T-cells to act, and oestrogen from the ovaries increases phagocytosis. Conversely oestrogen speeds shrinkage of the thymus and thus reduces T-cell formation. Perhaps it acts as a foil for thyroxine action, as the body has many ways of maintaining balance in all things.

Vitamins

● *Beta carotene* is a powerful antioxidant and so protects the thymus against damage and shrinkage. It strengthens immune barriers like skin and mucous membranes and has been shown to increase the following immune activity: helper T-cells, phagocytosis, antibody response, killer T-cell activity and destruction of tumours. An excess of vitamin A will decrease interferon production, whereas an adequate amount will increase it, which means that too much prevents surrounding cells from protecting themselves against invasion. The safety margin of beta carotene is very much higher than vitamin A but even so, studies indicate that gross excesses of it may reduce vitamin E by as much as 40%. Carrot juice is a good source of beta carotene.

- *Vitamin C* increases the chemical messengers, which is important in infections and cancer. It improves the rate of all immune cell production and interferon as well as raising the secretion of hormones from the thymus. Clearly the whole immune system requires vitamin C.
- *Vitamin E* improves the function of T-cells, B-cells and macrophages. It has been shown to increase T-cells by three to five times. The helpers are raised in laboratory tests if doses are below 150iu daily, which means that low dosage fights infection and cancer. The suppressors are raised if the dosage is at 400iu daily, which means that allergies and auto-immune diseases like multiple sclerosis benefit. However, researchers have not conclusively established the effect of vitamin E on these ratios in human studies. Vitamin E protects the thymus gland along with other antioxidant vitamins and minerals.
- *Vitamin B6* is needed by T-cells and B-cells and without it the spleen and the thymus shrink, so that less cells can be made and the quality is reduced. Folic acid, vitamin B5 and vitamin B12 are required for all white blood cell production and function.

Minerals
- *Selenium* increases B-cells, complement and lysozyme.
- *Zinc* regulates T-cell numbers, phagocytosis, thymic hormone and the function of complement. A deficiency of zinc can either cause low levels of T-cells (infections) or an excess (auto-immune disease). Zinc is anti-microbial in a broad sense and is of particular value in destroying genito-urinary microbes. It will also banish colds in many children. Zinc is rapidly used up in growth and development and this is why so many youngsters are deficient in this mineral.
- *Manganese* increases T-cell activity, but if the levels are too high it will depress the

messenger interferon.
- *Iron* deficiency means that our first line of defence is reduced, but an excess allows the invader to use it and therefore multiply its army. Iron balances the T- and B-cell ratio, and like all other supplements, the correct dosage is important.
- *Calcium* and *magnesium* are also essential nutrients for immune system competence.

Essential fatty acids
- *EPA* from oily fish enhances immune function, and it has been noted that a deficiency reduces the healthy inflammatory response instigated by the neutrophils, basophils and infected cells. If this happens, infection cannot be nipped in the bud. Those who eat harmful oils and margarines, block the activity of EPA in the body.
- *Evening primrose oil* is the precursor of the tissue hormone PGE1, which regulates T-cell function. It increases suppressor T-cells when necessary and is therefore useful for reducing antibodies in auto-immune disease and allergy. The suppressors modulate killer T-cells in these conditions so that they stop destroying self and concentrate on foreign invaders instead.

Amino acids
The immune system cells are made of protein so it is not unreasonable that individual components have specific effects on immunity. For instance, glutamine and ornithine are aminos which increase the immune response to bacteria by raising killer T-cells. Histidine regulates the helper/suppressor ratio in allergy and auto-immune disease and increases phagocytosis. The catabolic aminos, cysteine, methionine and glutamic acid inhibit viral replication and also act as powerful antioxidants. Tryptophan and phenylalanine stimulate antibody production. Arginine activates the thymus to produce T-cells, stimulates phagocytosis and increases the activity of

killer T-cells. In a test where an enormous dose was used for just three days, natural killer T-cells increased by 91%. Research in this area may lead to usage for AIDS and cancer, but the test dose used would almost certainly be toxic long term.

Herbs

There are a great many herbs in nature's pharmacy which act on the immune system. A few of the well-known ones are explained as follows:

- *Echinacea* protects the mucous membrane and tissue barrier, increases complement and interferon, enhances all phagocytic activity, activates T-cells and has a specific anti-viral, anti-bacterial and anti-fungal action – a virtual cure-all which is used in the case of a great many diseases.
- *Licorice* increases the antibodies IgA, IgG, IgM and memory cells. It also raises interferon levels, macrophage, and natural killer-cell activity. It is strongly anti-viral and will completely inactivate the DNA of the herpes virus, amongst others.
- *Golden seal* and other berberine plants increase spleen function and have an anti-bacterial effect against a very wide range of organisms.
- *Shitake mushrooms* and *reishi mushrooms* (*ganoderma*) increase interferon, T-cells and enhance macrophage and helper T-cell function. They are very powerful stimulants to the immune system and of great value in cancer and leukaemia.
- *Ginseng* is for allergies and the recovery stage of infections. At high doses it inhibits lymphocytes but the reverse is true in moderate doses. Phagocytosis is increased by the herb, and it inhibits tumours and their spread. It protects the immune system against radiation and chemotherapy, as do all the following Chinese herbs.
- *Astragalus* and *atractylodes* increase pha-

gocytosis, interferon, IgA and IgG. They enhance T-cell division and so are especially good for shortening colds.
- *Hoelen* and *polyporus* restore the anti-tumour immune surveillance system as does the reishi mushroom.
- *Ligustrum* works with astragalus and increases anti-bodies.
- *Schizandra* increases T-cell activity and is anti- viral and anti-bacterial.
- *Codonopsis* increases macrophages, phagocytosis, T- and B-cell activity and IgG. One Chinese study using this herb indicated a 55% cure rate in the auto-immune disease, psoriasis.

In auto-immune disease, astragalus, codonopsis, ganoderma, atractylodes and licorice go together well. Chinese herbs promote normal function of the immune system rather than having their effect by stimulating production of immune components.

- *Pau d'arco* strengthens the immune system and is strongly anti-viral, anti-parasitic and anti-fungal.
- *Suma* has an anti-cancer effect via the immune system. Both this herb and pau d'arco originate in South America.

General supplements

The choice and dose of supplements depends on whether you are treating allergies, auto-immune disease, cancer or infection. However, for general immune enhancement the following in adult doses are of great value:

- *Beta carotene* – 15mg daily;
- *Vitamin C* – 500mg three times daily;
- *Vitamin E* – 200iu daily;
- *Selenium* – 100mcg daily;
- *Zinc* – 15mg daily;
- *B complex* – 50mg daily;
- *Evening primrose oil* – 1500mg daily;
- *Flaxseed oil* – 1 tablespoon daily;
- *Iron phosphate* – 15mg daily;

- *Manganese* – 5mg daily;
- *Kelp* tablets for natural minerals every day;
- A *Lactobacillus acidophilus* supplement daily has a controlling effect on immune competence. For these supplements to flourish, a non-toxic, healthy bowel environment is essential.

Remember to follow the naturopathic diet and lifestyle, as supplements alone will not restore the immune system to health.

III: *2. FOOD ALLERGY*

Food allergy is an immunological response and the physical reactions can be anything from skin afflictions to vital organ malfunctions. The common signs of the existence of allergy in a person are puffiness or dark circles under the eyes, a blue tinge to the whites of the eyes or a horizontal crease in the lower lid. Although the symptoms of allergy are caused by the immune response to food, they can be triggered by physical trauma, stress, drugs like antibiotics, vaccinations and pollution.

There are many types of reactions to foods that are not mediated by the immune system. Intolerance involves an abnormal response such as vomiting the food within minutes of ingestion. An increased metabolic action is often produced in those taking caffeinated drinks. Many also mistake their reaction to monosodium glutamate for allergy but it is just a drug-like response in most cases.

True food allergies are either fixed or cyclic in nature. Fixed allergies tend to be those which have been present for years, and reactions may occur throughout life. Having said this, after an initial long period of abstinence, and as long as the immune system is strong, an offending food can sometimes be eaten on a weekly basis with no adverse symptoms. Cyclic allergies arise through eating a single food too often, over a long period of time. Avoidance for a few months is usually enough to overcome the problem as long as the food involved is not eaten too frequently again.

Although the incidence of allergy is increasing, it has been mentioned throughout time as a cause of illness. As far back as 400 BC, Hippocrates cited food allergy as a cause of disease. However in recent years the incidence has climbed dramatically, to the extent that *over 60% of the world's population has food allergies.*

The primary cause

It is an underlying faulty immune system that causes the body to form antibodies against a perfectly good food, which then becomes known as an *antigen*. Initially, antibody/antigen complexes form in the blood stream and then collide with specific white blood cells (basophils) in the blood, or pass into the tissues and attach to mast cells. The latter are just basophils that have moved out of the blood stream and changed their names. The result is that the mast cells disintegrate and release their histamine load. This instigates an inflammatory reaction, which means redness and swelling in affected tissues. The symptoms depend on where the reaction occurs. For instance, an asthmatic releases histamine in the bronchi of the lungs. Tissue damage is brought about by another part of the immune system destroying the antibody/antigen complexes on sight. Wherever the allergic reaction is occurring, malfunction is inevitable.

Allergic people have too many helper T-cells in relation to suppressors, and this leads to an over-production of antibodies. Consequently, allergic responses are very easily triggered. Other examples of allergy are frequent upper respiratory tract infections and glue ear, where the allergic reaction creates an excessive build up of mucous and fluid on which bacteria can breed and cause infection. Frequently-occurring sore throats which do not normally become colds are also an allergic reaction to food, as is a catarrhal throat. Chronic sinusitis is so commonly due to allergy that this should always be investigated before embarking on painful invasive surgical treatment. In the gut an allergic response can cause such diverse conditions as gastric ulcers, colitis, gall stones, colic, gas, diarrhoea or constipation.

The brain is very commonly affected by allergy, and histamine release may have wide-ranging effects. It causes insomnia in some, headaches or depression in others. Irritability and anxiety, poor concentration and learning difficulties may also result from allergic reactions. Frequent comment in my practice comes from teachers noticing a marked improvement in behaviour and learning skills once allergy foods are removed from a child's diet. Allergic response is a major feature in hyperactive children and clinging, whining, miserable youngsters can be transformed by removing an offending allergen. Many other conditions are partially or wholly mediated by allergy, such as eczema, asthma, psoriasis, fluid retention, glaucoma or bed-wetting. I have even seen some cases of arthritis, back pain and bursitis totally disappear with allergen avoidance. Vague pains in unusual places, if not due to stress, are often allergy-related. Food allergy has become a major cause of disease and should be investigated much more often than it is.

Immune system weakness

The increased incidence of allergy is due to disordered immune systems. A poor diet deficient in nutrients which are needed by the immune system is a primary cause. The widespread use of processed oils, margarine, white flour, sugar and food chemicals is also directly implicated. Over-eating and over-weight slows the immune function and stress hits it fair and square in the mid-rift. Drugs

including the contraceptive pill, cigarettes and antibiotics weaken in the same way as pollution. Toxic chemicals in the air, water and food chain inhibit normal immune response. Lack of exercise, living in climates in which one is not born, and vaccinations all have detrimental effects on our defenders. In children, increased incidence may be genetic, in that they inherit the *tendency* to allergy. However, a major feature is that they are weaned too early on to solid foods and then offered a limited variety. The other problem is that most common allergens are given not only too frequently but also too early in life. Wheat, cows' milk, eggs, citrus, potatoes and tomatoes should not be given to any child under 10-12 months of age. Even soya milk on a daily basis will quickly cause reactions in those who are born genetically prone to allergy. Breast-feeding is essential so that control of allergies can be initiated through the mother's diet. Her allergies will not necessarily be passed on to the child; he or she will develop their own if they are born prone to allergy.

Types of reactions

Immediate response is not so common but involves a histamine reaction occurring within an hour of an allergen being taken.

Delayed responses are most common, and occur more than two hours after exposure. Sometimes symptoms only happen after several repeated doses of an allergen.

Adaptation is a situation where the body is always trying to cope with an allergic condition, and in this case symptoms are subtle because antibody/antigen complexes are not reaching the tissues. Where the T-cell part of the immune system is strong the complexes will be destroyed in the blood stream and no harm done.

Cravings are a symptom of *adaptation*. In the early stages an allergen may cause a rush of adrenalin which makes the person feel good. Then the system demands a regular 'fix' of this food which is producing such rewarding effects and withdrawal symptoms occur when a dose is delayed. If you are in this stage you will subconsciously ensure regular doses of the allergen in order to continue feeling good. Additionally, an allergy to one food may cause an addictive reaction to another. For instance a chocolate addict is often allergic to dairy products but doesn't crave cheese or milk in any form, only chocolate. People in this type of adaptation who awaken in an aggressive state are improved by a breakfast which contains their particular allergen, whatever it may be.

Aversion is another symptom of adaptation. In this situation, addiction is still a feature but the doses now have to be frequent and larger to ward off unpleasant sensations. The period of being pleasantly stimulated by an allergen is now over. Eventually only the downside prevails, and aversion may develop. In this phase the body is biochemically unbalanced and many processes malfunction, but the person still has no obvious allergic responses. Addiction may lead to symptoms not thought of as being related to allergy, such as hypoglycaemia (low blood sugar). A high percentage of blood sugar problems disappear when allergic foods are removed from the diet. Late afternoon fatigue, headache, irritability, shakes or weakness may simply be symptoms of food addiction. Problems like aggression, destructiveness and general abusive behaviour are also seen in addiction.

Once adaptation fails there is no more adrenalin release, no more mopping up of antibody/antigen complexes in the blood, and finally they reach the tissues where an allergic response occurs. Many people never go through any form of adaptation because they are born with allergic tendencies and a disordered immune system. These individuals are very quickly sensitised to a food appearing in the diet too frequently and allergic reactions soon develop.

Growing out of allergies

Some children appear to grow out of an initial allergy which perhaps has caused a mild eczema, but when another condition develops later, like frequent colds, ear infections or asthma, the link with allergy is all too often ignored. It is a homeopathic maxim that suppression of the initial eczema with cortisone just drives the allergic reaction into a deep area from whence it will eventually produce symptoms. Childhood allergies, when suppressed, can remain dormant for years, and perhaps reappear as migraine in a twenty to thirty year old. An example of the child who appears to spontaneously grow out of his allergies is the one who initially hates milk. Later he starts eating dairy products regularly with no symptoms because the immune system is adapting to the situation. However, as he gets older, and stress, pollution and a poor diet conspire to weaken his immune system further, adaptation ceases and asthma or some other condition suddenly appears. That child never 'grew out of' his allergy. In another scenario where an allergy exists, a person may have no symptoms as long as the particular foodstuff is eaten infrequently. However if that substance suddenly becomes a daily staple food, a full blown allergic reaction will occur.

A very early sign of being allergy prone is the development of cradle cap on the scalps of infants. At this stage, great care should be taken with the diet because allergy invariably follows.

Other types of allergies

Contact dermatitis is mediated by the immune system but it involves T-cells and not antibodies. The inflammatory reaction is due to stimulation of overly sensitive T-cells and a reaction occurs one to three days later.

Leaky gut syndrome and allergy are discussed in chapter III:7 on Bowel Toxaemia, and the basic pre-determining factor is a toxic bowel. When healthy micro-flora or gastric acid and enzymes are deficient, then fungus, toxins, bacteria and pesticides are not destroyed. The walls of the intestines become porous to molecules of food not completely degraded, and this is even more likely in a vitamin A deficiency. Large food molecules pass into the blood stream where the immune system perceives then as foreign and sets up an allergic reaction. In those with multiple allergies, which are forever changing, leaky gut is heavily implicated and must be rectified to cure the problem. In infants, it occurs if solid food is introduced too early before the gut lining is fully developed.

A lack of bifidus bacteria in mothers' milk is another major cause, as this means that the infant's intestines become toxic and IgA is destroyed. The latter is an antibody which prevents a child from becoming allergic to food in the mother's diet. A supplement of digestive enzymes will ensure that food is properly broken down, and this alone will often prevent allergic reactions. Live acidophilus and bifidus maintain a healthy colonic environment in children and adults but infants must not be given acidophilus. Instead, they should take bifido bacteria alone as this is the only normal flora in the unweaned child.

Inflammatory chemicals at high levels in the body (*eg* in asthma) can alone cause mast cells and basophils to release histamine so that the inflammatory response looks like food allergy when it is not. The condition is exacerbated by using non-steroid anti-inflammatory drugs which suppress one inflammatory path in the body whilst allowing

another an uncontrolled run. Naturopaths are always aware of the need to remove the cause of increased inflammatory chemicals so that there is no need for suppression. This is done by manipulating the fatty acids in the diet – by reducing the fats which induce inflammatory chemicals and increasing those that subdue them.

Histamine and other amines

Many foods either contain high levels of histamine or cause its release. In someone who has not got an overload of inflammatory chemicals, the liver produces enough antihistamine to mop these up. However, there is a limit, which means that in those with existing allergies, histamine foods in the diet will adversely tip the balance. The most potent are strawberries, shellfish, tomatoes, chocolate, wine, tuna, sausages, spinach, banana, papaya and pineapple. A great many people who think they are allergic to shellfish are pleasantly surprised that there is no reaction to these once the real allergen is removed. The same happens with reactions to non-food allergens like dust, pollen and grasses. However, in rhinitis sufferers there is always an underlying food sensitivity and removal means that a person reacts much less strongly to her cat or the feathers in a duvet.

Vasoactive amines are chemicals which increase the permeability of blood cells and so allow immune complexes to more readily pass into the tissues from the blood. The best known are tyramine, serotonin and phenylalanine. Vasoactive amines are high in avocados, bananas, plums, citrus, cabbage, eggplant, potato, cheese, canned fish, aged meat, chicken liver, seafood, wine, beer and chocolate.

Many books written about allergy only highlight the very severe cases and leave readers feeling that they have little in common with themselves. In my experience with several thousand cases, removing the real allergen is enough. After that very few have to bother about histamine foods or vasoactive amines. It always helps to include foods in the diet which inhibit the release of inflammatory chemicals, and the best of these are onion, garlic, dill, asparagus, kale, Brussels sprouts, pears, apples and the herbs fenugreek, tarragon and eucalyptus. EPA (from oily fish), evening primrose oil and vitamin E have the same effect.

TREATMENT

- Allergy testing for foods;
- Follow a rotation diet if necessary;
- Reduce inflammatory chemical formation;
- Strengthen the immune system through sound diet and supplements;
- Treat any underlying cause such as leaky gut syndrome.

Allergy testing

Skin tests are only of value in environmental allergic reactions, and cytotoxic blood tests were somewhat discredited when it was discovered that one person's blood sent to several laboratories resulted in as many different conclusions. The RAST test, which measures immune response to allergens, is only of value for the immediate response conditions. RASP testing, which is similar but much more accurate, is not widely available except in USA.

Touch for Health (TFH) is a system which notes muscle response to foods put on the tongue, or against the skin. Some people get good results and others very poor. Reliability depends on the skill of the practitioner.

Vega and *Mora machines* have become very popular amongst alternative practitioners, but again the results can be very misleading. It is not known whether the fault lies with the machine or the operator. Certainly some people appear to get good results but I have seldom seen an accurate allergy test from one of these. They seem unable to distinguish between allergy, intolerance, idiosyncrasy or drug-like reactions, and the triggers like caffeine often show up as allergies as well.

Radionics is a system of allergy testing which is very well developed in Britain. It too, like the Vega machine is not scientific, and in this case, accuracy is dependent on the skill of the operator. Some are extremely proficient, and the results are at least 90% accurate. These people are quietly employed by many of the medical profession in Britain as well as by alternative practitioners. On the other hand, some operators are hopelessly inefficient, so one must go by word-of-mouth when looking for an accurate radionic tester.

The *Dr Coco pulse test* is one which can be done at home. Suspected allergens must be avoided for four days before testing as follows: sit quietly for fifteen minutes in a relaxed state, check the pulse rate and then eat a normal serving of the suspect food; take the pulse again after fifteen minutes, and if the rate is eight points higher or more over a one minute period, an allergic reaction is said to be occurring.

The most laborious method and perhaps the most accurate is to *avoid all known allergens for at least one week, and then introduce them one by one*, observing carefully when reactions occur. This is certainly necessary for those with multiple allergies. Some need to be fasted on water only as a preliminary to testing. Others can manage by starting on a few days of fruit or a mixture of pears, lamb, millet and mineral water, to which hardly anyone is ever allergic. After the initial fast, one new food family is introduced in normal servings for two to four days and the effect observed. Following this a second food is tested for a few days. Any allergic reactions are usually quite marked because when a food has been avoided for a period, adaptation is relaxed and an immediate response is more likely to occur.

Allergen avoidance and rotation diets

Avoidance for a substantial period is the ideal situation, as it allows memory antibody cells to forget and the immune system to strengthen, so that antibody production is reduced. However, this can be very difficult in social situations, when travelling or in buying from supermarkets full of processed foods. Many common allergens like eggs, soya, wheat and dairy products are hidden everywhere. These hidden sources must be avoided as well, or the allergy will continue. There are always excellent substitutes available for any type of food. A good naturopath or the staff of a well-stocked health food store will provide guidance in this area. Eventually, even though the allergic condition remains, food can often be eaten on a four-to-seven day rotation basis so long as the immune system is not weakened by the likes of stress or pollution.

For those with very mild reactions a rotation diet – whereby no food family is repeated in the diet more often than once every four days – can be used to great effect without long term avoidance. The same process is vital in those with multiple or shifting allergies but in this case, known allergens must also be totally excluded for a long period. In the case of cyclic allergies, the offending foods may be added to the rotation diet once reaction ceases and tolerance is observed. Maintenance of some semblance of rotation is necessary in allergy-prone people, as they may develop reactions to other foods being repeated too often.

Leaky gut repair

If gastric acid or enzymes are deficient these must be given in tablet form. Bowel toxins can be absorbed with use of the herb called sarsaparilla. Any fungus can be destroyed with a mixture of garlic, echinacea and golden seal. Flaxseeds or psyllium seeds may be necessary to clear the bowel of toxic waste. The next step is to repopulate the intestines with an acidophilus and bifidus supplement which has a guaranteed potency, and then heal the cells lining the intestinal tract with vitamin A and butyric acid or glucosamine sulphate supplements. People with debilitating allergic reactions have found it possible to tolerate their allergens whilst on glucosamine. Infants and children need only the lactobacillus in toxic bowel conditions although an IgA supplement may be necessary until the immune system strengthens. If stomach acid is not produced adequately, they will need a supplement when solid food is eaten.

Desensitisation

Many have tried this – the process involves making potencies of allergens and using them to neutralise symptoms. Test doses have to be experimented with to find the appropriate potency because some will induce symptoms whilst others will block them. The patient is either injected regularly or takes drops orally for months or years. Treatment is reasonably effective while ongoing, and some can eventually continue eating the offending allergens with no symptoms. Others receive no benefit at all or regress once the treatment ceases. This process will help a person overcome allergies quicker if he or she is avoiding the relevant food.

Allergic reactions may also be turned off with the following mixture sipped slowly. One teaspoon of soda bicarbonate and half a teaspoon of potassium bicarbonate in a glass of warm water. Selenium 400mcg daily inhibits chemical allergic reactions.

Natural anti-histamine products
• *Quercetin* – is a flavonoid which makes mast cells less sensitive and reduces other inflammatory chemicals.
• *Bromelain* – increases the absorption rate of quercetin and in its own right inhibits inflammatory chemicals.
• *Vitamin C* – in large doses is anti-histamine.
• *Selenium* and *zinc* – are needed to detoxify chemicals.
• *EPA* – blocks an inflammatory chemical cascade from animal protein.
• *Calcium* 0.5g, and the amino acid *methionine* – prevents a build up of histamine.
• *Ginseng*, *licorice* and *feverfew* – inhibit histamine release.
• *Ginkgo* – inhibits the eosinophils – white blood cells found in increased amounts at the site of allergic reactions. This herb is very effective against rapid allergic reactions.

Immune system repair
This is discussed in full in chapter III:1, but using supplements to alter the ratio between helper and suppressor T-cells is important. Allergic people have too many helpers, which increases antibody production.
• *Histidine* is an amino acid which regulates the helper/suppressor ratio by raising the suppressors. It is also effective in blocking reactions from absorbed undigested protein.
• *Glutathione* is an amino complex, which is important in regulating the function of T-cells as well as the B-cells from which the antibodies are formed.
• *Evening primrose oil* leads to an increase of suppressors, as does vitamin E.
• *Zinc* and *iron* regulate T-cells, as do many herbs, of which echinacea is especially notable. Chinese herbs used in immune system restoration also regulate T-cell activity, as does the African herb *Devil's Claw*.
• *Magnesium* is very important in immune competence.

Supplements of value
Adult doses:
• *Vitamin C* – 3-10g daily in divided doses depending on the degree of allergic reaction.
• *Quercetin* 500mg + bromelain 200mg + histidine 100mg – twenty minutes before each meal if necessary, to block reactions.
• *Selenium* – 200mcg daily.
• *Vitamin E* – 400iu daily.
• *Zinc* – 30mg daily.
• *Evening primrose oil* – 500mg 4 times daily, and avoid all processed oils and margarines.
• *L acidophilus* + *L bifidus* bacteria improve immune competence and prevent a leaky gut.
• *Ginseng* and *licorice root* tea – 3 times daily.
• *Ginkgo* extract – 40mg 2-3 times daily, for rapid response allergic reactions.

A quality supplement designed for immune system repair would contain some of the above as well as vitamins A, B-complex, a small amount of iron and some herbs. Children can take a multi-vitamin/mineral tablet plus evening primrose oil and acidophilus.

Preventing allergies is the real challenge and this can be greatly enhanced by maintaining a strong balanced immune system with a quality and widely-varied food intake, plenty of exercise, clean air, water and sunshine. Practising meditation, visualisation or some other form of relaxation technique greatly improves immune function. Be happy, enjoy life to the full, and ensure time each day for some creative pursuit.

III: *3. STRESS*

I am often asked what I can do to relieve stress. The person asking is clearly looking for a quick-fix pill to banish his feelings of tension rather than taking stock of his life-style and attitudes.

Stress is defined as anything that threatens the health of the body or has an adverse effect on its functioning, such as injury, disease, depression or worry. The presence of one form of stress diminishes resistance to other types. For instance, when a person is ill he cannot cope adequately with worry and will notice that minor upsets are blown out of proportion. Constant stress brings about hormonal changes in the body and also reduces the immune function. For instance, students close to exams who are studying night and day often develop streaming colds which clear quickly when the exam stress is over. Stress is associated with serious illnesses like cancer, cardio-vascular disease, rheumatoid arthritis, respiratory and gastro-intestinal diseases. These only develop in response to a stress level which is ongoing for an extended period without adequate release.

Stress in moderation is the spice of life and we would be very dull people without it. A certain level acts as an incentive in every aspect of our lives and as such is important to our survival. So positive stress is not harmful and is indeed necessary. What is important is the *response* to it. If a heavy workload is viewed as a burden, then stress is present. On the other hand, if it is viewed as a challenge or even a pleasure, then stress does not occur.

The response depends on the type of person. An A-type who is constantly on the move, drives himself hard, sets impossible deadlines, is ambitious and can't relax, will accumulate stress rapidly. A B-type person who is much more laid back in every way will not, although he may also be ambitious. What is a major stress to an A-type person is of no importance to a B-type – an example of this is seen when considering meeting impossible deadlines. The person who does not respond correctly to the stress will panic over being late, whereas the person who does react adequately will accept the impossibility with equanimity and just do his best to finish as soon as possible. Clearly everyone should endeavour to become more relaxed about life in order to prevent stress-induced illness.

Alternatively, where potential stress loads cannot be reduced it is important to react differently, so that tension is released instead of internalised. When anger is aroused over trifles, stop and examine the problem and deliberately put it in perspective. If the anger is due to a major event then be sure to remove it harmlessly by expressing your feelings appropriately or using a deep breathing exercise or some other relaxation technique. For some, a primordial scream may be appropriate.

Stress is cumulative, and we become less able to cope with its symptoms as time passes. Unless an adequate response is mounted every time, physical illness will eventually occur. For this reason it is also important to avoid the pitfall of no response, as stresses buried inside are as harmful as an uncontrolled flaring anger, anxiety or depression over small events. When unhappiness, anxiety, jealousy, fear or rejection is buried, it festers and becomes internal hostility or anger which is harmful. Feelings must be expressed and solutions found to these painful emotional events. Once the load has become heavy, a single minor event may tip the balance from adaptation to stress into physical illness.

It is important to accept that we have free choice as to how we react to events, people and emotions, because only then is it possible to make the necessary changes in attitudes, responses, personality and pace of life. The people who cope with stress well are not only the B-types. Those who are somewhere in the middle but have what is known as a 'hardiness factor' also respond well. These people have control over all aspects of their lives, which means that they (rather than others) determine their thoughts and actions. Outside influences are only secondary. These people have an inner sense of responsibility concerning their lives and know that they can chart their own course. Those who feel at the mercy of others, who don't make their own decisions and who blame someone else for life's misfortunes have a very low hardiness level.

Viewing life as a challenge and seeing it as something exciting also increases hardiness, as does feeling *involved* in life – being stimulated by events, people, places and situations outside one's immediate environment. Parents can do much to encourage these healthy traits in their offspring, but even adults can learn with the help of counselling and supportive friends and family. Just becoming aware of the need for change and accepting its possibility is a major step on the road to becoming a well person.

As you progress through this book, you will see that living with stress plays a major role in all the serious diseases of this century. Stress can trigger the immune system to malfunction and make antibodies against food (allergies) or its own tissue. The latter situation occurs in self-destructive diseases like rheumatoid arthritis, lupus erythematosus or multiple sclerosis. Cortico-steroid hormones (released from the adrenal glands in stress) not only increase fuel for energy – they deliberately depress the function of the immune system because it is not a necessary part of stress-control. Therefore, if you remain in a state of longterm stress, the immune system stays suppressed – the thymus, spleen and lymphatic glands cease to react to infection, or worse still, start recognising 'self' and perfectly good food as foreign.

Stress causes disordered hormonal releases of all kinds, including the female reproductive ones. It can also lead to peptic ulcers, chronic fatigue syndrome (ME), liver damage and insomnia, to name just a few conditions common in our modern world.

The release of stress hormones like adrenalin and cortisole sends messages to the whole body that all is not well. This results in unhappy cells, because every cell in the body can receive these hormonal messages. If they are on the receiving end of unhappiness longterm, then cells inevitably malfunction to the extent that serious disease develops. At first it was thought that only the immune system communicated with the brain on an emotional level, but it has become evident that every cell in the body can send and receive emotions, which means that cells contain some sort of intelligence. Cells receiving unhappy messages from cortisole not only become depressed themselves (and therefore sick) but they send negative messages to the brain. Equally, a relaxed smiling person sends happy messages throughout the body. When you feel low, try holding a smile on your face for a few minutes and notice how your mood lightens. The facial muscles are sending happy chemical messages to the brain. Just as we as a whole cannot function properly when we are depressed or anxious, the cells of every organ also malfunction if they are depressed by stress hormones over a long period.

The causes of stress

There is an endless list of things which have the potential for causing stress, and it is interesting to note that even happy events can be perceived as stressful. A rating system for lifestyle changes was developed by the researchers Holmes and Lake in the 1960s, whereby stressful events were allocated specific numbers according to the degree of harm they could cause. Death of a spouse has the highest score of 100 and divorce rates 73. A happy event like marriage is more stressful than losing a job or retiring, and pregnancy is rated the same as sex problems. In fact, anticipating changes in lifestyle is actually worse, in terms of stress, than dealing with the reality. For instance, the fear of losing a job is worse than getting on with finding a new one.

Dangerous jobs are stressful. Police and firemen have high stress levels, and men who have to climb dangerous scaffolding for a living pump out lots of stress hormones. A traffic jam and no phone in the car is a problem to many, because the thought of being late is stressful.

Emotions such as guilt, resentment, self-pity, self-loathing, anger, depression, anxiety or brooding over conflicts are all causes of cumulative stress unless they are harmlessly discharged. An inability to defuse emotions by talking them through is very harmful.

Once stress leads to physical illness, the anxiety engendered by the symptoms further increases the problem, unless attitudes and coping skills are drastically altered. Treating symptoms and then carrying on as usual just deepens the stress. It is no use swallowing antacids to alleviate ulcers or taking antispasmodic drugs to relieve irritable bowel syndrome – the hardiness factor has to be

increased so that the disease can be healed completely.

The physical effects of stress

The body has adaptation systems for coping with all excesses – for instance, when we are overheated we sweat, when we are cold we shiver to increase internal heat, and when we are low in nutrients the body conserves what it has more carefully.

The hypothalamus in the brain responds to stress by initiating the general adaptation syndrome (GAS) via two pathways. The first is the sympathetic nervous system, which affects internal organ function and adrenalin release. The second is via the brain hormones which stimulate the release of a variety of other hormones from the outer rim of the adrenal glands.

This first response is rooted in the fact that human beings are animals and our bodies are physically prepared to run from danger or stand up and fight back. Children do this instinctively. Lashing out with their fists in anger or frustration frees the stress. Adults on the other hand over-ride the instinct because it is anti-social, and in this way the stress is internalised, where it becomes cumulative and leads to physical illness.

The alarm response

When stressful events occur, the following sequences happen.

All the muscles tense so that a person can run or fight. The tense muscles increase lactic acid buildup (as in exercise) and anxiety levels rise. Sugar is released for extra energy and the adrenal glands secrete more adrenalin to increase the heartbeat and its strength. An increased flow of blood provides more nutrients to the muscles and improves alertness. The blood supply to non-essential areas like the skin and internal organs is reduced by constriction of the small arteries, and this raises the blood pressure. The spleen puts more blood into circulation, which further increases blood pressure. The rate of respiration increases so that blood oxygen levels rise, because the muscles of the extremities, brain and heart all need extra oxygen for increased activity. The pupils dilate to see better in the dark and the pores of the skin open to cool the body, because increased blood flow and energy production raises internal heat.

Look back at an instance where fear was great and you will recognise that all of the above events occurred. During the alarm response, non-essential body functions such as digestion are reduced. The salivary secretion dries up so that a dry mouth ensues, acid and digestive enzymes are not secreted and peristalsis (the movement of the intestines which makes food travel through the system) stops. The kidneys slow down in producing urine because the blood flow for a non-essential function has been restricted. Immune system activity is also reduced, which means that we don't fight infection adequately.

Where an adequate response occurs, then everything returns to normal. In the face of a charging bull it is normal to run, but an adequate response to anger or misery could be to evaluate it, calmly discuss it or free it by some other method.

The resistance reaction

If stress is not released then the body enters what is known as the *resistance stage*, whereby many of the alarm responses become chronic. This reaction is also mediated by the hypothalamus in the brain, but this time it does so via hormone regulators from the pituitary gland and adrenal glands rather than via the nervous system.

When alarm reactions become chronic, muscles remain tense in some areas and anxiety may become constant. Hormones remain altered and the adrenal glands conserve so-

dium to maintain a normal blood pressure. Infections become chronic or occur frequently because of the constantly lowered immune response and wound-healing becomes slow.

Blood sugar disturbances may become a regular feature because sugar and fats are being continually broken down for energy that is required to meet the emotional crisis. This means that blood sugar levels see-saw, causing periodic sugar craving, irritability, weepiness, headaches and even shakes. The insulin response to sugar surges damages blood vessels, as do the stress hormones. Other symptoms of being in the resistance stage are:

• chronic fatigue and disturbed sleep patterns. Those who can't go to sleep easily or who wake and do not go back to sleep are stressed;

• eating disorders – either over-indulgence or loss of appetite. Some people will even turn away from a previously healthy diet and start routinely reaching for the worst kinds of junk food.

• nervous disorders like nail-biting, being unable to sit still and relax, twitching muscles, a tight chest, headaches and palpitations. When the nervous system control of organs goes awry, excessive sweating, irritable bowel syndrome, constipation or diarrhoea may occur. Cystitis or urethritis are frequently caused by stress rather than an infecting organism.

• emotional disturbances such as suppressed anger or crying too easily, feeling unloved, misunderstood, being fearful and anxious. A lack of self-esteem, irritability out of proportion to the event and a feeling that things frequently go wrong;

• being unable to plan or follow a schedule for coping with a workload. Not making time for self and worrying about the future;

• unexplained pains occurring anywhere in

the abdomen or chest;
• allergies or an auto-immune disease develops, whereby the body destroys its own tissue;
• a low sex drive or periodic hot flushes. Feeling uncomfortable or irritable about touching or being touched.

As the adrenals weaken further they tire of constantly conserving sodium, which means that potassium collects instead, causing fluid retention, weakness, cramps and even weight loss. As sodium levels decrease, the skin dries and thirst develops. Dizziness and low blood pressure become a feature. Emotional and nervous system disturbances worsen along with the fatigue and sleep disorders. Exercise programmes become impossible to continue because low sodium causes muscle pain. When the blood levels of sodium drop, blood vessels constrict in an effort to maintain normal blood pressure. This decreases blood supply to the tissues, and therefore causes poor oxygenation and a lactic acid retention. Lactic acid in muscles causes pain and it also increases anxiety, tension, irritability and depression. By this stage, serious efforts to combat stress become essential.

Chronic stress damages blood vessels and leads to them being clogged up with cholesterol. It also makes platelets sticky, which is believed to play a central role in initiating cancer. Anyone in the adaptation phase because of accumulated stress would be well-advised to take stock and change whatever is necessary in order to prevent future serious illness.

An interesting side note on cholesterol is that it is needed by the adrenal hormones, and a person under stress is constantly making new supplies of cholesterol for conversion to hormones. This is one of the reasons that stressed people often find that they also have high serum cholesterol. To dramatically reduce it would be harmful under these circumstances, and in any case the level goes down naturally when the stress is dealt with. However, after a long period in the resistance stage, the constant higher levels of the LDL type of cholesterol would trigger atherosclerosis.

The resistance stage allows the body to continue fighting a stressor after the effects of the alarm stage have worn off. This is very valuable when we need extra energy to see us through a very stressful period. However we should then allow our bodies to return to normal so that disease does not develop. Fortunately this stage is reversible if attention is paid to diet, exercise, stress release techniques and building hardiness. The length of time it can last depends on the strength of the constitution, degree of stress, quality of diet and many other factors. Some people may remain in this state for ten to twenty years before resistance stops. However, if drugs are used to suppress stress symptoms, then the onset of the *exhaustion stage* will be more rapid. Aspirin, tea, coffee and cigarettes are all recognised by the body as drugs.

The exhaustion stage

This occurs when the body gives up and no longer adapts to stress. A major cause of the onset of this stage is the loss of potassium, and without sufficient levels of potassium in the cells they start to die. The adrenal glands are also worn out by this time and don't secrete the sugar-releasing hormones for organ function. The heart and blood vessels are weakened anyway after a long period of working overtime at resistance. Unless this stage is rapidly reversed, the prognosis is serious indeed – heart attacks, strokes, ulcers, diabetes and cancer are strong possibilities.

Diet

Someone who is stressed has a major need for

an increased amount of vitamins, minerals and enzymes. To this end, everything that is eaten should be of top quality in terms of nutritional value. Many people think that eating processed food is all right because it won't actually do any harm. However, if you eat a bowl of processed breakfast cereal (which is not much better than a bowl of sugar), you will be full without ever having a food rich in nutrients, and the body will have to wait another few hours in the hope of receiving good food.

Follow the naturopathic diet in part one of the book and make sure that 65% of the food is raw in the form of fruit, vegetables, seeds, nuts and cereals. Remember that raw cereals should be soaked, sprouted or fermented, so that minerals are not leached from the body. Green vegetables in particular, contain an important source of natural sodium for the resistance stage.

Make real efforts to avoid white flour and all sugar and everything made from them. This means avoid even bread that is partially made from white flour, pizza, pasta, cakes, crumpets, pancakes and pastry. Avoid jams, soft drinks, squashes, tea, coffee and the many cocoa-type drinks. Everything eaten should be made from natural fresh food and not come from packets, cans or the freezer section of the supermarket. Sweet treats can be made from wholewheat flour with honey or maple syrup used in place of sugar. Buy brown rice instead of white, muesli or porridge oats, instead of pretty packaged cereals, whole grain flour – and make your own cakes, pizzas and pancakes. Wholewheat, cornmeal and buckwheat pastas are widely available.

I never understand someone choosing white pasta when wholegrain pasta has the enormous advantage or never going sticky. Some brands taste better than others, so experiment. Change from crisps and processed snacks to eating raw fresh nuts, olives, cru-

dités and home-made dips, such as hummus and live yoghurt-based varieties. In restaurants choose salad with beans or cottage cheese, eggs and an olive oil/lemon juice dressing. Skip the white pasta and potato salad covered in thick poor quality mayonnaise and definitely skip the croutons. Choose fresh fish with a variety of vegetables and a side salad, and ask for wholewheat bread when the white rolls arrive. Freshly made soups make good starters and fresh fruit or cheese and wholewheat bread/crackers can finish a meal. A glass of wine with the evening meal is permissible, but drink a mineral water with a squeeze of lemon otherwise. Herbal teas can replace tea and coffee and dandelion and barley grain 'coffees' are available.

TREATMENTS

Flower remedies

Bach flower remedies are taken to rebalance emotions which are out of control and these help stressed people enormously. Some of the useful ones are detailed below, but there are 38 flower remedies, and a stressed person would be wise to read up on this and choose up to five which are the most appropriate.

• *Impatiens* is for the impatient individual who is always in a hurry and would rather do something himself than take the time to teach another. These people react quickly, are irritable, difficult to please, nervy, intolerant of restraint and restless. They don't tolerate fools and cannot wait for events to take there course. Recognise yourself here?

• *White chestnut* is for those who cannot put aside problems. They prey on the mind and even prevent sleep. This is for mental tension, teeth grinding, chronic headaches, fatigue and depression. It is also for those people who have constantly whirring minds which cause great mental and physical ten-

- *Olive* is for complete physical and mental exhaustion after a long period of strain. The person feels washed out with no reserves and everything is an effort.
- *Heather* is for the self-centred person who has reached the stage of making mountains out of molehills, weeps easily, and is full of self-pity.
- *Elm* is for those who feel temporarily overwhelmed by responsibility. These people are normally very capable.

Australian bush flower remedies have been developed by Dr Ian White and although some overlap with Dr Edward Bach's flowers, many are unique and useful for the problems we face in modern life. *Black-eyed Susan* is Ian's equivalent of Edward Bach's *Impatiens*.

- *Crowea* is for those who constantly worry or experience anxiety. It is also appropriate for that 'not quite right' feeling. It is for those who always have something to worry about but never have specific fears. It is also good for worriers with stomach upsets.
- *Bottle brush* is for those who are going through major life-changes which are stressful. The remedy brings calm and the ability to cope.
- *Banksia robur* is for the weary, disheartened, frustrated person who is low in energy. This remedy is for those who are normally very dynamic but are temporarily burnt-out.
- *Paw paw* is for those who are feeling overwhelmed with problems and burdened by the decisions which have to be made. It brings calmness and clarity of mind and goes well with Crowea.
- *Macrocarpa* has an affinity for the adrenal glands. It is for exhaustion and burn-out and acts as a pick-me-up.

Vitamins and minerals to support the adrenal glands

- *Vitamin B-complex* – 50mg daily, or

brewer's yeast, 1-2 tablespoon daily.
- *Pantothenic acid* (vitamin B5) – 500mg daily.
- *Vitamin C* – 1g twice daily.
- *Beta carotene* – 6mg daily.
- *Vitamin E* – 200iu daily.
- *Selenium* – 200mcg daily.
- *Zinc* – 25mg daily.
- *Manganese* – 5-10mg daily.
- *Kelp* tablets for natural sodium and other minerals.

An immune-stimulating formulation will contain many of the above in similar dosage. Some people may need higher doses of the B vitamins such as B3, B6 and B5.
- *Calcium* and *magnesium* – 400mg daily of each as citrate, aspartate or amino acid chelate.
- *Celloids® PPMP* (see appendix 1) – 1 tablet three times daily is the food of the nervous system, and stressed people use up this combination very quickly.
- *Inositol* – 250mg three times daily of this B vitamin has an anti-anxiety effect on brainwaves, similar to valium.
- *L-tyrosine* – 500mg twice daily, for the formation of adrenalin and to regulate emotions and moods.
- *Celloids® SP* (sodium phosphate – see Appendix 1) – 160mg three times daily, if you have reached a stage of sodium depletion.

Herbs
- *Ginseng* – 1-2g three times daily, to tune the adrenal cortex to respond correctly to stress.
- *Licorice root* – 400mg three times daily, reacts with the part of the adrenal gland controlling sodium and fluid levels and reduces stress damage to the adrenal cortex. This herb affects potassium balance in long-term usage. Deglycyrrhizinated licorice does not deplete potassium and is safe to use in the long term.

• *Chinese thoroughwax* – 2-4g three times daily, increases adrenal hormones and enhances their effect.

The Brazilian herbs guarana and suma also support adrenal function.

See chapters III:4 on Anxiety and III:6 on Insomnia for appropriate herbal teas and essential oils.

Exercise and breathing

Aerobic exercise four times weekly is a very good way of discharging accumulated stress. This can be brisk walking, jogging (for the fit), swimming, skipping, skating or using a rebounder in the home. Exercise at 60-80% of maximum – which means being able to talk whilst exercising, and if you are puffed, then slow down the pace. Tennis and squash are not aerobic, as movement is not sustained. One of the reasons that people feel so refreshed after aerobic exercise is because adrenalin is released in much greater amounts. Additional benefit is derived from the fact of improved circulation, lymph flow, and the freeing of tight muscles.

Yoga exercises are good for muscle-stretching and learning important breathing techniques, which can be used to de-stress the body. Spend a little time each day breathing slowly so that the abdomen is pushed out first followed by the expansion of the lower ribs and finally fill the upper part of the lungs. Exhale slowly and repeat at a pace which doesn't produce inner tension.

Sunshine through the eyes (no specs on) daily is important for healthy hormone function and general wellbeing. In climates with little sunshine, full-spectrum lighting in the house is a substitute. Winter depression occurs in many people simply because of the lack of ultra-violet light, and using full-spectrum lamps has been found to markedly decrease depression, anxiety, hyperactivity,

nervousness and other emotional disturbances.

Relaxation

Sleep is vital to health, and disturbed sleep patterns need to be rectified as soon as possible. Exercise, a warm bath at bedtimes, flower remedies and mineral supplements with chamomile tea should help a lot, but see the chapter on insomnia for additional ideas if necessary. Everyone, whether stressed or not, should practise a relaxation technique daily. It can be a progressive muscle relaxation, autogenics, abdominal breathing or a biofeedback technique. There are many books on the market which teach these techniques. Try out several methods and follow the one that suits you best.

Most people find the autogenic method very relaxing, and Dr Kay Kermani has published an excellent book on the subject. Very briefly the technique is as follows:

• lie down, take a deep breath and then roll your eyes to look at your third eye in the centre of your forehead, and then close them;

• instruct your arms and legs to go heavy and spend fifteen to twenty seconds on each limb in turn – the instruction is *"my arm (or leg) is getting heavier and heavier"*. Focus your entire attention on feeling and mentally seeing the instruction but don't force it. Do not allow your mind to stray elsewhere – and if it does, gently bring it back to what you are saying to yourself;

• then continue the instruction to the buttocks, lower back, right up to the shoulders and neck before relaxing the stomach, chest and face;

• next, instruct all four limbs to become warm – *"my arm is getting warmer and warmer"*;

• and then, cool the forehead, which refreshes the mind;

• finally, lie still and enjoy the feeling of

relaxation, while mentally saying "*I am completely relaxed and at peace with myself*".

The whole process takes fifteen to twenty minutes, and for those who can't get off to sleep this works very well. For those who go to sleep easily, relaxation techniques are better done during the daytime. Everyone to whom I have taught this technique has felt immediate benefit, and I have noticed that the rate of breathing and the pulse always becomes slow and regular.

Regular massage to free knotted muscles is very beneficial, and if essential oils are used at the same time the effect is even greater. Touch is comforting and relaxing in its own right so make the time for a weekly massage.

Meditation

There are many different types, and again you need to find what suits you best. Buddhists and Raj Yoga people teach very good methods free of charge and Transcendental Meditation (TM®) is taught for a fee.

Meditation involves concentrating the mind gently on a single thought, word or vision, which stills the chattering thoughts to bring an oasis of peace and calm. It is a chance to listen to your inner self. This should follow on directly from a brief relaxation period and it needs to be done three to four times weekly. Even ten minutes a day has a beneficial effect which is cumulative.

Christians who are adverse to Eastern meditation techniques can meditate on a saying from the teachings of Jesus such as "I am the way, the truth and the light". This phrase will rapidly take you into a deep meditative state. Meditation is not the same as prayer. Persevere with the technique, because even if thoughts do crowd the mind there is benefit from having sat down with the intention of meditating, and in time it becomes easier.

Changing habits and attitudes

Everyone can change, and those who don't accept this will stay in a state of stress until ill-health strikes. However, this is the hardest part of all the treatment, as real commitment is necessary to alter stress – inducing habits of a lifetime. Here are a few suggestions:

● take one day at a time and do one thing at a time as far as possible;

● make lists of what needs doing, schedule them so that you can cope without feeling stressed, and tick them off as you go. This will prevent panic, produce a feeling of control and prevent you from going round in circles without achieving your goals;

● stop making impossible deadlines – delegate and build in some flexibility to schedules;

● always take at least a full day away from work at the weekend;

● don't ignore fatigue or illness, as your body is telling you to slow down;

● take regular holidays so that some are occasionally three day breaks. The long holiday should be no less than two weeks in duration;

● meditate or practise a relaxation technique every day;

● exercise four times weekly;

● eat regularly in relaxed conditions and avoid stimulants and snacks in place of meals;

● spend time each day at a relaxing pastime, be it reading a book not associated with work, watching TV, being social with friends, or doing a creative hobby. Say no to anything which impinges on this area, and always ensure adequate sleep at night;

● look at each day in advance with the sole view of finding part of it which generates pleasure in your mind. This develops a positive outlook and optimism equates with being happy and relaxed;

● resolve anger and emotional problems through discussion or expression. Don't suppress them, as it is important to discuss painful emotions. Work at not over-reacting to small irritations, and where these exist, solve the problem instead of reacting to it;

• develop hardiness, by first accepting that you alone are responsible for everything in your life and no one else is to blame for situations you don't like. Only then will you be in charge of your life and able to change that which disturbs your equilibrium. Work towards being an optimist, solving your own problems and not being a doormat within the home or workplace;

• recognise the point where duty becomes self- sacrifice, and call a halt;

• where your expectations conflict with the realities of life, stop and examine ways of living with the reality, instead of reacting against it. For instance if an irritating noise is going to wake you at 6am every morning, instead of feeling uptight, use ear plugs or get into the habit of taking your daily exercise in the early morning. Alternatively, discuss the problem with the perpetrator.

• it is acceptable to express your feelings accurately in order to resolve a problem. In this way you control events and do not allow them to damage your health.

Finally, if you like yourself and feel self-confident, your self-esteem will be in good shape, and this also increases your hardiness factor. Remember that stress powerfully depresses immune function and that developing hardiness forms a valuable buffer against this, and therefore against many serious diseases.

III: *4. ANXIETY*

Anxiety is a normal response to threat. Its purpose is to mobilise the *'fight-or-flight'* reaction controlled by hormones from the adrenal glands. However, many people suffer constant anxiety as a reaction to prolonged stress or even as a response to something which is clearly non-threatening. This is an unpleasant feeling of dread or fear called *anxiety neurosis*.

Sometimes the reason for the anxiety is because of a previous situation which triggered the 'fight-or-flight' reaction, and then a constant dread of it recurring remains deep in the mind. A more common and less severe example is that of a highly-disciplined child feeling subconscious anxiety as an adult because she is no longer constantly busy, or the mother who is forever anxious about her family when there is absolutely no need.

People with anxiety neuroses have high blood levels of lactate resulting from glucose metabolism. Panic attacks have been initiated by infusing lactate into anxious people, but the same infusions have no effect on normal people. This indicates that some actually accumulate lactate, and an added amount then pushes them into panic. Anxious people also have much higher lactate levels after exercise than others, and should therefore avoid strenuous or prolonged types. Lactate normally accumulates with exercise but is slowly cleared from the blood when the exercise ceases.

A lack of B vitamins or minerals such as calcium or magnesium can cause the lactate accumulation. However, there is increasing evidence that food allergy plays a major role in causing high lactate. The adrenalin produced by the anxiety further increases the reaction.

Yet another cause of anxiety is poor liver function. The liver detoxifies all the junk and chemicals we ingest and breathe. If its function is below par, the brain can be adversely affected by toxic chemicals circulating in the bloodstream.

Clearly there are many diverse reasons for anxiety which need evaluating. There is no point in spending hours meditating to relieve it if an allergic reaction may be responsible for the problem.

TREATMENT
Diet
- Avoid foods to which you are allergic.
- Avoid all sugar, honey, sorbitol, refined grains and cereals, milk, caffeine and alcohol, as they increase lactate levels.
- Reduce fruit and avoid fruit juice, as fructose also increases lactate.
- Follow the naturopathic diet (chapter II:13), but increase protein levels and reduce even healthy complex carbohydrate such as grains until you improve. Lactate accumulation responds to this combination.

Supplements of value
Adult doses:
- *Inositol* – 250mg three times daily of this B vitamin, has an anti-anxiety effect on brain waves similar to valium.
- *B-complex* – 50mg twice daily.
- *Niacinamide (B3)* – 400mg twice daily in addition to B-complex. It stimulates the normal conversion of lactate to pyruvic acid.
- *Magnesium* – 250-750mg daily, also converts lactate to pyruvic acid.

- **Calcium** – 250-750mg daily.
- **Histidine** – 200-500mg daily, half an hour before food, with a little vegetable juice. This amino acid is reduced in stress, especially in the central nervous system. The result is increased nervous activity, increased adrenalin and low alpha waves in the brain. 200mg a day may be sufficient to calm the mind.
- **Celloids® PPMP** (see appendix 1) are nerve nutrients.
- **Bach** and **Australian flower remedies** matched to emotions – for example, *crowea* for a constant feeling of anxiety.

Herbal teas

- **Chamomile** – calms the nervous system.
- **Lemon balm** – for panicky feelings with palpitations.
- **Betony** – for stress, anxiety and tension headaches.
- **Skullcap** – for anxiety and tension. It's good for aggressive children and those who throw tantrums.
- **Vervain** – for irritability, depression and nervous fatigue.

Herbs to strengthen the adrenal glands

Adult doses:
- **Ginseng** – 1g three times daily, as a tea.
- **Licorice** – 1g three times daily, as a tea. If using this amount of licorice long term, take a potassium supplement or drink a glass of freshly-made vegetable juice 3-4 times weekly. Deglycyrrhizinated licorice does not cause a potassium loss.

Essential oils

- Lavender.
- Marjoram.
- Bergamot.
- Basil.
- Neroli.
- Ylang ylang.
- Juniper.

See chapter III:6 on insomnia for notes on the individual oils, and use those above which suit best. For a bath use 10 drops in total to half a bath and soak in it for twenty minutes. As a massage oil use 15 drops in total to 30ml of carrier massage oil.

Homeopathy

Adult dose: 6c twice daily, or take one dose of 30c and see how long it lasts.
- **Kali Phos** – symptoms are often caused by overwork and worry. Apprehension, nervous dread, irritability, tearfulness, flying into passions easily. Everything seems to be an effort.
- **Aconite** – great fear, anxiety, anguish of mind and forebodings. Emotional, physical and mental tension.
- **Ignatia** – if caused by grief. Tearfulness, sighing and sobbing.
- **Lycopodium** – anxiety about an impending public ordeal. Especially for people who crave sweets and have digestive upsets.
- **Phosphorus** – feeling very strung-out, or having a deep sense of anxiety even on awakening. For those who are extremely sensitive to the needs of others.
- **Tarentula** – an overactive mind, can't relax, can't get off to sleep. Symptoms caused by overwork.
- **Arg Nit** – tearfulness, trembling, anxiety, mentally too weak to handle a challenge. Tormenting fears which may cause sweating or diarrhoea.
- **Nat Mur** – for chronic worrying about the future. Vulnerable to emotional pain but mentally strong. Absorbs the suffering of others. Always tries to avoid being hurt by emotional injury. May be impatient and irritable.
- **Picric Ac** – stress caused by mental overwork and anxiety. Brain fatigue, headache and the least mental effort is exhausting.
- **Nux Vomica** – irritability, overworked, stubbornness, reproachfulness, sullenness, fault-finding. Can't bear noise and wants to

be left alone.
- *Pulsatilla* – anxiety, emotional, inclined to weepiness but not irritable or subject to mood-swings. A good-natured mild personality.
- *Arsenicum* – anxiety or habitual worrying. A restless perfectionist type.

III: 5. FATIGUE

This has to be the most common condition presented in my clinic, but it is only a *symptom* of an underlying problem. There is no quick-fix pill to raise energy levels permanently – rather the source of the symptom has to be found and eliminated. Sometimes the causes are many and interlinked within a person, but the first area to investigate is the diet. *You are what you eat* – meaning that what you eat turns into you – so if poor quality food is eaten, poor quality *you* results!

Causes

• *Iron deficiency* is the best known cause of fatigue and is more common in menstruating women than others. Iron is necessary for the formation of haemoglobin, which transports oxygen in the blood for delivery to the tissues. Low oxygen levels equate with fatigue. Iron is also essential for resistance to disease, as the bone marrow uses it for producing white blood cells. When replacing iron, use iron phosphate, as it is non-toxic, rarely causes side-effects or constipation, and it absorbs well. Dietary sources of iron should be increased. Meat-eaters can get it from lamb's liver/kidneys, other meats and dairy products. This type of iron is organic and is of the 'haem' type, which means that it is absorbed as it is. Vegetarian sources of iron have to be changed by the body to the ferrous type before absorption can occur, and vitamin C is needed for its uptake. Green vegetables are high in iron, but it is poorly absorbed, so vegetarians must rely on food sources lower in content but high in availability, such as kelp, brewer's yeast, molasses, walnuts, sunflower seeds and sesame seeds, soya beans, other pulses and fruit. Grains must be soaked, sprouted, fermented or cooked, or the phytates will prevent the absorption of many minerals, including iron.

• *Folic acid deficiency* may cause anaemia because this vitamin is necessary for the formation of red blood cells. With deficient numbers of these, oxygen-carrying capacity is reduced. Vegetarians rarely suffer from this type of anaemia, as folic acid is high in green vegetables, brewer's yeast, soya products, asparagus, lentils, oats, wheatgerm, fresh nuts, wholegrains and avocados. This is one of the many vitamins washed out of the body by the contraceptive pill, and research points to the value of folic acid in preventing birth defects, if the mother takes it before conception and for the first three months. Unfortunately many young women go straight from the contraceptive pill to becoming pregnant. The recommended dose is 400mcg daily for adults.

• *Hypoglycaemia* causes fatigue because of low blood sugar levels, which mean no energy sources for the cells. If fatigue is clearly related to certain times of the day, such as late afternoon and before breakfast and if there is accompanying irritability, mood swings, weepiness or headaches, then follow the diet for hypoglycaemia.

• *Hypothyroidism* can cause fatigue because when the thyroid gland is working too slowly, metabolism (energy production) is decreased. A slight hypothyroidism is common and will not show on a blood test. Diagnosis is according to symptoms, and several of the following will be present: difficulty in losing weight, fluid retention, a low body temperature, increased sensitivity to cold, dry skin or hair, puffy eyes in the morning, callouses on the feet, a slow pulse, lethargy and poor digestive function. Getting a thyroid gland going again requires aerobic exercise and a largely raw diet, which supplies all the nutrients needed by the thyroid gland. Where pure sources are available, thyroid glandular supplements are known to be absorbed intact, and the active ingredients are taken up by the thyroid and utilised. Glandulars are made from freeze-dried animal glands, but it is important that these are extracted from healthy stock. The amino acid tyrosine stimulates thyroid function – this is readily available in most protein foods and as a supplement. Sometimes, enough thyroxine is produced by the thyroid gland, but it is not activated. It is known that zinc and selenium are necessary for changing thyroxine to its active T3 type.

• *Stress* is a direct cause of fatigue because it eventually weakens the adrenal glands. This means that the adrenalin supply is reduced, and therefore the normal conversion of stored sugar (in muscles and the liver) to glucose happens very slowly. The human body holds stores of sugar in the form of glycogen, and it can be quickly converted to glucose when extra energy is required. Slow conversion leads to low blood sugar levels and fatigue. After long periods of anxiety, overwork or tension, the adrenal glands will become exhausted and say 'enough is enough'. The symptoms depend on which part of the adrenal gland is affected, because different hormones are secreted by different parts of the gland. If the glucocorticoids are reduced then sugar supply is slow, with resulting symptoms of sugar craving, irritability, headaches, mood swings, weak muscles or tremor. If cortisone release is slow, allergies, auto-immune disease and infections occur more frequently. After menopause, sex hormones are produced in the adrenal glands, and if this is prevented, menopausal flushes and a low sex drive result. The medullary portion of the gland, which is the central part, secretes adrenalin and noradrenaline, which affects metabolism and all internal organ functions. Low levels may result in such things as constipation, obesity and sluggish liver function. Support for the adrenal glands is supplied by vitamins A, C, E, B complex, pantothenic acid, zinc, omega-3 fatty acids, ginseng and licorice herbs.

• *Heavy metals* accumulating in the body can affect brain function and energy levels. It is well known that aluminium, mercury and lead can have toxic affects on the brain. The early symptoms of mercury poisoning are anxiety, depression, headaches, fatigue, poor concentration and poor memory, spaceyness and muscle tremor. Later muscle weakness and poor co-ordination develop. Numbness and tingling of the extremities or visual or speech difficulties may occur as well. In fact mercury poisoning looks rather like M E (see chapter III:29).

• *Lead, aluminium, copper* and *nickel* all affect brain function, and the best method of determining body levels is through hair analysis, as blood tests are inaccurate. Vitamins, minerals and amino acids can be used to remove heavy metals.

• *Chronic constipation* is a major cause of fatigue, as the brain is poisoned by the reabsorption of toxins through the bowel wall. Modern diets high in junk food, processed food and animal protein are low in fibre, so that the bowel contents are not cleared quickly enough. Healthy bowel microorganisms are deficient in most people and these are needed for detoxification of anything ingested. The use of laxatives, poor habits, lack of exercise and constant worry all contribute to chronic constipation with its resultant fatigue. Treatment and prevention is outlined in chapter III:7 on bowel toxaemia. Diarrhoea, lack of digestive enzymes and malabsorption problems also cause fatigue by virtue of preventing nutrient absorption.

• A *lack of nutrients* is another major cause of fatigue. Usually it is not a deficiency of the common vitamins at fault, but a lack of the trace and macrominerals, which should be plentiful in the diet. There are twelve basic minerals of which the body is largely composed, and if any are unbalanced a chain reaction of symptoms occur. It is now recognised that minerals are more important than vitamins, in that they are required to metabolise vitamins correctly. The only way to pinpoint specific mineral imbalances is to take a holistic view of a person, but the rewards for doing so are very great. A high percentage of fatigue can be cured very quickly once the basic mineral balance is readjusted, because other nutrients like B vitamins are then better absorbed. You need to see a naturopath or nutritionist for professional guidance in this area.

• *Allergic reactions* to common food is, in my experience, the most usual reason for fatigue. It happens to children, adolescents and adults and can be quite devastating. I always do an allergy test on my 'tired' patients, because even if other factors are involved, allergy at least contributes to low energy levels. People who are stressed have compromised immune systems, and this is often enough to tip the balance from adaptation to allergens into producing allergic symptoms. When a person is in adaptation, allergic complexes are removed from the blood by the immune system and symptoms are prevented. This is why many people are not even aware of being allergic to a food. However, the blood brain barrier, which protects the brain from toxicity in the blood, is permeable to histamine released as a result of an allergic reaction. This is why so many people with food allergies suffer variations of mental effects.

• Other causes of fatigue are depression, boredom, anxiety and lack of exercise, and of course many diseases have fatigue as one of the symptoms. An early warning of rheumatoid arthritis is fatigue when any sort of effort is made. Candida, M E, liver and kidney diseases, infectious fevers and cancer all make people tired and lethargic.

TREATMENT

Supplements
The cause must be found and treated at the same time as improving the diet, so follow the naturopathic lifestyle detailed in part two of this book. In addition there are supplements which will enhance energy production. These are explained as follows:

• *B vitamins* – are of undoubted value. Use a quality brand, or take brewer's yeast as a source of natural Bs. Any multi tablet should contain all of the B vitamins, and not just 4-6 as is found in so many brands. Vitamin B12 by injection often produces extraordinary levels of energy.
• *Co-enzyme Q10* (CoE Q10) – occurs naturally in the body as part of energy production, but as we get older, supplies diminish. When taken in tablet form, it has the effect of oxygenating the system and therefore increasing energy. The dose is 30-50mg daily, but benefit is not felt until treatment has been ongoing for a month or so.
• *Antioxidant vitamins and minerals* improve energy for some, and can be bought as a single supplement containing vitamins A, C, E, B- complex, and minerals selenium, zinc and manganese.

The amino acids following are useful for increasing energy:
• *L-glutamine* – 250mg three times daily acts as brain fuel, and also enhances brain function and intelligence. This amino is useful for those who are studying, as it relieves

brain fatigue and increases concentration.

• **Phenylalanine** – 200-500mg daily forms another amino acid called tyrosine, which then makes adrenalin and the thyroid hormone thyroxine. A deficiency of this amino acid causes stress symptoms, depression, PMT, poor memory and slow thyroid function. The use of this product is contra-indicated in pregnancy, high blood pressure and where MAO type anti-depressant drugs are being taken. If you are on drugs, check with your doctor for the type of anti-depressant.

• **Arginine** and **lysine** release 'growth hormone', which increases energy production to relieve fatigue. They also improve memory and concentration.

Amino acids must be taken half an hour before food and require B complex and vitamin C to function properly.

Herbs

• **Ginseng** prevents insomnia, exhaustion and headaches, and can be taken from time to time as a tea to improve stress tolerance.

• **Guarana** is a Brazilian herb renowned for its rejuvenating effect. It has a similar molecular structure to caffeine but is absorbed slowly so that alertness is long-lasting. The dose is a half gram at breakfast and lunch, but don't take it at night or sleep patterns will be disturbed. The herb is not addictive.

• **Gentian** – 0.5-2g three times daily invigorates the whole system, and if taken half an hour before food it will stimulate the appetite.

• **Gold thread** and **poplar** herbs also stimulate the whole system and are regarded as universal tonics.

Essential oils

These can be used as massage oils or put in the bath. Put a total of 10 drops in half a tub of water and soak for twenty minutes to absorb the oils through the skin. A selection of the oils which relieve fatigue are:

• Rosemary.
• Lemon.
• Lemon grass.
• Eucalyptus.
• Peppermint.
• Jasmine.
• Black pepper.

Homeopathy

Dose: 30c once or twice daily if necessary.

• **Arnica** – for muscular aches, pains and exhaustion. This remedy stimulates the vital force and encourages rest, relaxation and a sense of well- being.

• **Arsenicum** – severe exhaustion following an infection. The person is very restless and cannot mentally relax.

• **Carbo Veg** – extreme exhaustion, cold extremities, clammy, sweating and extreme pallor. Sluggish, worn out and debilitated. Sudden loss of memory.

• **China** – for fatigue following a prolonged exhaustive illness or a prolonged period of nursing an invalid. Person is apathetic, taciturn and despondent and may have sudden crying spells. Pain in limbs and joints, great debility, trembling and numbness of limbs. Headache, digestive upset, coldness in the stomach.

• **Nux Vomica** – spasm pain and weariness. Trembling and numbness in the legs. Cannot sleep after 3am. Normally a quick, active, nervous, irritable person. For fatigue from mental strain and over-study. Person likes rich food and suffers digestive upsets.

• **Opium** – when collapse is imminent and there is drowsiness and extreme inertia.

• **Phos Ac** – general weakness, anxiety about one's condition, fatigue, cold clammy sweats, weakness on exertion. Debility is very marked, producing nervous exhaustion which may be due to chronic illness. This is good for young people who are overtaxed mentally and physically and who are normally constitutionally strong. The person is listless, apathetic, indifferent and may even stumble easily. The fatigue is better after a short sleep.

• *Picric Ac* – mental and physical fatigue, great weakness of the legs and feels compelled to lie down. A washed-out feeling and lack of willpower to do anything. No anxiety, person is very calm. Disturbed sleep patterns which are not refreshed by sleep. Cold, clammy sweats.

III: 6. *INSOMNIA*

Insomnia is one of the most common complaints. Everyone suffers from it at least occasionally but if the problem occurs frequently then the cause must be ascertained. Taking sleeping tablets is *not* the answer.

The problem may be due to the consumption of stimulants such as tea, coffee, chocolate or alcohol. Oral contraceptives cause insomnia in some women because they wash out many vitamins and minerals. Other common causes are a lack of exercise or being unable to switch off at the end of the day.

I have seen all manner of sleep problems caused by food allergies. One person suffers sleep-onset insomnia, while another gets off alright, but wakes around 2am and has to read for an hour or two. I have even seen foods cause sleepiness to occur throughout the day.

Sometimes a deficiency of the minerals that feed the nervous system play havoc with sleep patterns. These may be calcium, magnesium or potassium bound to phosphate. Many a child has had insomnia cured with a mix of potassium phosphate and magnesium phosphate. Stressed people also use up these minerals at an increased rate. Stress is a major reason for disturbed sleep patterns.

Amongst older people, restless leg is a cause of frequent waking. High doses of folic acid may sort this out, especially in those with malabsorption problems. Vitamin E is also of benefit, and essential fatty acids such as evening primrose oil. Jerking of the limbs just as sleep overtakes or during the night can cause insomnia. This will be helped by calcium and magnesium supplements or homeopathic remedies.

Hypoglycaemia may be a culprit, because if blood sugar levels drop, adrenalin is released to add sugar to the blood from stores and this chemical stimulates alertness. Chocolate, desserts and alcohol late at night may trigger hypoglycaemia.

To facilitate sleep, a release of specific chemicals must occur in the central nervous system. One of these is serotonin, but it is dependent on the amino acid tryptophan, which is derived from protein foods. Unfortunately, this amino acid is quite a large molecule which does not pass easily through the blood brain barrier (BBB) when other smaller aminos are competing for transport. Only those with sleep-onset insomnia are short of tryptophan. At this moment the product is not available as a supplement because of a world-wide ban, due to a single supplier in Japan having widely distributed poisoned stock. When and if tryptophan returns to the stores, the dose is 2-3g half an hour before bedtime, with a little fruit juice to encourage central nervous system uptake. Any protein food such as milk is to be avoided in the evening so that competing amino acids do not block food sources of tryptophan from entering the brain. The other amino acids found in protein foods are smaller and pass through the BBB in preference to tryptophan. It is a good idea to eat some carbohydrate like cracker biscuits at bedtime, as this indirectly ties up the small amino acids and allows tryptophan to pass through. Better still is a complex carbohydrate evening meal as well, but no simple starches like white flour, white rice or sugar.

Meantime, insomniacs could try inositol, a

B vitamin. Studies in USA show that it has an anti-anxiety effect on brain waves similar to that of addictive tranquillisers, and that those on valium or librium could stop once established on inositol. This is best taken with a low dose B complex, vitamin C and some fruit juice. Again, no milk. A 100g (3oz) serving of brown rice at dinner provides 300mg of inositol, and 100g (3oz) of vegetables or bread contains 100mg. Add an orange at bedtime for another 200mg and you have 600mg of inositol in a single evening. The B vitamin niacin may also be of benefit, as it does encourage the degradation of food tryptophan into serotonin. If niacin causes an uncomfortable flush use niacinamide instead.

Some other major causes of insomnia are anxiety, tension, depression, external noises, pain or discomfort, climate or environmental changes, jet-lag or even fear of sleeplessness. The key to successful treatment is finding the cause and dealing with it.

TREATMENTS
Diet and lifestyle
- No stimulants or sugar in the evening.
- No protein after the evening meal.
- A glass of fruit juice at bedtime.
- Exercise during the day.
- Meditate or practise some other form of relaxation technique during the evening.

Supplements of value
Adult doses: Choose from the following, and take 45 minutes before bed.
- *Tryptophan*, 2-3g with vitamin B6 50mg and magnesium 250mg.
- *Niacin*, 100mg for sleep-onset insomnia, and for those who wake in the night and can't get back to sleep.
- *Calcium* 250mg + *magnesium* 250mg.
- *Inositol* 250-750mg, with a B complex tablet and vitamin C 100mg.
- *Flower remedies* for emotional imbalances

(see chapter III:3 on Stress).

Herbs
Adult doses:
- *Passiflora* – 0.25-1g of the dried herb for those with sleep-onset insomnia.
- *Betony* – 2-4g dried herb for stress, anxiety and tension headaches.
- *Valerian* – 0.03-1g dried herb improves sleep-latency. However in some people this herb doesn't degrade properly and acts as a stimulant instead.
- *Hops* – 0.5-1g dried herb. This is contra-indicated in cases of depression.

Blends of some of these can be bought in tablet form.

Herbal teas
- *Linden* tea for chronic insomnia, especially in the elderly and young children.
- *Balm* (melissa) for sleep-onset insomnia, anxiety, depression and panicky feelings with palpitations.
- *Chamomile* calms the nervous system and sedates it.
- *Catnip* strengthens the nervous systems of children. Add *fennel* for fractious babies with colic.

The last three can be mixed together.

Essential oils
For massage or adding to the bath.
- For *nervous tension*: bergamot + lavender, or neroli + marjoram, or lavender + ylang ylang + juniper + basil. All these recipes are very relaxing.
- For *anxiety* and *depression*: bergamot + basil + clary sage.

To prepare a bath add a total of 10 drops of essential oils to half a tub and relax there for 15-20 minutes, to allow the oils to penetrate the skin. To prepare a massage oil add a total of 25 drops to 50 ml of a carrier oil such as avocado or almond. Massage this into the back in preference. Children and babies love a massage.

- **Bergamot** – for tension and depression.
- **Lavender** – for insomnia, depressions, headaches, palpitations, faintness, aches and pains, fatigue, anxiety, panic and hypertension.
- **Neroli** – for panicky people who get over-wrought about nothing, anxiety, depression, palpitations and nerve spasms.
- **Marjoram** – for insomnia and anxiety, muscle aches and pains.
- **Ylang ylang** – for insomnia and anxiety, depression, tension, hypertension and tachycardia.
- **Juniper** – for stress, anxiety and the chronic worrier.
- **Basil** – to refresh the mind. It treats depression and nervous exhaustion.
- **Clary sage** – a wonderful nerve tonic in depression. For nervous, weak and fearful types who are inclined to panic.

The olfactory lobe in the brain, which interprets smell, is connected to our emotional brain (the limbic system). The latter plays a central role in senses such as pain, pleasure, happiness, sadness, joy, anger, fear and sexual feelings as well as in memory and interpreting experience. For this reason, just the smell of some plants or their essential oils can directly affect our emotions. This is why the choice of an oil can also be made according to whether its smell is pleasurable.

Homeopathy
There are as many remedies for insomnia as there are sleepless people! Here are some useful ones. Dose 30c and repeat if waking in the night.
- **Arsenicum** – anxiety or worry, very restless especially from midnight to 2am.
- **Arnica** – if mentally or physically over-tired, bed feels too hard.
- **Coffea** – overactive mind, can't switch off.

- **Chamomilla** – irritable about not being able to get off to sleep, restless, anxious, moaning during sleep.
- **Cocculus** – too tired to sleep because of having to get up often to a child, feeling giddy.
- **China** – ideas crowd the mind and prevent sleep.
- **Lycopodium** – the day's work preys on the mind and prevents sleep. Dreams a lot, legs jerk in sleep, inclined to sleep during the day and early evening.
- **Nux Vomica** – mental overwork or over-indulgence in food and drink, wakes at 4am and drops off just as it is time to get up. Drowsy in early evening or after food. Better for a short nap.
- **Opium** – feels sleepy but can't fall asleep, bed feels hot and person moves around for a cool place. Hears every dog bark, clock chime or car going by.
- **Pulsatilla** – if insomnia is due to nervous exhaustion. Restless sleep in the early night, or unable to fall asleep until midnight. Sound asleep when it is time to get up, and then sleeps on late. Alternately hot and cold during sleep. Person inclined to weepiness.
- **Ignatia** – if caused by emotional upset. Legs jerk in sleep, yawns a lot but can't go to sleep.

Children's homeopathy
Dose 30c, and repeat if child awakens.
- **Ant Tart** – very light sleeper, talks and moans in sleep.
- **Calc Carb** – head sweats, frequent waking and nightmares. Starts at every noise.
- **Chamomilla** – tired sitting up, but not when put to bed. Wakes in the night and is cross and complaining, must be held by mother.
- **Cina** – ill-humoured, very cross child who doesn't want to be touched or carried, grinds teeth, limbs jerk, may have worms.

- **Coffea** – can't sleep because of too much excitement beforehand.
- **Kali Brom** – nightmares and sleep-walking.
- **Lycopodium** – can't get to sleep, and keeps everyone awake by singing and talking, active mind, hungry at night.
- **Nux Vomica** – wakes 4am crying, and refuses to be consoled.

III: 7. BOWEL TOXAEMIA AND BOWEL DISEASE

The health of the bowel is central to the health of a person as a whole, because toxins abound in the colon in unhealthy situations. The walls can become more permeable and toxins are then re-absorbed into the blood. There is now a wealth of documented evidence linking many of today's chronic diseases with bowel toxaemia.

The colon contains billions of bacteria and there are several hundred species. When the colon is unhealthy, or drugs like antibiotics are taken, undesirable bacteria release poisons called endotoxins which are harmful to all body tissue. Unfortunately a toxic bowel is usually also associated with increased permeability of the colon wall, and so endotoxins get to circulate freely in the body causing all manner of diseases. Psoriasis, pancreatitis, liver disease, rheumatoid arthritis, systemic lupus erythematosus, Crohn's and ulcerative colitis are all conditions associated with endotoxins – almost any less serious illnesses can also be attributed to a toxic colon. Many cases of psoriasis are completely cleared when the patient is given the herb sarsaparilla, which binds endotoxins while they are still in the bowel.

Probiotics

The healthy bacteria (micro-flora) of the colon, such as L acidophilus and bifido bacteria, digest food, produce energy from fibre, make some B vitamins, detoxify chemicals and pesticides in food and water and make important fatty acids like butyric acid, that helps prevent cancer in the bowel. These micro-flora produce antibiotic-like chemicals to destroy bacteria, fungi and parasites. Additionally they also make hydrogen peroxide, which destroys unwanted organisms. Furthermore, the immune surveillance in the body is increased by the presence of the healthy bacteria. Some strains of lactobacillus have displayed powerful anti-cancer properties – not directly but by the stimulation of immune function.

Immunoglobin A (IgA)

Locally, cells of the intestinal lining contain thousands of antibodies known as IgA. These stimulate immune system recognition and destruction of the unhealthy flora, endotoxins and parasites. IgA is also the most common antibody found in breast milk, because the infant needs a steady supply (along with bifido bacteria) to protect him or her against developing allergic reactions to foods appearing in mother's milk.

IgA binds compounds escaping through the bowel wall and oversees their passage to the liver, where they are disposed of. However when IgA levels are low, these complexes pass through the bowel wall freely to the circulation and the numbers can be so great that the liver cannot cope. Thus, immune complexes are formed which then circulate freely and enter the tissues to cause allergic reactions. A deficit of IgA is extremely common because of low levels of beneficial micro-flora in modern people's colon and also because of weakened immune function. IgA deficiency is heavily implicated in auto-immune diseases like lupus and rheumatoid arthritis, as well as eczema, asthma and all sorts of allergic conditions.

Increased permeability

Some of the less desirable micro-organisms in the bowels of modern people form toxic complexes that damage the bowel wall. This leads to an increased permeability and the absorption of toxins and large molecules of food into the bloodstream. When food particles escape into the circulation in appreciable amounts, there is an immunological response and allergic reactions then occur elsewhere in the body. At the same time there is a constant low grade inflammation of the colon wall.

The well known E coli, which often escapes externally to pop in through another door and cause cystitis in women has also been implicated in serious diseases like maturity-onset diabetes, Hashimoto's disease and myasthenia gravis. Proteus and klebsiella, which are common undesirables in modern people's colons, contain protein similar to human tissue. These are often involved in causing rheumatoid arthritis, simply because the body, forming immune complexes against these bacteria, also mistakenly forms antibodies against its own tissue, which is almost identical to the bacteria. Studies done in Britain have found that over 80% of rheumatoid arthritic patients have antibodies to proteus, which means that they are destroying their joints in the process of destroying the organism.

Fungal conditions like candida albicans which are allowed to flourish in a toxic bowel eventually put down roots into the wall and then readily pass into the bloodstream to spread to all parts. Re-absorbed toxins can lead to symptoms in any part of the body, from headaches and fatigue to asthma, hepatitis or even high blood pressure. However,

the healthier the colonic environment, the more the good guys crowd out the undesirable micro-organisms. For this reason, a healthy diet is of great importance.

Glucosamine

This is an amino sugar which our bodies make as a precursor to many types of tissue. It is the first step in the composition of collagen, cartilage, tendons and ligaments, blood vessels, skin, hormones, many enzymes and all sorts of fluids for body linings and joints. It is also the precursor of molecules that transport fats, vitamins and minerals. As far as the gut is concerned, glucosamine is the starting point for the fluid which coats the mucous membrane to protect the lining cells from irritants such as bacteria, parasites and fungus. It is even needed for making the IgA which live in the cells of the gut lining. The formation of chondroitin sulphate requires glucosamine, and this substance, along with the amino acid glutamine, forms two-thirds of the structure of the mucous membrane lining the whole intestinal tract. Chondroitin sulphate is a mucopolysaccharide, which also has anti-inflammatory properties.

Where tissues are under attack because of inflammation, injury, toxins or allergens, the repair mechanism is strained and new tissue is often not synthesised quickly enough. By providing the initial ingredient in abundance, the body can more quickly repair damaged tissue and fluids throughout.

In the bowel, glucosamine supplements block fungus and E coli from adhering to the lining, prevent partially digested foods from passing through the wall, encourage bifido bacteria to attach to surface cells and inhibit inflammatory diseases like Crohn's and ulcerative colitis.

The role of diet in colonic health

The modern diet is the prime cause of problems because it is high in fat, protein and simple depleted carbohydrates like white flour products and sugar. When people eat this type of diet over a period of time, the lack of fibre causes a very stagnant situation. More serious is the effect on the digestive activity. Intestinal changes occur which inhibit the flow of stomach acids and digestive enzymes. The food is then not broken down completely, and large molecules remain in the colon undigested. This stimulates the formation of undesirable flora, and IgA becomes depleted, with a consequent tendency to allergic reactions. Avoiding processed foods and eating whole, natural varieties is critical to proper function of the intestines.

Signs of disturbed colonic flora

Failure to maintain a healthy digestive system results in any of the following: constipation, gas formation, indigestion and bloating, diverticulosis, diarrhoea, bad breath, parasitic infestation, mucous colitis and ulcerative colitis, fatigue, depression and mood swings, chest pains, palpitations, excessive sweating and IgA deficiency. These are all quite aside from the more serious problems that can occur outside the colon.

Prevention

• Follow food combining to ensure the full breakdown of food.
• Eat slowly and chew very thoroughly.
• Do not eat when tired, ill or emotionally distressed.
• Eat a high fibre diet of wholegrains, pulses and lots of fresh fruit and vegetables, including garlic. Fibre decreases the transit time of food so that digestion can be completed. It also stimulates digestion, and decreases toxic reabsorption. However, do not eat wheatbran (bran flakes etc) stripped out of the whole grain as it decreases food digestion, irritates the gut lining and leads to toxic bowel conditions. Ricebran or oatbran are safe, as these brans bind endotoxins and do not act as irritants.
• Ensure that essential polyunsaturated oils are part of the diet as they prevent E coli from attacking the intestinal lining.
• Drink 4-6 glasses of water daily, plus an abundance of high water foods like fruit and vegetables.
• Reduce fat to the minimum and take only moderate amounts of protein. Reduce dairy foods also as they are mucous-forming.
• Avoid laxatives, antibiotics, antiseptics and other drugs.
• Form regular bowel habits.
• Exercise on a regular basis.
• Short-term fasting restores digestive function, IgA and healthy flora as well as destroying immune complexes and allowing the bowel wall to heal. It is a regular 'cure-all' for a wide variety of conditions.

Treating toxic conditions

Following the prevention outline is essential, but many products are available to mop up toxins, replace healthy flora and IgA and clear existing pockets of waste products.
• Begin with a juice fast and daily enema.
• Correct any digestive deficiencies by using betaine hydrochloric acid supplements and digestive enzymes if necessary from a health food shop.
• Use a colon cleansing product to clear waste for a limited period. These are also bought in health food shops and should contain fibre and herbs to cleanse the bowel, bind toxins and cleanse lymphs. The herb sarsaparilla binds endotoxins very effectively and golden seal, walnut, wormseed, fennel

and fenugreek herbs, as well as garlic and grapefruit seed extract destroy unhealthy bacteria, fungi and parasites. Yucca prevents their absorption. Later, natural unpasteurised aloe vera juice can be taken daily to maintain a healthy function and environment.

Treating Leaky Gut Syndrome

If the intestinal wall becomes permeable to toxins, the following outline needs to be implemented in addition to the above regime. Some indications of a leaky gut are: multiple or shifting allergies, unexplained diarrhoea, bowel gas, low zinc levels and burning, thin skin.

• *Bromelain* – 500mg three times daily with meals, clears mucous from the bowel so that it cannot provide a safe haven for parasites.
• *EPA* and *evening primrose oil* to provide the anti- inflammatory prostaglandins that protect the gut lining, and they also prevent E-coli from attaching itself to the mucosa.

Restoring normal gut lining and probiotics

• Replace bowel flora with a quality *lactobacillus* and *bifidus* product.
• *Glucosamine sulphate* – 0.5-3g daily, restores the gut lining, promotes the adhesion of bifido bacteria and prevents fungi from attaching to the lining.
• *Chondroitin sulphate* – 100mg, three times daily.
• *L-glutamine* – 250mg, three times daily.
• *Butyric acid* – 8g daily, to restore the individual cells lining the gut.
• *Vitamins A, C, B-complex* and *zinc* daily, for the proper function of the gut lining and essential fatty acids.
• *Oil* – 1 tablespoon daily of fish oil or even olive oil is important in healing the mucous membrane.
• *IgPlex* is a product which lines the gut

with IgA to provide control of bacteria, parasites and fungus.

Colonic irrigation

This is not an enema but a system whereby the whole colon is continually flushed over a lengthy period. It is carried out in a clinic using a closed circuit system. Believe it or not, the process is quite relaxing and will not cause embarrassment. Several treatments are sometimes necessary, and each session lasts 30 minutes. The process removes pockets of waste and old peanuts that may have been present for years, and the bowel is cleansed so that endotoxins cannot be systemically absorbed. Irrigation of the intestines also dramatically increases beneficial bile flow so that the immune complexes can be more quickly removed.

Probiotic supplements

There are many strains of lactobacilli, but the one used as a supplement is L acidophilus. This is usually combined with another important inhabitant of the colon called bifidus. These bacteria can be used to treat all toxic bowel conditions as well as a wide range of auto-immune related conditions. The supplements have been shown to be effective in systemic E coli and parasitic conditions, cancer, high cholesterol, vaginal infections, candida, eczema, asthma and psoriasis, to name a few. An incredible number of bacteria are strongly inhibited by acidophilus, and the immune response in infections is also greatly enhanced.

It is important to use bacteria which will colonise the bowel effectively. For this reason the product must be resistant to acid, bile and digestive enzymes. Supplements should be freeze-dried, require refrigeration and have a stated minimum potency. They should also be manufactured from human sources so that the affinity for the human mucosal lining is very high. In this manner the bacteria will multiply rapidly as long as the diet is high in fibre and contains B vitamin food sources. If not, then acidophilus activity is greatly reduced.

Because people most in need of acidophilus are those with allergies, the supplement should be free of lactose, sugar, wheat and soya products. There are some excellent brands on the market which do comply in this manner. Infants should only be given bifido bacteria until weaned as they do not have acidophilus in their colon until eating solid food.

Although some yoghurt labels state that they contain the correct bacteria (L bulgaricus and S thermophilus) it is important to establish that you are getting a live product. If fruit is present it is just a dessert and not a live yoghurt, and even some plain yoghurts are pasteurised to destroy the healthy bacteria and therefore increase shelf-life. These products are pre-digested milk but definitely do nothing to increase lactobacilli in the bowel. If a yoghurt is live you will be able to use a spoonful of it to turn fresh milk into yoghurt or at least into a sour milk drink.

III: *8. CANDIDA ALBICANS*

This is a fungus which is present inside everyone. It normally inhabits the bowel and does no harm, as it is kept in control by the immune system and normal healthy intestinal micro-organisms. However, when the immune system is damaged and the micro-flora wiped out by antibiotics or other drugs, candida is no longer held in check, and so proliferates. The speed at which this happens depends on the health of the person and his or her diet. If the latter contains processed foods, alcohol, sugar and white flour, candida will spread rapidly because it just loves junk food.

Eventually the fungus changes shape into a form which puts down roots into the intestinal wall. This makes the intestines too porous, and allows partially digested food, fungus and toxins to readily pass into the bloodstream. The immune system then recognises them as foreign and an allergic reaction occurs. Once the candida has penetrated the colon wall, it can spread to any part of the body via the bloodstream and cause havoc to its human host, with a variety of unpleasant symptoms.

These symptoms vary, depending on which area is invaded. For instance, candida is known to interfere with adrenal hormones, leading to stress symptoms, fatigue, blood sugar disturbances and fluid retention. It can also bind the thyroid hormone so that metabolism is slowed and the spirit is depressed. Should toxins reach the brain, all manner of mental powers can be disrupted. Premenstrual problems arise when the fungus interferes with the normal metabolism of polyunsaturated oils and vitamin B6. If the pancreas is affected, blood sugar control is altered, and when the toxic level is very high, liver function is inhibited. Should the candida become established in the lymphatic system, the fungus can recolonise the bowel at will. This means that treatment of the bowel only can be self-defeating – the whole body must be cleansed.

An added insult is that the body becomes sensitised to all other forms of fungus, and a wide variety of even natural foods must be avoided, quite aside from the simple carbohydrate on which candida lives. By this time a person feels exhausted to say the least, if not 'sick all over'.

Candida of the vagina has increased dramatically in the past decade until it now seems to be one of the most common causes of discharge. A study in the 70s found that all cases also had a proliferation of candida in the intestines. The contraceptive pill, antibiotics, steroids and a junk food diet are all heavily implicated in causing this condition.

Research has highlighted a very sinister side of candida over-growth. It has become clear that if a staphylococcus infection occurs simultaneously, the bacteria take on a high-powered virulence, against which antibiotics have no effect; cases of toxic shock syndrome have resulted.

Diagnosis

Because we all have candida inside us, laboratory tests are of little value in diagnosing systemic infestation. Rather the total symptom picture is important. The following are symptoms of candida, but a person needs to have several at one time before a diagnosis is positive, as other conditions such as post-viral fatigue syndrome can also cause some of these symptoms.

• Intestinal bloating and flatulence, nausea, abdominal pain, diarrhoea or constipation. All of these symptoms are worse after eating sugar, yeast or refined carbohydrate.

• Vaginal thrush, persistent itch or burning, menstrual problems, endometriosis, PMT, recurrent cystitis or urethritis.

• Depression, fuzzy-headedness, poor concentration and memory, fatigue, dizziness, mood-swings, confusion, anxiety, headaches, irritability or erratic vision.

• Itchy nose, oral thrush, pains and tightness in the chest, sore throats, bad breath, nasal congestion or a post-nasal drip.

• Aches and pains in muscles unrelated to exercise. Joint-swelling, tingling, numbness or burning sensations.

• Feeling unwell in damp or mouldy conditions and reacting strongly to chemicals, perfumes, fumes, synthetics or tobacco smoke.

• Athletes' foot, rashes or fungal patches on the skin.

• Multiple allergies and cravings for sugar, alcohol and bread.

• Slow metabolism, low body temperature and weight gain.

The symptoms depend on which part of the body has been infiltrated by the candida. In addition to several of the above conditions being persistent, there should be a history of one of the following: taking of antibiotics either for a month at a time or a few short courses within the past year, use of the contraceptive pill for over one year, or a short course of cortisone-type drugs.

There is no point in treating candida at a local level and ignoring the systemic aspect. Using anti-fungals for a vaginal infestation and not treating the gut just ensures repeated attacks, and in the long run there is a risk of the whole body becoming affected.

Some people are very ill with candida, and in fact some have their lives completely disabled by it. The condition is easy to treat, but results take time and even when symptoms disappear, a very long period of dietary restriction is essential while the bowel wall heals, and once again becomes a barrier against fungus and toxins. In serious illness the adrenal glands will be stressed and the immune system severely weakened. *Unless both systems are strengthened the anti-fungal/ anti-parasitic treatment will not hold for long.*

TREATMENT
• Starve the fungus.

• Destroy it.

• Destroy any parasites which are probably also present in the gut and perhaps the lymphatics.

• Strengthen the immune system and liver function so that they can destroy the candida and detoxify the body. No one develops candida unless the immune system has first been damaged.

• Ensure a healthy intestinal environment.

• Heal the bowel wall.

Diet
• High fibre, high complex carbohydrate, moderate protein and low fat.

• Abundant vegetables twice daily, especially asparagus, broccoli, beetroot, cabbage, peppers, onions, garlic and cucumber.

• Juiced vegetables daily, as the diet must be 75% alkaline-forming to inhibit fungus.

• Fruit in moderation, after the first three weeks of treatment.

• Live plain yoghurt in moderation.

• Wholegrains such as oats, millet and rice, to be used liberally. Toasted 100% black rye bread is all right in moderation, but restrict wheat, as the carbohydrate ferments easily.

• Pulses, lentils, chickpeas, soya beans, pinto beans and so on.

- Sprouted peas, beans, seeds and grains, especially mung and alfalfa.
- All seeds, plus almonds, walnuts, fresh co-conut and buckwheat.
- Oily fish and white fish, egg and low-fat cottage cheese, meat in moderation, but only if free of hormones and antibiotics.
- Lamb and organic chicken, or game, are the safest.
- Extra-virgin olive oil – two teaspoons daily as a dressing.
- Herbal tea, vegetable juices, mineral water and vegetable broth as drinks. Take two pints daily.
- Cinnamon, thyme, lemon balm, rosemary and garlic are destructive to candida.

All food should be organic and as much raw as possible.

Avoid

- Chemicals such as contraceptive pills, anti-biotics, cortisone, preservatives, colourings, flavourings, perfumes, fumes, MSG and chemical cleaning products.
- All sugar, white flour, white rice, and everything made from them. For instance, jams, pickles, frozen and canned vegetables, cakes, biscuits, crackers, pasta, pizza and processed breakfast cereals.
- All refined, canned, processed and packaged food, as sugar or yeast is often involved.
- Alcohol, tea and coffee, as they stimulate the release of sugar from the liver.
- All carbonated drinks, squashes, fruit juices, dried fruit, bananas and sweet grapes, even after some fruit is again permitted.
- All foods where fermentation occurs: tofu, soya sauce, vinegar, and everything made from them – dressings, mayonnaise, pickles, sauces, and Indian or Chinese tea, except green tea.
- Smoked fish and processed meats – salami, sausage, bacon and hamburgers.
- All moulds: left-over food, dried fruit, and all peanuts. Any other nuts that are not fresh and mould-free, mouldy cheese, mushrooms, damp basements, mouldy bathrooms, cupboards and rugs. Even some herbal teas may be mouldy, so buy herbs from reliable medicinal suppliers.
- All yeasts: bread, pizza, commercial cakes, biscuits, crackers and bread-crumbed food. Brewer's yeast, Marmite and Vegemite. All vitamins and minerals that are not guaranteed yeast-free.
- All malted products: cereals and malted milk, etc.
- All honey and maple syrup.
- All fruit for three weeks, and then only in moderation, because of the sugar content. Avoid low-fibre fruit like melons.
- Milk, because of the milk-sugar content.
- Meat that is not organic, as the antibiotics and hormone residues will increase candida growth.
- Foods to which you are allergic.
- Oils except olive oil and guaranteed cold-pressed polyunsaturates, otherwise the immune response to candida is inhibited.
- Microwave cooking, as enzymes are inhibited and the molecular structure of foods altered.
- Where candida symptoms are very mild, it may not be essential to avoid perfumes, moulds, yeasts or ferments for long. Candida lives on sugar, not moulds and yeasts. The reason for avoiding the latter is that in more serious conditions, the body becomes sensitised to them.

Candida diets

For those who wonder if there is *anything* they can eat, here are some menu ideas!

Breakfast

- Raw muesli (sugar and fruit-free), add chopped fresh nuts and seeds, fresh coconut and wheatgerm.

• Oatmeal, millet, brown rice or buckwheat porridge. Serve all cereals with sugar-free soya milk, nut milk, or plain live yoghurt.
• Cooked eggs and yeast-free bread, wholegrain Ryvita or rice cakes.
• Wholewheat or buckwheat pancakes, with a little butter or sugar-free jam and yoghurt.

Lunch
• A herbal or Spanish omelette.
• Low-fat cottage cheese.
• A baked potato, with yoghurt dressing that has lemon juice added.
• Dishes made from dried peas and beans.
• Dahl made from lentils and spices.
• Salads made from brown rice, brown pasta, buckwheat, barley or millet, with added flavourings like yoghurt and horseradish or garlic, oil and lemon juice. Add chopped vegetables to this, or stir in curried vegetables.
• Home-made soups with vegetables, beans or grains.
• Nut roasts or patties.

Any of the choices for lunch should be served with a large salad and sprouted peas, beans or seeds. Dressings are made of extra-virgin olive oil, lemon juice, garlic and herbs.

Dinner
• Fish, especially salmon, mackerel, sardines or trout.
• Lamb or genuine free-range poultry.
• Lamb's liver or kidney.
• Vegetarian protein, as at lunch. If not eating animal protein be sure to combine beans and grains or nuts/seeds in the same day, to make complete protein.

The above suggestions should accompany a large plate of vegetables, lightly-steamed or stir-fried, and a salad. Use a great variety of vegetables every day.

If eating out, starters could be salads or plain asparagus, the main course fresh salmon

and vegetables, and the dessert, fresh fruit – once it is again permitted. Remember, no roasting or frying.

Wash all fruit and vegetables thoroughly, as they often have mould on them. Yeast will grow on stale grains and nuts, and pistachios grow it particularly easily. The peanut crops in the world are infested with a toxic mould, so *no one* should eat them. The amount of raw vegetables eaten would depend on your digestive system. You may need to slowly increase the amount rather than suddenly start eating large servings.

Snacks
Raw vegetable sticks, seeds (pumpkin, sesame, sunflower, linseed), yoghurt with herbal tea or mineral water.

The above dietary programme starves the fungus, so that it begins to die off.

Supplements of value
Adult doses:

Anti-fungal supplements
• *L acidophilus*, in capsule form or as a powder. The product must be guaranteed potent, it requires refrigeration and must have an expiry date. L acidophilus repopulates the bowel with healthy bacteria, makes the B vitamin biotin and controls the fungus.
• *Candex 30c*, daily, is the homeopathic treatment.
• *Biotin* – 400mcg daily, and two teaspoons of *olive oil* daily. Both of these prevent the candida from changing to the invasive form. Excessive biotin has the opposite effect.
• *Garlic* – 1-2g three times daily, raw, or the equivalent in dried form. One very large clove weighs 5-6g.
• *Aloe vera juice* – two tablespoons daily.
• *Fibre* as guar gum, psyllium or flaxseeds – one tablespoon at night, to flush toxins from the colon.
• *Betaine HCl acid tablets* and *digestive*

enzymes with meals if necessary to increase stomach acidity and prevent the fungus spreading upwards. The enzymes ensure complete digestion of food.

● Bromelain – 500mg three times daily with meals, to clear away intestinal mucous which shelters parasites.

The following should be added after an initial period of starving the candida through dietary control. Depending on the severity of the condition, one or more would be used.

● *Tea tree oil* or *German chamomile oil* – 1-3 drops three times daily, orally.

● *Capricin*, *mycopryl* or *mycocidin* – in capsule form, according to the manufacturer's instructions. Usually the dose is gradually increased to reduce die-off symptoms which worsen conditions, like fuzzy heads. The capricin and mycopryl are coconut derivatives which go through the gut destroying yeast. The mycocidin is very similar to caprylic acid but is extracted from castor bean oil, and this also effectively destroys fungus.

● *Citricidal* (grapefruit seed extract) – according to manufacturer's instructions.

● Licorice + golden seal + walnut leaves + fennel, or golden seal + bayberry + echinacea. Mix either of these herbal blends in equal weights, and make a tea of 1oz (30g) to a pint (6dl) of water, and drink one cup three times daily. Alternately make a tincture from the blend, and take one teaspoon three times daily.

● *Pau d'arco* – 20g to one pint (6dl), and boil five minutes. Infuse another 10 minutes, and drink this herbal tea in one day.

Immune System Support
Look for a supplement designed for immune system repair. It will supply the first eight listed below, in similar amounts, in a full day's dosage, and possibly some herbs as well. These nutrients will also restore tired

adrenal glands, but in that case, add 500mg pantothenic acid and ginseng tea. Additionally, all the following nutrients are important in preventing the candida from damaging various glandular functions, such as may occur in the thyroid, pancreas and ovaries.

● *Beta carotene* – 6mg, or *vitamin A* – 10,000iu daily.

● *Vitamin C* – 500mg, three times daily.

● *Vitamin E* – 200-400iu daily.

● *Vitamin B-complex* – 25-50mg daily, with B6 as pyridoxine-5-phosphate.

● *Selenium* – 200mcg daily.

● *Zinc* – 30mg daily.

● *Manganese* – 5mg daily.

● *Iron* – 5mg daily.

● *Evening primrose oil* – 500mg three times daily.

● A *calcium/magnesium supplement*, supplying 250mg of each daily.

● *Béres Drops Plus*.

Liver Support
This is important, as the liver has to detoxify the candida.

● *Red beet* and *green vegetable juice*, daily, before food, increases liver function.

● *Silymarin herbal extract* – 50mg three times daily, regenerates the liver and powerfully protects it.

● *Dandelion tea* improves liver function, as does golden seal, used to destroy candida.

● *Molybdenum* is necessary for forming the liver-detoxifying enzymes, and will often clear the debilitating brain symptoms of confusion, poor concentration and fuzzy feelings.

Heal the bowel wall
This is vital so that the colon ceases to be porous to fungus and foods that are not properly digested. The acidophilus has some effect of course, together with the zinc, pantothenic acid (vitamin B5), folic acid and vitamin A, already indicated for immune competence. See chapter III:7 on Bowel

Toxaemia for the complete regime.

Vaginal candida treatment choices

- *Betadine*, *citricidal* or *tea tree oil* dou-
ches daily, for 2-3 weeks at a time. Add a
kyolic garlic capsule to the solution.
- *Boric acid* 600mg, put into capsules and
inserted nightly for seven doses is a very
effective treatment, or make a solution with a
little water and soak a tampon which is already inserted.
- Two *L acidophilus* capsules should be inserted nightly, once the boric acid treatment
is finished - use concentrated solution if it is
easier.
- Studies indicate that the herb *echinacea*
will prevent the recurrence of vaginal candida
in those who are frequently affected.
- Calendula + golden seal as a douche is
healing and soothing.

It is possible for symptoms to clear reasonably quickly with the above treatment, and
this tempts people to relax the diet. It is very
important to resist this, as the condition will
recur until the fungus is under complete control, the immune system is doing a good surveillance job and the bowel has healed, and
has been re-populated with the correct micro-
organisms. In some cases this takes two years
or more. For those with less severe conditions, control may be possible with diet alone,
although a general immune system supplement and lactobacillus is advisable.

Seek guidance

It is wise to see a naturopath for initial guidance, as we all have different requirements.
No two people are ever treated in exactly the
same manner, and some require higher doses
of certain nutrients than others.

III: *9. VAGINITIS*

Vaginal infections are one of the most common conditions in young women. This is probably due to a mixture of being sexually active, taking the contraceptive pill, and eating an inadequate diet that is nutritionally deficient.

Vaginitis needs to be taken seriously as it may be associated with a chronic inflammation of the cervix or a sexually-transmitted disease. If not treated adequately, infection can spread into the uterus and fallopian tubes, causing endometriosis salpingitis or pelvic inflammatory disease. Some women have a discharge at various times during the menstrual cycle which is caused by hormonal stimulation, but inflammation is not involved here and treatment is unnecessary.

Predisposing factors

If the pH of the vagina is changed, infection can readily develop. 'The pill', and a diet containing white flour products and sugar will make the vagina too alkaline. The healthy micro-flora which normally inhabit the vagina are important, since without them, mucous secretion is increased and a fertile breeding-ground for organisms occurs. If the immune system is strong, infection is prevented. However, immune function is readily inhibited by a poor diet, 'the pill' and other drugs, unhealthy lifestyles, stress, illness and allergies.

Candida albicans (Monilia)

This is by far the most common reason for vaginitis. It causes itching or burning and may be so thick that it looks like cottage cheese. Small patches are white with a red border.

The increased use of the contraceptive pill, antibiotics and a poor diet causes the fungus to proliferate, and treating only the local symptoms ensures constant recurrence of the condition. If candida is present in the vagina it is also flourishing in the gut, so a general systemic anti-candida treatment is required, as well as ensuring that any existing predisposing factors are removed.

Topical treatment choices

See chapter III:8 on Candida Albicans for candida treatment.

Trichomonas

This is a sexually-transmitted protozoa which may be found in the vagina, urethra and surrounding glands. It causes itching and burning, and there is a frothy yellow/green discharge, sometimes with a fishy odour. It is often associated with gonorrhoea, and is a major cause of cervical erosion. It is one of the reasons for the high rate of false positive cervical smears.

TREATMENT

Outline

• Stimulate the immune system with a diet of whole natural foods, an abundance of fruit and vegetables and avoidance of sugar, white flour and all refined packaged food.

• Avoid the contraceptive pill and other drugs.

• Practise safe sex.

• Take the following natural supplements to strengthen the immune system, destroy the infection and improve the vaginal environment.

Supplements
- *Beta carotene* – 15mg daily, for a healthy vaginal lining resistant to infection.
- *Vitamin C* – 1g four times daily.
- *Vitamin E* – 200iu daily.
- *Selenium* – 100mcg daily.
- *Zinc* – 15-25mg daily, as citrate or picolinate.
- *B-complex* – 50mg daily.
- *Garlic* – 1g three times daily.
- *L acidophilus* – 2 capsules daily, of a guaranteed potent type.
- *Glucosamine* – 1g twice daily, to quickly restore the normality of cells and fluids lining the vagina.

Herbs
- *Golden seal* – 0.5g, three times daily.
- *Echinacea* – 1g, three times daily.

These can also be made into a decoction and used as a douche.

Topical treatment
Insert two *L acidophilus* capsules nightly, or use a live yoghurt, and choose from the following for douching twice daily for two to three weeks:
- *Tea tree oil, peppermint oil* or *lavender oil*.

Use 5-10 drops of one of these essential oils to 5oz of water.
- *Betadine* douche.
- *Zinc sulphate* 2%, as a douche. Use one tablespoon to 16oz (4.5dl) of water.

Tampons may be soaked in douche solutions with garlic added, and inserted during the day. Kyolic garlic is good and effective, as well as odourless. In the case of essential oils, 5-10% solutions may be used on a tampon twice weekly all day. Add squeezed garlic or garlic powder to all douching solutions, as it is effective against all infecting agents in vaginitis. Added chlorophyll is very soothing.

Chlamydia
This genital infection is sexually-transmitted, and often associated with urethritis and inflammation of the cervix or fallopian tubes in women. In men there may be proctitis or epididymitis.

Chlamydia is a parasitic bacterium which usually infects the cervix in women and the urethra of men, and is often asymptomatic. Any discharge is like a thick mucous, and there may be some burning on passing urine. The eyes and respiratory tract can be infected with chlamydia, and in the case of newborn infants from infected mothers, the eyes must be carefully treated immediately. Treatment should be vigorous as there is a risk of pelvic inflammatory disease, tubal scarring and infertility. Antibiotics may be needed as well as the herbs, but studies have shown that recurrence is more common in those taking antibiotics alone.

Because chlamydia tends to be symptom-free, it is one of the most potentially harmful sexually-transmitted diseases. This is because it is often detected only after pelvic inflammatory disease or sterility already exists. Chlamydia can remain undetected in cells for years, and passed to any sexual partner during that time. When the immune system is weakened, or a woman undergoes gynaecological surgery (including I U D insertion) the bacteria can spread to the uterus and fallopian tubes. Anyone at risk should have regular checks so that treatment can be instigated early.

TREATMENT
Use the same supplements as in trichomonas.

Herbs
- *Golden seal + barberry + oregon mountain grape* (berberine). Mix these together in equal proportions, and take 1g three times daily of the powdered root, or one teaspoon of tincture.

Topical

- Douche with **betadine** or 2% **zinc sulphate** solution twice daily, and berberine tea once daily.
- Add 2 drops of **Lugols solution** and **garlic** to a tea tree oil douche.

Gardnerella

This is sometimes asymptomatic, but often the discharge has a foul odour. The treatment is the same as for chlamydia.

Homeopathy for Vaginitis

For any of the infections. Dose 6c. 4-6 times daily for 10 days.

- **Borax** – for an egg white discharge which irritates or itches.
- **Kreosote** – for milky discharge which is corrosive, burning or itchy. Pain in the lower back and great weakness.
- **Alumina** – for chronic copious yellow discharge which hardens on underwear. Itching which is better for washing in cold water.
- **Bovista** – for thick green discharge, especially after periods.
- **Carbo Veg** – for green discharge which burns, especially before periods.
- **Nit Ac** – for stitching pain in the vagina, flesh-coloured, watery, smelly discharge.
- **Mercurius** – for a foul-smelling green discharge which burns or itches. Better after washing with cold water. Pain in the ovaries. Person sweats easily and may have bad breath.
- **Sepia** – for yellow/green discharge and a stitching pain in the uterus. Itching worse when walking.

III: *10. SLUGGISH LIVER*

The liver has the following major functions:
- making bile salts for the emulsification and absorption of fats, and making heparin for the blood-clotting process;
- storage and filtering of blood;
- destruction of any bacteria, bowel toxins, allergic complexes, old red and white blood cells and any poisons which have escaped into the blood;
- involvement in the metabolism of fats, carbohydrates and proteins, vitamins and minerals; it stores glucose, vitamins A, D, E and K, the minerals copper and iron, and even chemicals which cannot be broken down;
- removal of used hormones and cholesterol from the blood, and their excretion into the bile for removal from the body. Drugs, pesticides and other toxic food additives are also dealt with and excreted.

In this age of chemically-polluted air, water and food, the liver has to work much harder and is in constant need of nutritional support. It is an incredibly complex organ, which is capable of self-regeneration. A liver firing on all cylinders is central to our health, but most people subject their liver to unacceptable levels of toxins. The diet contributes, with its load of rich food, alcohol, high-chemical diet drinks, strong spices, heavy metal content (lead, aluminium and mercury), and the amazing load of chemicals used in processed and packaged foods found in supermarkets. Governments add all sorts of toxic chemicals to the water supply, and factories belch clouds of poisonous air for us to breathe. The liver has to deal with all of these in addition to other very important functions.

A sluggish liver will not register on blood tests – only more serious dysfunction shows up. However, moderately poor liver function can be so long-term, that in itself it becomes serious. For instance, it can no longer deal with bowel toxins and they travel freely in the bloodstream to all parts of the body. In this way, brain function may suffer, joints become congested and varicose veins develop, as well as a host of other serious organ malfunctions. Bowel toxins can even directly damage liver cells by initiating a free radical attack. This means that destructive forces are released within the liver cells, which set up chain reactions of damage. Where liver function is reduced, allergic complexes are not destroyed and illness affecting any part of the body may then occur. If the liver is too overworked to remove oestrogen from circulation at the proper time, P M T becomes a reality. All the tissue waste is taken away by the lymphatic system and bloodstream to the liver, and if this is poorly-detoxified the whole body becomes very sluggish. Blood sugar disturbances also occur when the liver is too tired to release stored glucose as needed, and an efficient liver is vital for removing cholesterol from the blood.

A diminished bile flow results from alcohol-induced fatty deposits, toxins from the bowel, drugs including the contraceptive pill and liver disease itself, such as hepatitis. Pregnancy also reduces bile flow and many pregnant women will notice red liver spots being deposited, in particular in the palms of their hands or on the arms. When bile flow diminishes, toxins remain in the liver, and if the enzyme systems are damaged the position is serious indeed. In aging, a liver under free radical attack deposits brown spots in the skin on the backs of the hands as well as elsewhere inside the body. The antioxidant vitamins and minerals protect against this. It is well to remember that outward signs are indications of internal problems.

Improved liver function depends on many factors and needs working on from several angles. A colon cleanse is of initial importance so as to prevent liver poisoning from reabsorbed toxins. A juice fast is very effective here and will at the same time cleanse every other part of the body as well as the liver. In addition, various supplements and herbs can be utilised to improve the liver function and protect it against damage.

Treatment Explained

• *Antioxidant vitamins and minerals* protect the liver against free radicals; *vitamins A, C, E* and *selenium* with co-factors iron, zinc, manganese and B vitamins.

• *Magnesium* is also an important element for most liver functions.

• *Lecithin*, ready-made in the food chain, is found mainly in egg yolks and soya beans. However, the body makes its own lecithin, given the necessary ingredients. This substance is vital to liver function, as it helps in the processing of fats and cholesterol as well as protecting every liver cell wall against damage. It is also believed to break down fibrous tissue which has formed as a result of scarring. In 1991 a 10-year study of beer drinkers was reported, indicating the enormous benefit of lecithin as protection against alcohol damage to the liver. The subjects were divided into two groups, and daily given several cans of beer each. Only one group took lecithin as well. At the end of eight years, the ones drinking beer only, had considerable liver scarring and two already had full-blown cirrhosis. Those taking lecithin with their beer developed only traces of scar-

ring. When the lecithin was removed from a few in this same group, cirrhosis developed within two years. This study was carried out on baboons – which is unacceptable to a growing number of people. However, it did highlight the protective properties of lecithin. This nutrient is made in the liver and intestinal walls, with the B vitamins choline, inositol, folic acid and vitamin B6, as well as the amino acid methionine. Essential polyunsaturated oils from nuts, seeds and oily fish are also required, but these oils must be unprocessed to be of any use.

• *Methionine*, a sulphur amino acid, is responsible for protecting the level of a compound amino acid called glutathione. This compound combines with toxic elements in the liver in order to neutralise them. Methionine is also responsible for inactivating oestrogen after ovulation. The dose is 500mg, twice daily, half an hour before food, with juice. Studies have indicated a 50% improvement in liver function tests within six days of starting treatment with methionine, and after three weeks these tests are often completely normal.

• *Carnitine* is the other important amino acid for liver function, as it increases fat-burning, and therefore reduces any fatty accumulation in the liver cells. Extra carnitine is always needed in high fat and alcohol diets. The dose is 500mg, twice daily, taken in the same way as methionine.

• *Dandelion* is a very valuable herb as a liver remedy, but it also has a lot of other uses, some of which are diuretic, anti-rheumatic and laxative. The nutrient content of dandelion is very high, as it contains vitamins A, B, C, D, the minerals potassium, calcium, sodium, silica and manganese as well as pectins, protein and insulin. The vitamin A content is even higher than that of carrots. Dandelion increases the flow of bile in the liver and through the gall bladder to the bowel, thus improving any liver congestion. It is used with very good effect in diseases such as hepatitis and gall-stones. The root is the best part to use, but young dandelion leaves daily in salad protect against hepatitis. The dose is 4g three times daily of the dried root.

• *Globe artichoke* is another herb which improves the flow of bile in the liver and to the gall bladder, but it also possesses liver-regenerating and protective properties. Both this herb and dandelion significantly reduce the synthesis of cholesterol by the liver, and increase the removal of this fat from the blood to the gall bladder for excretion. *Turmeric* has the same actions as globe artichoke.

• *Catechu black* is ten times more powerfully antioxidant to the liver than vitamin E. This herb also improves bile flow and has immune-enhancing properties. It is used very effectively in alcohol-induced liver disease, and will prevent damage to liver cells. The dose is 1g three times daily of the extract (catechin), for an acute or chronic liver disease.

• *Milk thistle* contains the most powerful liver antioxidant known. It stabilises liver cell walls, stimulates the production of new liver cells, prevents free radical damage and inhibits the production of inflammatory chemicals. Silymarin is the flavonoid extract of milk thistle herb, and it is this part which has the protective effect. The dose of silymarin is 50-150mg, three times daily.

• *Yellow dock* improves liver function and acts as a blood cleanser. It is used in the type of obstructive jaundice which is caused by liver congestion and this herb is often combined with dandelion. The dose is 2-4g three times daily of the dried root.

• Some other herbs which improve liver function very effectively are: blackroot, pulsatilla, balmony, golden seal, fringe tree bark, wahoo bark, boldo and butternut bark. Any of these can be made into a tea, and a cup

taken twice daily.

• *Coffee enemas* are very effective in causing the liver to dump its toxic load into the gall bladder. The recipe is three tablespoons of ground coffee added to two pints of water, simmered for three minutes and then left to stand for fifteen minutes before straining. 8oz (2dl) at body temperature is used at one time, and should be retained for fifteen minutes. It is a good idea to drink liver-cleansing juices for two days beforehand. The enema may be repeated several times a week until you are feeling better. Drinking coffee is harmful, but using it as an enema flushes the liver very quickly.

TREATMENT
Supplements of value
• An *antioxidant blend of vitamins A, C, E*, and *selenium*.
• *Silymarin* or *catechin*.
• *Dandelion* alone, or with other herbs.
• *L-methionine* – 1g twice daily.
• *L-carnitine* – 0.5g twice daily.
• *Lecithin* granules – 1 tablespoon twice daily.
• *Brewer's yeast* – 1 tablespoon twice daily.

Liver diet
• This should be high in fibre. Water soluble fibre foods like oatbran and ricebran, pectin and guar gum increase the flow of bile and cholesterol through the liver and gall bladder.
• Fruit and vegetables in abundance, and as much raw as possible, especially lemon, grapefruit, papaya, grapes, beetroot, endive, artichoke, cucumber, garlic, onion, radish and greens of all kinds.
• Sprouted grains, seeds and beans.
• A serving of seeds and walnuts daily on top of fruit at breakfast.
• Tahini (sesame seed paste) is high in methionine, calcium, protein and polyunsaturated oil. Use it in small amounts for flavouring.
• Wholegrain bread and pasta, muesli,

wheatgerm, cornmeal, millet and brown rice.
- Dried peas, beans and tofu for their high sterols and fibre.
- White fish and occasional oily fish like fresh salmon or sardines.
- Replace cow's milk with soya milk.
- Drink dandelion coffee, herbal tea, sugar-free fruit juice and mineral water.

Avoid
- All fats and oils for several weeks, except for the essential polyunsaturates in raw seeds and walnuts.
- Processed foods and chemical additives.
- Salt and spices.
- Sugar in any form, and refined bread or cereal.
- Alcohol, coffee, chocolate, and restrict tea to two cups daily.
- Meat, fowl and eggs for several weeks, as they are high in fat.
- All dairy products except very low-fat, live yoghurt.
- Nuts, except almonds and walnuts.
- Restrict dried fruit to use in muesli.
- Drugs including 'the pill' and aspirin.

Menu ideas
Breakfast
- Fresh fruit and low-fat plain yoghurt with chopped seeds and walnuts.
- Oatmeal porridge, raisins and soya milk.
- Sugar-free muesli and soya milk.
- Mushrooms or tomatoes on wholegrain toast.

Lunch
- Salad and sprouted seeds, or beans with any of the following: wholegrain pasta, buckwheat, hummus, tofu, millet burgers, brown rice salad, polenta, thick homemade vegetable soup with lentils or barley, bean casseroles, jacket potato, wholegrain bread with vegetable paté, lentil spread, Marmite or a fruit spread.

Dinner
- Lightly-cooked vegetables with any of the lunch choices. Fish may be served three times weekly and textured vegetable protein (TVP) twice.
- Follow vegetable protein combining on the days that no fish is eaten.

Dessert
- Fresh or stewed fruit – no sugar; grain puddings with soya milk, and sweetened only with chopped raisins or carob powder.

Drinks
- Juices as listed below. Start the day with lemon juice in hot water and drink a vegetable juice three times weekly.
- Herbal tea, dandelion coffee, rooibosch tea, mineral water, grain coffee.

Juices
- Lemon, grapefruit, papaya, grapes.
- Beetroot, green vegetables, radish.
- Fasting on juices for three days is very beneficial. Add a little honey to a daily lemon juice and mineral water.

III: *11. FEVER*

Naturopathy views fever as an expression of the body's self-healing mechanism, which must be managed and not suppressed. High temperature inhibits bacterial and viral growth and speeds the body's reaction for killing organisms and repairing tissue.

Fever begins when infecting organisms and the immune response cause the body's set point for temperature to be raised. The anterior hypothalamus in the brain controls many body activities, most of which are related to homeostasis (balance). One such function is heat-loss and heat-production. However, when an infection is present, the control mechanism is turned up and maintained until micro-organisms are eliminated.

Imagine that the thermometer was reset to 103°F (39.4°C). The autonomic nervous system responds by causing physical changes designed to raise the body's core temperature to the new setting. Firstly the pores of the skin as well as the blood vessel walls are constricted to keep heat in. Adrenalin production is increased, which in turn stimulates metabolism to speed heat-production. At the same time, the nervous system causes increased muscle tone, so that an involuntary stretch and contraction occurs in rapid succession. This induces shivering. So the cold skin and shivering, called a chill, is the body's method of raising its core temperature. When it reaches 103°F the chill goes, because no further heat increase is required. However, this temperature is maintained until the infection is destroyed. At this stage the heat-loss centre in the hypothalamus is activated to return the body temperature to normal. Heat is lost by relaxation of the muscle fibres in blood vessel

walls and dilation of the pores of the skin.

The fever, besides inhibiting toxins, also clears waste from the tissues, lymph and blood, on which bacteria feed and multiply. Iron is used up in retarding bacterial growth during fever, but the temperature needs to be very high to kill microbes. It is not the heat alone at work, rather that the raised temperature stimulates an increased immune response. Killer T-cells are increased, as are neutrophils and macrophages, which are the white blood cells responsible for destroying invaders. At the same time, tissue-repairers like fibroblasts and collagen are formed at an increased rate.

Sometimes the thermometer appears to be set too high, and only then do we intervene to lower the temperature to a reasonable level by natural means. Studies have shown that children receiving antibiotics treatment have fevers of longer duration that those on placebo, and considerably longer than those on herbal teas and bed rest alone. Putting out the flame prematurely reduces the response to an infection which is still present. Studies have also shown that infections requiring urgent treatment will respond to fever-reducing drugs faster than less serious diseases. This may induce a false sense of security, especially in the case of smouldering meningitis, because the fever is gone but the disease remains. So what is a safe level of fever? 103°F (39.4°C) is generally acceptable in adults, and at this level immune response is enhanced. However, in a child of six months or less, it is too high and must be reduced. The cause also needs immediate investigation. Infants cannot localise infections easily, and so infections are more likely to spread at this age and precipitate meningitis. Serious note must be taken of any localising signs or symptoms accompanying fever, such as a stiff neck or joints, and medical treatment should be sought immediately.

It is thought that the body has a built-in mechanism that limits fever to 106°F (41.1°C), which a healthy adult body can tolerate for several hours. Cells do not die off until 110°F (43.3°C) is reached. However, if a patient fasts on water alone, it is rare for a fever to go over 104°F (40°C). Individual safety margins must be assessed, because much has to do with a person's normal vitality levels.

In some diseases, such as cancer, fever is deliberately induced to raise core temperature and stimulate the immune system to destroy malignant cells. This destruction begins at 106°F (41.1°C).

Outline of fever management

• Assist the fever to natural completion so that it is resolved as quickly as possible.
• Intervene only if the temperature is over 101°F (38.3°C) in an infant, 103°F (39.4°C) in a child or 104°F (40°C) in an adult, or if there is some other health factor which contraindicates fever, such as pregnancy, heart disease or low vital energy.
• Never use aspirin, and only reach for paracetamol if the temperature stays too high for more than two hours in an infant, or six hours in a child, in spite of natural interventionist methods.
• Prevent dehydration.
• Strengthen the immune system in the long term.

General
• Bed rest, and keep the patient warm and free from draughts.
• No cold drinks, as the fever is to be encouraged. Lowering the core temperature with cold drinks means the body has to work harder to raise the temperature again.
• A warm mustard bath, hot drinks and a night's sleep will often ensure a quick resolution of a smouldering fever. After the bath, the patient must be tucked snugly into bed.
• Only intervene if the temperature goes too high.

TREATMENT
Diet
• No food, as digestion is reduced at a body heat of 100°F (37.8°C) and comes to a grinding halt at 103°F (39.4°C). Fasting on mineral water initially is best, and in fact most feverish patients choose to do this quite naturally. Drink a glass of water every hour.
• Diluted, sugar-free electrolyte drinks, alternated with water, are of value in preventing dehydration. Mineral water should contain potassium and magnesium as well as sodium.
• No sugar in any form, including fruit juice and honey, until the fever is reduced. Studies have shown that in the first 56 hours of a fever, one teaspoon of sugar will cause a 50% drop in phagocytosis (bacterial/viral destruction) within half an hour, and the effect lasts for five hours. Fruit sugar also has the same action.
• After 56 hours, introduce dilute fruit juice, although vegetable broths and dilute vegetable juice may also be given earlier if desired.
• Introduce a light diet as the appetite returns.

Supplements of value
Adult doses:
• *Vitamin C* – as powdered ascorbic acid (one teaspoon = 4g). Put one teaspoon in a glass of water and sip through a straw over a four hour period.
• *Celloids® IP* (see appendix 1) – 1 tablet, 1-2 hourly helps to control the fever, or use

the cell salt **Ferrum phos**, one tablet 1-2 hourly.
• **Echinacea** tincture – 1 teaspoon of this herb 2-4 hourly, or half a teaspoon powdered root.
• **Garlic** perles – 3 capsules three times daily.

To reduce fever
Only if too high.

Herbs
• **Elderflower** + **yarrow** + **peppermint**, as an infusion. One cup two-hourly if necessary.
• **Fresh ginger** + **prickly ash herb**, as a tea.
• The following herbs are from the berberis group and have a safe and much greater fever-reducing effect than the potentially-deadly aspirin: **mountain grape**, **barberry** or **golden seal** – make a tea with half a teaspoon to a cup, or buy tablets/capsules, as these herbs are very bitter.

Hydrotherapy
• Cold compresses to the head, and tepid sponging of the arms, chest and neck.
• An immersion bath is best. Run a bath which is a little cooler than the patient. Total immersion with even the back of the head in the water, if possible. A child must be held at all times so a third person needs to control the water. A feverish patient must never be left alone in a bath. Gradually add colder water so that the temperature is eventually lowered to about 83°F (28.3°C).
• Friction should be applied to the skin during bathing to increase the heat-loss from the body. Take the patient's temperature whilst in the bath, and stop treatment when it is almost down to a safe level. The body's core temperature will be 1°F (0.6°C) lower than the oral reading at the moment of recording.
• If shivering occurs, stop the treatment immediately and wrap up the patient warmly. Just as heat passes from a radiator into a room, so heat will radiate from the body into cooler water if immersion is total. The reason for a *gradual* reduction in water temperature is that if very cold water is used initially, the body may raise the core temperature in response to the suddenly-chilled skin.

Homeopathy
6c four hourly, or 30c 4-8 hourly.
• **Aconite** 6c – in the case of sudden onset of fever after exposure to cold. It starts in the middle of the night, usually with a dry cough, and often a swinging temperature. Dry skin, red, not sweaty, and person wants a lot of cold water. Worse in the evening.
• **Belladonna** 30c – sudden onset, throbbing head, fast pulse, burning hot, dry, no thirst, feet icy cold, red face, won't be held by mother. Sensitive to light, touch and pressure.
• **Apis** 30c – sudden onset but stays on a plateau. Skin red, dry/moist, no heavy sweat, frequent chills. Sleeps after fever. A shrill piercing scream. Very hard to please, worse in stuffy heat. Won't drink.
• **Arsenicum** 30c – excessively restless and agitated. Extreme prostration, out of proportion to the fever. Thirsty for sips only. Worse from midnight to 2am.
• **Baptisia** 30c – specific for enteric fever and typhus fever. Rapidly becomes gravely ill. Temperature irregular. Worse after 11am.
• **Bryonia** 30c – onset gradual, shivery. Irritable and wants to be left alone. Profuse perspiration. Sour sweats, pulse full, hard, tense and quick. Thirsty for large amounts of cold water. Won't move.
• **China** 30c – three-phase fever. Chills and shakes, great heat, profuse sweat, plus intense thirst.
• **Rhus Tox** 30c – extremely weak and very restless. Complains of pain and tosses and turns to change position and get comfortable. Sweating, but not on the face. Thirst for cold

milk or water.

• *Mercurius* 30c – flu type. Chills and burning heat. Profuse sweat which brings no relief. Worse in the night. Extreme thirst, foul breath, and sour perspiration.

• *Gelsemium* 30c – violent shivering, chills. Aching muscles, no thirst, headache and worse with least movement. Heavy eyelids.

• *Phosphorus* 6c – no thirst, but hungry and looks well in spite of fever. Bright eyes which occasionally water. May crave cold drinks and vomit soon after. Eyes may be anxious and watch doctor's every move carefully.

• *Ferrum Phos* 30c – onset gradual and not very high. Pale, tired but inclined to be red faced at times.

Febrile fits

These are greatly feared by parents, but there is no medical evidence that they cause brain damage. In fact studies indicate that neurological defects are no more common in those who have had fits than those who do not. They will however often recur in a susceptible child within the next year or two. The following homeopathic remedies may be given every minute for three doses if necessary, while you call your doctor. The symptoms given below precede a fit:

• *Aconite* 30c – fevers of sudden onset, cold and heat alternate, dry skin and red face, patient restless and anxious. This may be effective if given at the first sign of a fit.

• *Belladonna* 30c – violent fever of sudden onset, red faced, staring eyes and excited behaviour. Hot dry skin, great thirst.

• *Stramonium* 30c – red hot face, staring eyes, raging fever in spite of profuse perspiration. Delirium. The fever is not as high as for belladonna, but the functional excitement of the brain is more marked in this remedy.

• *Aethusa* 30c – fever and profuse sweat plus diarrhoea and vomiting.

III: *12. UPPER RESPIRATORY TRACT INFECTIONS*

Children with compromised immune systems may develop a syndrome whereby they suffer frequent attacks of fever, colds, coughs, bronchitis or ear infections. Medical practices are inundated with the very young and their frequent bouts of infection. Traditional treatment involves course after course of antibiotics, adenoidectomy, and in the case of ear infections, the surgical insertion of grommets to allow drainage of fluid from the middle ear.

Antibiotics, which are actually just pesticides, cause serious harm by disrupting the growth of the healthy gastro-intestinal micro-flora. These bacteria maintain the ecological balance in the bowel and have a profound controlling effect over the immune system, especially in the young. In fact it is becoming increasingly evident that acidophilus and bifido bacteria are essential for preventing allergies, infections, eczema and asthma in children. Destroy them and fungal overgrowth is encouraged, with the consequent effect of the bowel wall becoming permeable to incompletely-digested foods, bacteria, pesticides and other chemicals. It should not be forgotten that candida albicans (a fungus) leads to a serious debilitating condition *which is directly caused by traditional medical treatments* of other diseases.

Many children on antibiotics have to endure diarrhoea and the consequent loss of vital minerals like magnesium, potassium and zinc. Eventually the therapy simply makes the child feel more ill than he or she was before the treatment began. At this stage, surgical intervention is considered. However, research indicates that the adenoidectomy performed to relieve ear infection helps only a small percentage of children. The grommets which come next, frequently caused hardening of the eardrum. Why put in drains for fluid rather than determining the cause of the condition and then instigating preventative therapy? The many studies which have been reported, indicate that those being treated by antibiotics and/or grommets do no better than those who have neither treatments. In fact, clinical studies show that children not treated with antibiotics have fewer recurrences of infection. One study within medical practices showed that in 60% of all cases of otitis media, the child had already had his adenoids removed!

The whole upper respiratory syndrome responds very well to nutritional and allergy management with herbal, vitamin and mineral therapy to treat symptoms initially.

TREATMENT

- Food allergy tests (see chapter III:2 on Allergy).
- Correct the diet and give supplement nutrients where applicable, to restore the immune system to health.
- Treat acute symptoms with natural products.

Diet
- Follow a four-day rotation diet if several allergies are present.
- Eat a diet of natural wholefoods, and not easy-packaged things from supermarkets. The naturopathic diet should form the basis of the regime.

- Abundant fruit and vegetables.
- Oily fish, three times weekly.
- Natural nuts and seeds, especially walnuts, sun flower, sesame and pumpkin seeds, daily – grind to a powder for young children, and sprinkle on breakfast cereals.
- Dried peas, beans and lentils added to tasty sauces and soups.
- Grains such as brown rice, corn meal, spelt, quinoa and millet. Buy some vegetarian cook-books and learn to cook dishes which children enjoy.
- Sprouted products greatly enhance children's immunity.
- Home-baking, using a little butter rather than margarine or vegetable shortening – and use carob in place of chocolate. Make biscuits, cakes and pancakes from wholegrain flour, and exchange sugar with molasses, maple syrup or honey. Any frying should be done with only a little virgin olive oil or coconut oil.

Avoid
- All your food allergens.
- White flour and sugar products.
- Processed food which involve oils or fats.
- All processed pretty-packaged cereals – use soaked muesli or porridge instead, and add dried fruit to sweeten.

Limit
- Animal fats and dairy products.
- Gluten grains, such as wheat, oats, barley and rye, as they sensitise the air passages.

Any specific indications will be listed under individual sub-headings.

Immune system repair
- Béres Drops Plus work like magic in restoring proper immune function in those with frequent upper respiratory tract infections. T-cell ratios are returned to normal very quickly.

- Bifido bacteria supplements for infants, and children should also be given L acidophilus.
- A multi-vitamin/mineral supplement, or higher doses of individual immune stimulants (see chapter III:1 on the immune system). In those who are prone to colds, daily vitamin A and C, zinc and garlic are very protective.
- Avoid anything which damages the immune system – stress, drugs and a poor diet.
- Exercise regularly, as this removes stress hormones that depress the thymus gland.
- Avoid getting chilled, as this also reduces immunity.

III: *13. SORE THROAT*

Streptococcal infection accounts for 10% of sore throats, and is a self-limiting disease, although usually much more painful than a viral infection. Almost all cases respond very well to herbal and nutritional treatment. Most sore throats are viral in origin; again the condition responds really well to natural treatment. Sore throats remaining in spite of treatment, and those which do not become colds, almost always have an allergic background which must be evaluated.

TREATMENTS

Diet

• Eliminate all sugar sources including honey, fruit juices, dried fruit, molasses, maple syrup etc. After 56 hours dilute fruit juice may be introduced, but in the early stages any form of sugar reduces immune function.
• Increase fluids to one glass hourly if possible. Drink herbal teas, water or vegetable juices.
• Avoid all other food initially, but add vegetable and fruit when improvement begins, and then move on to the diet for upper respiratory tract infections.

Supplements of value

Adult doses:
• *Celloids® PCIP* (see appendix 1) – 1 tablet two-hourly.
• *Vitamin C* – 1g 1-2 hourly to bowel-tolerance. Beyond this, some diarrhoea will occur. Cut back only to the level where this stops. In some infections, huge doses of vitamin C can be taken without ever reaching bowel-tolerance.
• *Vitamin A* – 25,000iu daily for one week, and then reduce to 10,000iu until well.

5,000iu daily is a maintenance dose. This vitamin protects the health of the mucous membrane so that microbes can't breed. For long-term use, it should be taken in the form of beta carotene.
• *Zinc* – 25mg daily as citrate or picolinate.
• *Garlic* – 3 perles three times daily (nature's antibiotic).
• *Propolis* – 500mg three times daily (bee-antibiotic).
• *Quercetin* – 400mg three times daily inhibits replication of respiratory viruses.

Herbal teas

• *Yarrow + elderflower* – 1 teaspoon of each to a cup of boiling water.
• *Boneset* – 1 teaspoon to one cup of water.
• *Ginger* – use the fresh root to make a tea.

Choose from these to induce sweating if high fever is present.

Herbs

Adult doses:
• *Echinacea* – 1g three times daily.
• *Golden seal* – 0.5-1g dried herb three times daily.

These two are specific against streptococcal or staphylococcal infections, as well as being anti-viral. The echinacea inhibits the replication of the bacteria and therefore the spread of infection, and the golden seal destroys them. Both enhance immune function.

Gargle

• *Golden seal*, *myrrh* or *echinacea* tincture or tea are effective gargles – see appendix 2.
• 5 drops of homeopathic *hypericum* + five drops of *calendula* in half a pint of water is also an effective gargle.

Homeopathy
With the following, *dose 30c 4-6 hourly, for 2-3 days if necessary.*

• *Aconite* – burning, smarting, tingling, red throat. Sudden onset. Fever.

• *Apis* – burning, red swollen throat and uvula (the fleshy extension of the palate, hanging above the throat).

• *Baryta Carb* – develops slowly. Recurrent tonsillitis. Lymph nodes in neck swollen. Feels as if there is a lump in the throat.

• *Belladonna* – burns like fire, bright red colour, red-hot face, dilated pupils, no thirst.

• *Causticum* – sore, raw, constricted feeling and must keep swallowing. Hoarseness relieved by expelling mucous.

• *Gelsemium* – swallowing is very painful. Bad taste in the mouth. Hot and cold chills. Person is weak and shaky.

• *Mercurius* – deep redness of whole tonsil area. Bad breath and glands swollen.

• *Phytolacca* – dark red and congested, glands swollen, sensation of red-hot ball in the throat. Swallowing causes shooting pain into the ears.

General
• Bed rest and sleep.
• Avoid getting chilled.

In my experience, a mix of Celloids® PCIP, vitamin C, garlic and herbs will quickly bring relief. Propolis in place of herbs is very useful for some. Homeopathy correctly matched is equally effective.

At the first sign of a developing upper respiratory infection, it can often be aborted as follows:

• To a mug of hot water add a squeeze of lemon juice, 1oz of grated ginger root, a cinnamon stick and a good pinch of cayenne pepper.

• With this drink, take several grams of vitamin C, garlic capsules, 25,000iu of vitamin A and 25mg of zinc.

• Add two tablespoons of dry mustard powder to a hot bath and soak in it for ten minutes and finally tuck yourself up in bed with extra blankets and sweat out the infection.

III: *14. COLDS*

Should a sore throat or that initial flu-like feeling not be arrested in the early stage and a full-blown cold develops, then homeopathic remedies may well change according to altered symptoms, but other treatment remains similar. If colds occur more than two-to-three times a year, take steps to strengthen the immune system by removing allergic foods and taking supplements.

TREATMENTS

Diet
• Follow sore throat guidelines in chapter III:13.
• Do not eat if feeling unwell or if fever is present.

Supplements of value
• Continue the *vitamin C*, *vitamin A*, *zinc*, *garlic* and *echinacea*, as outlined in chapter III:13.
• *Celloids*® *PCIP* and *Celloids*® *PSMP* (see appendix 1) – 1 of each two hourly. Children two years and under, take half dose.

These minerals or their tissue salt equivalents are anti-bacterial and anti-viral, but their great value is in removing and preventing catarrhal formation upon which bacteria and viruses can feed and multiply. With mucous removed, organisms cannot breed, and so they are destroyed. Reduce the frequency of dosage as symptoms improve.

Homeopathy
There are dozens of remedies for colds. Here is a selection. *The dosage is 6c 4-hourly if necessary.*
• *Aconite* – feverish, frequent sneezing and a clear hot drip from the nose. Thirst, colds coming on suddenly from exposure to cold winds or drafts, worse in stuffy conditions.
• *Gelsemium* – flu type with chills and fever alternating. Watery discharge which hurts the nose. Headache and heavy-lidded. Tearing, tickling cough. Better near the fire.
• *Arsenicum* – frequent sneezes, painful thin watery discharge which burns. The nose is stuffed, and sneezes don't relieve it. Better with heat and hot drinks.
• *Allium Cepa* – paroxysms of sneezing and streaming nose, burning discharge, nose and lips raw. Left nostril more blocked than the right. Worse in a warm room.
• *Belladonna* – violent onset after exposure, red face, hot skin, restless. Full pulse, cold extremities, raw throat, thirst, headache. Alternate with aconite if caused by a chill.
• *Nat Mur* – the cold begins with frequent sneezing, an egg-white discharge for 1-3 days, and then the nose is blocked. No fever, but smell and taste are lost.
• *Pulsatilla* – thick yellow mucous which is bland. Patient needs comfort. Pains in the face and nose. Better in the open air.
• *Euphrasia* – streaming eyes and nose.
• *Hepar Sulph* – lots of sneezing, which is watery but becomes thick yellow and offensive. The nose is painful and swollen. Sweaty, rattling breath and worse for the least draught.
• *Bryonia* – slow to develop, lots of sneezing, eyes red and watery, lips and mouth dry, thirsty. Dry stuffy nose. Person is irritable and hates to be moved.
• *Nux Vomica* – sniffles, drips in the day, stuffy at night and outside. Lots of sneezing,

Patient feels hot and cold, and the nose is alternately blocked and running. Patient is extremely irritable. When the nose runs it pours.

Remember that the body is eliminating toxins. Do not suppress the process with drugs.

III: *15. COUGHS AFTER COLDS*

This is a situation where the body is expelling mucous, and treatment is aimed at assisting the process as well as inhibiting further excessive production.

TREATMENT

Supplements of value
• Continue *vitamin A* and *vitamin C*, *zinc* and *garlic* but in reduced doses.
• *Celloids® PCIP* (see appendix 1) – 1 tablet two hourly if mucous is clear or white. *Celloids® PSMP* – 1 tablet two hourly if mucous is yellow, or use both together two hourly.

Herbs
• A hot lemon, honey and ginger drink.
• *Elecampane + horehound + pleurisy root + yarrow* – make a tea using equal weights and drink one cup three times daily. This recipe is bactericidal, expectorant, soothing and healing as well as fever-reducing.
• Mrs M Grieve gives a very pleasant drink as follows: one teaspoon *flaxseeds* + 1oz *licorice root* + quarter pound of *raisins* + two quarts of water. Boil until reduced by half and add lemon to taste. Drink 8oz at bedtime.

Homeopathy
Dose 30c, 4-hourly for 2-3 days.
• *Aconite* – constant short dry cough. Dry hard ringing cough. Sudden onset from cold exposure.
• *Ant Tart* – rattling, excessive sticky phlegm and a suffocating sensation.
• *Arsenicum* – wheeze, frothy phlegm, can't breathe. Restless, anxious, weak and ex-hausted. Worse midnight to 2am.
• *Bryonia* – for acute bronchitis. Hard dry spasmodic cough, difficulty in breathing, tough mucous. Patient has a sore chest and must hold it while coughing. Bursting headache, must sit up. Peevish and wants to be alone.
• *Causticum* – hard cough which racks the body. Cannot expectorate (cough up phlegm), excessive mucous.
• *Drosera* – tickly in the throat, leads to a coughing fit and retching. Pain below the ribs. Worse at night. This is a good whooping cough remedy.
• *Hepar Sulph* – a choking cough, loose rattling, yellow mucous. Patient is chilly, sweaty and wants hot drinks. Better in warm moist weather. This is a good croup remedy.
• *Ipecac* – spasmodic, rattling, wheezing. Person may go blue and stiff during cough bouts. Nausea which is not improved by vomiting.
• *Phosphorus* – dry hard tickling cough, racks the body and is exhausting. Coughing causes a bursting headache. Worse in temperature changes, laughing, talking, eating, cold drinks, vomiting and lying down.
• *Pulsatilla* – dry persistent cough which is worse when taking a breath. Stuffy feeling. Patient is tearful and intolerant of heat. Better in open air.
• *Spongia* – noisy, rasping, no wheeze or rattle. Wakes choking with a violent cough. Patient is anxious and worse talking, swallowing or when the head is low. Better with hot drinks. This is also a croup remedy.

III: *16. ACUTE BRONCHITIS*

This is normally a complication of colds, but in some it occurs frequently with no other upper respiratory infection. In the latter situation, food allergy is heavily implicated.

Bronchitis is more likely to occur at changes of season and in cold damp weather. It may begin as an acute tracheitis, with a dry and painful cough, but soon after, infection spreads to the bronchi. Once there, a wheeze or breathing difficulty occurs before the infection precipitates a sticky mucous, which quickly becomes profuse and yellow as secondary bacterial infection occurs. A slight fever is usually present.

Treatment is designed to clear and prevent mucous production, heal the mucous membrane and remove the infecting organisms.

TREATMENT

Diet
- Eliminate all sugar sources, including fruit juice and honey, until the fever subsides, although diluted fruit juice may be introduced after about 56 hours.
- Drink a glass of fluid every hour in the form of water, freshly pressed vegetable juice, vegetable broth or herbal teas.
- If fever is present, you may use the herbs discussed in chapter III:11.
- Initially, eat only if hungry, and concentrate on alkaline-producing foods – fruit and vegetables, millet and soya products like tofu.

Supplements of value
Adult doses:
- *Celloids® PCIP* and *Celloids® PSMP* – 1 tablet of each two-hourly.
- *Garlic* perles – 3 capsules three times daily.

- *Vitamin C* – 500mg 1-2 hourly, to bowel-tolerance.
- *Vitamin A* – 25,000iu daily.
- *Zinc* – 25mg daily as citrate or picolinate.

Herbs
- *Thyme + grindelia + marshmallow + eucalyptus + cowslip* – make a tea of two parts of thyme and grindelia to one part each of the remaining herbs. Drink one cup three times daily.

Homeopathy
Dose 6c-30c, 2-4 hourly for a few days.
- *Bryonia* – hard dry spasmodic cough. Difficult quick respiration. Sore chest, tough mucous. Bursting headache. Chest pain, relieved by holding the chest, must sit up.
- *Arsenicum* – wheeze, frothy phlegm and can't breathe easily. Restless, anxious and weak. Worse midnight to 2am.
- *Ant Tart* – for the rattly phlegm stage. Difficulty coughing up.
- *Ipecac* – coughing spasms, rattling, wheezing. Nausea not improved by vomiting.

Change the remedy as symptoms alter.

III: *17. SINUSITIS*

A condition whereby the linings of sinuses become inflamed because of a spreading cold or an allergic reaction, causing a release of histamine. Excessive mucous is then produced, which blocks the narrow sinus cavities and causes pain. A secondary bacterial infection will change the mucous to a thick yellow colour. If the frontal sinuses are affected, the headache may be quite severe. Where the blockage is chronic and not necessarily associated with a cold, food allergy is probable, and if colds are a frequent occurrence, then the sinusitis following on will also have an allergic background.

TREATMENT

Diet
• Avoid common allergens such as dairy products, wheat, eggs, citrus and soya products, if specific allergens are unknown.
• Avoid all processed, refined and junk foods.
• Eat plenty of fruit and vegetables and drink a lot of fluids in the form of mineral water, herbal tea and vegetable juices.

Supplements of value
Adult doses:
• *Celloids® PSMP* and *Celloids® S79* (silicea – see appendix 1) – 1 tablet of each two-hourly, drains the sinuses.
• *Vitamin A* – 50,000iu daily for a week, and then reduce to 25,000iu until improvement is clear. Beta carotene is preferable on a long term basis.
• *Vitamin C* – 1g, 2-hourly, to bowel-tolerance.
• *Zinc* – 25mg daily as citrate.

• *Garlic* – 3 perles three times daily.
• *Propolis* – 500mg three times daily.

Herbs
Adult doses:
• *Echinacea* + *golden seal* – half a teaspoon of each to a cup three times daily as a tea, and douche the nasal passages as well.
• *Eucalyptus* inhalations – a few drops of essential oil in boiling water.
• Sniffing up *salt water* also clears the sinuses.

Homeopathy
Dosage as below, and take two-hourly if necessary.
• *Kali Bich* 6c – clear stringy mucous and a feeling of congestion.
• *Belladonna* 30c – sudden onset, flushed face, temperature raised. Worse lying down, severe headache over the eyes.
• *Hepar Sulph* 6c – yellow catarrh which is offensive, nose feels swollen and painful. Worse with the least draught. Patient is irritable and chilly.
• *Pulsatilla* 6c – yellow catarrh, frontal headache. Worse in the evening and craves fresh air.
• *Silicea* 6c – when the pain feels as though it is in the bones surrounding the sinuses.

III: *18. INFLUENZA*

An infection caused by an ever-changing variety of viral strains. The condition is characterised by fever, headache, aches and pains and sometimes sore throat or chest pains.

TREATMENT
Complete bed rest and as much sleep as possible. A mustard bath, a hot drink and sleep may abort the 'flu, if caught early enough. Put two large tablespoons of dry mustard in a hot bath and soak in it before wrapping up warmly and going to bed.

Diet
- No food.
- Hourly drinks of 8oz of mineral water, herbal tea or vegetable broth/juice. Alternate these drinks. A loss of minerals contributes to the aches and pains of flu.
- Eliminate all sources of sugar, including honey and fruit juice for fifty six hours and then reintroduce in dilute form.

Supplements of value
- *Vitamin C* – 1g hourly to bowel-tolerance. Add ascorbic acid powder to a glass and sip frequently through a straw. One teaspoon equals 4g vitamin C.
- *Celloids® PCIP* and *Celloids® PSMP* (see appendix 1) – 1 tablet of each, two-hourly.
- *Garlic* perles – 3 capsules three times daily for adults.
- *Quercetin* – 400mg three times daily inhibits respiratory viruses.

Herbs
Adult doses:
- *Echinacea*, 1g of dried root, three times

daily. In the winter it pays to have a tincture made up and stored in the fridge. Take one teaspoon 2-4 hourly.

Herbs for fever
- *Peppermint* + *yarrow* + *elderflower*, as a tea.
- *Peppermint* + *yarrow* + *pleurisy root*, as a tea.
- Fresh *ginger* tea.

Homeopathy
Adult doses:
- *Oscillococcinum* 30c – every 2-3 weeks during the winter, as prevention.
- *Influenzum Co* 30c – 4-hourly, may arrest the flu if started quickly.
- *Bacillinum* 30c – every 2-3 weeks, is often an effective prevention for those prone to upper respiratory tract infection.
- *Gelsemium* 30c – 2-4 hourly, for slow-developing flu, shivering then hot, aching all over, heavy-lidded, muscle weakness, occipital headaches.
- *Bryonia* 30c – 2-4 hourly, everything feels dry, very thirsty at intervals, hard cough, splitting headache. Patient is very irritable and wants to be left alone, lies still and is pale. Onset is slow. This remedy may be alternated with gelsemium.
- *Arsenicum* 30c – 2-4 hourly, severe chills and exhaustion. Thirsty for sips only. This remedy may be alternated with gelsemium.
- *Pyrogenium* 30c – temperature goes up and down, bed feels hard, weak rapid pulse, aches all over, chills.
- *Belladonna* 30c – sudden onset, high temperature, flushed face, excited behaviour.

III: *19. CHRONIC OTITIS MEDIA*

Glue ear develops after a child has had several bouts of ear infections, which may or may not cause pain and fever. The condition is characterised by a build-up of fluid in the middle ear and a painless hearing loss.

In most cases, abnormal function of the eustachian tube is the underlying factor. The job of this tube, connecting the naso-pharynx and the middle ear, is to regulate the air pressure in the middle ear and clear secretions from it. In otitis media, the tube becomes obstructed, fluids remain and may become colonised by bacteria. However, the underlying cause of eustachian tube obstruction is usually allergy to food and chemicals, so if we are to cure the condition, treatment begins with food allergy tests.

Allergy

Most studies done in the past few years indicate that approximately 90% of glue ear patients have food allergies. Treatment involving avoidance of the offending allergens, plus nutritional support, results in a 92% success rate. No antibiotics or surgical intervention are normally necessary. The alarming increase in cases of otitis media in the past few years parallels the rise in the incidence of allergy in the population. Allergic reactions to a food may be occurring because the immune system is mistakenly recognising it as foreign.

On the other hand the immune reaction may be caused by a permeable intestine, leaking large protein molecules into the blood. The immune system will automatically recognise those as foreign, because protein should be reduced to individual amino acid components before absorption occurs. This leaky gut syndrome arises because antibiotic treatment destroys the essential healthy bowel micro-flora, and allows candida albicans (a fungus in the colon) to flourish and put down roots into the intestinal wall. So you can see that by using drugs to treat the infection, you just exacerbate the original allergic reaction and increase the incidence of ear infections.

The most common allergens are dairy products and gluten grains, although there are usually other foods involved as well. Gluten has been shown to initiate hypersensitivity of upper respiratory tract tissues, and casein in milk causes allergic complexes to collect in the upper respiratory tract. If these foods were not introduced into a child's diet until the age of one year it would prevent a lot of health problems.

Inflammatory chemical mediation

See the quick reference chart in chapter II:6 on Fats and Oils.

Studies have indicated that 75% of children with otitis media have no bacteria in their middle ear secretions. The inflammation and fluid are a result of an excessive release in the body of inflammatory chemicals such as histamine, leukotrienes and prostaglandin E2 (PGE2). An allergic reaction results in the release of histamine, but the reason for the excess of leukotrienes and PGE2 is quite simply an imbalance in the fatty acid components of the diet – between animal and seed sources of fats. There are several reasons for the imbalance. One is a glut of processed oil present in the diet. This elbows out the essential oils from walnuts, seeds and oily fish. The result is that anti-inflammatory hormones (PGE1 and E3) cannot be formed from these natural oils.

Processed fatty acids are found in vegetable shortening, margarine, oils that are not genuinely cold-pressed, mayonnaises, dressings, hydrogenated peanut butter and anything fried in these oils, such as crisps, nuts and other snacks. They are also found in most commercial biscuits and cakes. In fact the list is endless, and modern people eat an enormous amount.

The second reason for the imbalance is that once the good guys are pushed aside, inflammatory chemicals (originating from meat and dairy products) are produced in excessive amounts, because the controls are not present. These are PGE2 and leukotrienes, amongst others.

Thirdly, we simply don't eat enough foods containing the essential omega −3 and −6 oils in natural form. These are found in oily fish, flaxseeds, walnuts, pumpkin, sesame seeds and soya beans. Put differently, there is too much in the way of meat and dairy products, sugar, food made from white flour and processed oils and fats. Concurrently there is too little in the way of oily fish, raw nuts and seeds in the daily diet. The result of this, plus histamine from the allergic reaction, causes ear infections.

Where foods containing natural oil form a proper part of the diet, inflammatory chemicals are blocked, and putting fish in the diet automatically reduces meat content as well. In terms of food choices, a simple method of addressing this imbalance is to avoid processed oils and everything made from them, avoid most white flour and sugar, limit meat and dairy foods, eat small amounts of nuts and seeds daily and use oily fish three times weekly. Sweeteners can be found in molasses, honey, maple syrup and dried fruit. Never

cook with a polyunsaturated oil such as walnut, canola, flaxseed or sunflower, as heat damages them easily. Use a little coconut oil or a monounsaturated oil (virgin olive) instead and keep the heat low.

Breast-feeding is very important, in that it has a prophylactic effect. Recurrent otitis media is much more prevalent in children who are put onto bottle-feeding too soon. Breast milk contains high levels of GLA, which is the substance found pre-formed in evening primrose oil, and as you can see from the chart in chapter II:6, it leads to the formation of PGE1, the powerful anti-inflammatory tissue hormone which also has a beneficial effect on the immune system. GLA is not present in milk formulas or cow's milk. Breast milk is a source of bifido bacteria, if the mother's diet consists of organic foods and mineral water. These organisms also control immune function and help prevent allergies.

Nutritional deficiencies

Low levels of vitamin A and zinc predispose children to upper respiratory tract infections, and once they have an infection, it in turn further depletes those nutrients, as well as vitamin C. Other mediators of immune response which are of value here are vitamin E and the mineral selenium. It is interesting to note that children exposed to tobacco smoke have a four-fold increased risk of otitis media – this may well be due to the smoke using up their supply of antioxidants such as vitamins A, C, and E and the minerals selenium and zinc.

TREATMENT

Food allergy testing is essential, and then total avoidance of the food for as long as necessary.

Follow the dietary recommendations for frequent upper respiratory tract infections (chapter III:12).

Supplements of value

Children's doses:

• *Beta carotene* – 4mg-15mg daily depending on age. High doses only for short periods and under qualified supervision.

• *Vitamin C* – 500mg x age in divided doses daily – *ie* two years old = 1,000mg daily (250mg four times daily).

• *Bioflavonoids* – separately or with vitamin C. 50mg x age daily.

• *Zinc* – 2.5mg x age daily (maximum 15mg).

• *Evening primrose oil* – 500mg x age daily.

• Cold-pressed *linseed oil* – 1-3 teaspoons daily.

• *Béres Drops Plus* – for restoring immune system function. Take these for 2-3 months.

• *Bifido bacteria* for infants. This as well as *L acidophilus* for children.

Homeopathy

• *Mercurius Dulc* – for blocked eustachian tubes, especially in very pale children. 30c *weekly or monthly*, depending on symptom improvement.

• *Kali Mur* – chronic catarrh in the middle ear with some deafness, cracking, snapping noises in the ear on swallowing or nose-blowing. Nasal catarrh which is white, and a tendency to swollen glands. Dose as above in chronic conditions.

III: *20. ACUTE OTITIS MEDIA*

This may occur as a result of an acute flare-up of a chronic condition, or follow on from colds, sore throats or tonsillitis. Treatment involves rest, treating symptoms by natural means and manipulating the diet.

TREATMENT

Diet
In an acute attack with fever, restrict the diet to fluids only. These should be herbal teas, mineral water, vegetable broths or vegetable juices. Fruit juices, honey and all sugar sources are to be avoided in the first 56 hours of a fever, as they inhibit the immune system's ability to fight infection. In a less acute attack, just increase fluids and give fruits and vegetables primarily. Avoid all dairy products and gluten grains (wheat, oats, barley and rye).

Try to keep the child warm in bed and getting plenty of sleep.

Supplements of value
Children's dose:
- *Vitamin C* – to bowel-tolerance. Try 100mg x age hourly. A two year-old will take 200mg hourly. Put a morning's dose of powdered ascorbic acid in a glass of water and allow the child frequent sips through a straw.
- *Bioflavonoids* – 50mg x age daily, to unblock the airways.
- *Celloids*® *PCIP* and *Celloids*® *PSMP* (see Appendix 1) – 1 tablet of each two-hourly until pain subsides, and then three times daily for a few days. Half dose for children under 2 years.

Herbs
Adult doses: See appendix 2 for calculating the dose for children.
- *Echinacea* – 1 teaspoon of tincture 2-4 hourly.
- *Golden seal* – 0.5-1g dried root three times daily.

These are fairly unpalatable herbs, and are better taken in tincture or tablet form. The herbs fight any infection and strengthen immune response.

Herbal ear drops
Any one of these will reduce inflammation quickly.
- *Golden seal*, *pulsatilla* or *plantain* tincture – 2-3 drops, three times daily.
- *Mullein* oil – 2-3 drops three times daily.

Homeopathy
Half-hourly if necessary, for 6-10 doses.
- *Aconite* 30c – sudden onset, and after exposure to cold. Patient very restless and anxious.
- *Belladonna* 30c – violent symptoms of high temperature, flushed hot skin, dilated pupils and very excitable, no thirst.
- *Chamomilla* 30c – snappy, irritable and wants carrying. One cheek red sometimes.
- *Myristica* 30c – for middle ear pus formation, this acts better than hepar sulph or silicea.
- *Pulsatilla* 30c – a pressure pain behind the ear drum, as though it is being forced outwards. A full-stuffed feeling, redness and swelling, worse in warmth and the evening. Child is weepy and clinging.

After an acute attack, follow the regime for the chronic condition and repair the immune system function with diet and nutritional supplements.

In my experience a mixture of dietary control, vitamin C, bioflavonoids, herbal tinctures orally, ear drops and Celloid minerals (or tissue salts) will cure even a severe attack. Homeopathy is also very effective, but using the correct remedy is vital – the symptoms must be closely matched.

III: *21. ECZEMA (Atopic Dermatitis)*

This is a very common condition which often begins before the age of two years in children. The prime cause is food allergy. A child who is born with a tendency towards allergy can become sensitised to any number of foods through breast milk. For the infant who is not breast-fed, the situation is very complicated if he or she becomes allergic to cow's milk at an early stage. Breast feeding is important to an infant for many reasons, and any dietary changes can easily be made through the mother's food-intake. That is, any food to which the child is allergic can be removed from the mother's diet until he or she is weaned.

Skin abnormalities, such as dryness or a tendency to thickening when scratched, may predispose a child to eczema. Some people have skin which feels itchy with the least irritation and others have a tendency towards heavy bacterial levels. The latter indicates poor immune function.

Stress leads to eczema outbreaks in susceptible people, but this is largely due to the fact that it weakens the immune system, which then ceases to adapt to an allergen that has probably long been present. Certainly a sudden severe stressful situation or an accumulation of constant moderate stress will often trigger the start of eczema, and at this stage it becomes necessary to find the offending food causing the underlying problem.

Fats versus oils

In atopic eczema, a common problem is the imbalance of fatty acids in the body. This imbalance is identical to that found in asthma and all upper respiratory tract infections.

Some fatty acids lead to the production of inflammatory chemicals (PGE2 and leukotrienes), and some make controlling anti-inflammatory chemicals (PGE1 and PGE3). (In the very comprehensive chapter II:6 on this subject, prostaglandins are clearly explained in 'lay' terms).

Where the diet contains adequate levels of oily fish, raw walnuts, flaxseeds, sunflower and pumpkin seeds and soya products, they form the anti-inflammatory chemicals which block the troublemakers that are made from meat and dairy products. Do remember that besides reducing animal protein in the diet, it is vital to avoid using oils in processed form, because they will rudely trample over the natural oils in nuts, seeds and genuine cold-pressed oil. This means that these important oils will be unable to function in the body.

EPA is a supplement made from oily fish, and evening primrose oil is a supplement made from seeds. Both of these are ready-made precursors of the two essential anti-inflammatory prostaglandins, E1 and E3. Both of these should be taken by eczema sufferers until the skin improves and the diet has been adjusted.

Nutritional deficiencies

Vitamins and minerals involved in immune system function are often deficient in people suffering from eczema. Children in particular are frequently low in zinc, vitamins A, C, E and the Bs, calcium and magnesium. The body's production of anti-inflammatory prostaglandins E1 and E3 requires not only the natural oils, but a range of nutrients like zinc, magnesium, B and C vitamins. In some patients it is a deficiency of some of these nutrients that causes the lack of anti-inflammatory fatty acids, rather than a lack of the oils themselves.

A quality natural multivitamin/mineral product may be enough for mild cases of eczema. It is important to buy natural products from health food stores, as the drug companies make synthetic vitamins which are of little value in human nutrition. Our cells are intelligent and recognise the difference.

Allergy

In eczema there is an excessive release of histamine, another inflammatory chemical, but this is reduced by avoiding food allergens. Some flavonoids prevent histamine release from cells. Quercetin has been found to be the most effective, but the following herbs and berries contain very powerful flavonoids as well: rue, blackthorn, hawthorn and blueberry.

Research has shown that all children with food allergies have low levels of the healthy acidophilus and bifido bacteria, with a parallel overgrowth of harmful bacteria in the intestinal tract. Where such toxic bowel conditions exist, as a result of poor diet or the taking of drugs, the antibodies (IgA) lining the gut are reduced, and this means that allergic complexes form more easily. Low IgA levels are often found in eczema patients, and these days it, as well as bifido bacteria, tends to be absent from mother's milk. The IgA and bifida in breast milk are there to protect the infant against developing allergies, and she needs the IgA until her own immune system develops. Processed foods, pesticides, fertilisers and chemicals in meat are destroying both bifida and IgA in mother's milk.

TREATMENT
- Food allergy test.

- Correct the diet.
- Strengthen the immune system.
- Inhibit inflammatory chemicals.
- Deal with the itch, to prevent secondary infection from scratching.

Diet
- 80% fruit, vegetables and freshly-pressed juices. Half of this should be raw. Include plenty of onions and garlic. Other foods are treated as side-dishes to the main serving of fruit or vegetables at every meal.
- Grains should be unprocessed – brown rice, yellow corn meal, millet, wheat, oats, barley and rye. This means wholegrain bread, pasta and cereals. The latter can be porridge or soaked muesli. Infants should be given flaked millet or brown rice.
- Low animal protein, but twice a week eat cold-water fish such as fresh salmon, trout, cod or even canned sardines and mackerel for the EPA content. Good quality calcium is found in green vegetables and oily fish. Children who are breast-fed, until they are old enough to eat adequate quantities of these, have no need of cows' milk for calcium.
- Genuine cold-pressed oils – flaxseed, sunflower, walnut etc. Use these for dressings only as heat damages polyunsaturates.
- Organic honey.
- Pulses – a variety of soya and other dried peas, beans and lentils, 2-3 times weekly. Add them to soups, casseroles and salads.
- Pumpkin, sesame and sunflower seeds, or walnuts, daily.
- Follow the vegetable protein-combining guidelines on the days when you are not eating fish, in order to get adequate complete protein.

When the eczema is better, try reintroducing allergens, but on a strict four-day rotation programme only.

Avoid
- Foods to which you are allergic.
- All processed and refined foods in cans and packets.
- Meat, eggs and dairy products should be eaten in very small amounts only, in order to reduce inflammatory chemicals.
- Tea, coffee, alcohol and chocolate. Margarine and oils that are not genuinely cold-pressed. Reduce saturated fats to a minimum.
- Cosmetics, harsh soap and shampoo.
- Stress, and get adequate rest and exercise.

Juices
- Carrot, celery, spinach, beetroot and cucumber.
- Blackcurrant, blueberries and grapes.

Skin care
- Use oatmeal-filled bags to wash, or detergent- free soap.
- Do not use products containing mineral oil.
- Make a herbal calendula cream.
- Cold-pressed aloe vera gel is soothing and healing.

For the itch
- Make a herbal cream from *chickweed* or dried *stinging nettles*.
- *Zinc oxide* cream.
- *Epsom salt* wash, or use a corn-starch wash, for its anti-inflammatory effect.
- *Whey,* in which grated carrot and horse-radish have been soaked for an hour.
- The herb *rue* – one cup three times daily as a decoction.

Supplements of value
Adult doses:
- *Beta carotene* – 30mg daily for a month, and then reduce to 15mg.
- *Vitamin C* – has an antihistamine effect. 3-6g daily, in divided doses.
- *Vitamin E* – 400iu daily.
- *Zinc* – 50mg daily as citrate or picolinate,

and reduce to 25mg as the condition improves.
- *B-complex* – once daily, or brewer's yeast.
- *EPA* – 3-4g daily for a month, and then reduce to 1g daily.
- *Evening primrose oil* – 500mg, 3-6 capsules daily.
- *Bifido bacteria* for infants, as well as *L acidophilus* for children.
- *Quercetin* – 500mg twenty minutes before meals, to block histamine-release, if allergy foods are unknown.
- *Glucosamine* – 0.5-1g twice daily, to replace the damaged surface skin more quickly.
- *Magnesium* – 400mg daily, plays a role in controlling inflammatory chemical release.
- *Calcium* – for children not eating enough vegetables and fish.
- *Kelp* tablets – for organic multi-minerals.
- *Spirulina* powder, for organic vitamins, minerals and protein.
- *Rice bran oil* capsules – to soothe the skin.

Herbal teas
- *Burdock* + *yellow dock* + *red clover* + *Oregon mountain grape*.

Homeopathy
Constitutional treatment is preferable, as it will strengthen the person as a whole. The following remedies may be helpful. *Dose is 6c three times daily.*
- *Arsenicum* – dry skin with fine white scales.
- *Alumina* – very dry itchy skin, inclined to constipation and itchy eyes.
- *Graphites* – weepy itchy eczema, a honey-like discharge, worse on the palms and behind the ears.
- *Petroleum* – cracked sore skin, worse in winter.
- *Psorinum* – child is also prone to infections, skin has a greasy unwashed appearance, irritation inside knees and elbows.
- *Mezereum* – intolerable itch, crusty vesi-

cles on the scalp.

• *Rhus Tox* – blisters, itch especially on hands and wrists, worse in damp weather and at night. Better with warmth.

• *Sulphur* – red dry rough skin. Itch is worse with heat and washing.

If there is no improvement in two weeks, there is no point in continued use of a remedy, and if there is an aggravation also, stop immediately and see a homeopath.

Many eczemas clear very quickly with a mixture of removing allergenic foods, adding acidophilus, improving the diet and taking vitamin and mineral supplements for a period. For those in relatively good health a quality multi-vitamin/mineral tablet plus oil capsules is enough. However, some children have very weak immune systems and are also prone to upper respiratory tract infections or skin infections. These children will steadily improve with the above treatment, but it is also wise to add constitutional homeopathic treatment and to strengthen the immune system.

I have seen children covered from head to toe in red, raw, intolerably itchy eczema, with constant colds and ear infections, and sometimes hyperactivity as well. All have made steady progress towards recovery of health with regular guidance from a naturopath and homeopath. Children covered in little boils along with eczema have also been cured, without ever resorting to antibiotics. Strengthening the immune system is a key to success, but it is also essential to treat each person as an individual with unique requirements.

III: *22. SEBORRHEIC DERMATITIS*

This may be described as a very low-grade infected eczema, associated with both an excessive sebum secreted from the skin glands and dandruff. The scale is usually yellowish, and is known as cradle cap in infants. Eczema is sometimes also present inside the joints such as elbows, knees, groin and axillae (arm-shoulder joints). A food allergy test is essential, because this condition occurs in allergy-prone children who often go on to develop some other allergic condition.

The major underlying cause appears to be a biotin deficiency (a B vitamin) caused by low levels of bifidus and L acidophilus in the bowel. These micro-flora are largely responsible for our biotin supplies and are involved with other B vitamins such as PABA, folic acid and pantothenic acid. I have often seen children with seborrheic dermatitis, and also with patches of pigment loss, which disappear when PABA and a bowel flora supplement is taken.

In adults, where the condition is unusual, biotin supplements are usually ineffective, but high dose B-complex plus zinc and essential fatty acids have proved valuable. The B-complex must contain all of the B group including B12 and folic acid.

TREATMENT

Remove foods to which the person is allergic. If breast-feeding, the mother must stop eating whatever causes allergic reactions in the infant.

Supplements of value
Adult doses:
- **Bifido bacteria** and **L acidophilus** – this combined supplement must be live, have a guaranteed potency, an expiry date and must require refrigeration.
- **Biotin** – 3mg twice daily.
- **Zinc** – 25mg daily as citrate or picolinate.
- **Flaxseed oil** – 1 tablespoon daily.
- **Evening primrose oil** – 1000mg daily.
- **B-complex** – 50mg twice daily.
- **Magnesium** – 400mg daily.

Children's doses must be according to age.

Children have been given 10mg daily of biotin with no ill effects, but 500mcg twice daily is adequate for all ages. Zinc dosage is 2.5mg x age daily, to a maximum of 15mg until over 12 years old, and magnesium is taken at 100mg (under 1 yr), 150mg (1-3 yrs), 250mg (7-10 yrs) and adult dose (from 15 yrs).

Topical
- **Vitamin B6** ointment, or crush a 50mg tablet into aqueous cream and apply daily in the morning.
- **Evening primrose oil** rubbed into the scalp at night.

Homeopathy
Dose 6c three times daily, adults and children.
- **Graphites** – for weepy and encrusted skin that is easily infected.
- **Viola** – for thick crusts on the scalp which may ooze. As a herb, wild pansy (viola) may be made into an infusion, taken internally and used as a wash.

III: *23. ASTHMA*

Bronchial asthma is a condition of airway hyper-sensitivity whereby a person suffers attacks of wheezing, difficulty in breathing and cough. This is due to broncho-spasm, swelling of the air-passages and the formation of excessive amounts of sticky mucous. There are two forms of asthma: extrinsic and intrinsic.

Extrinsic asthma is also known as allergic asthma. The major factor is a release of histamine in the bronchial tubes as a result of an allergic reaction to an external factor. This may be a commonly-eaten food, pollens, grasses, moulds, dust or household pets. Food allergies are always involved.

Intrinsic asthma is caused by a bronchial reaction to such things as emotional upset, respiratory infections, physical exertion, cold air, chemicals, excitement, laughter or weather changes. Food substances which naturally contain high levels of inflammatory chemicals can also trigger asthma.

Chemical mediators

In both types of asthma there is a release of inflammatory chemicals in the bronchi and it is these chemicals which cause the swelling, mucous formation, and broncho-spasm. In chronic asthma there is a persistent inflammation of the bronchial mucous membrane, but in sporadically-occurring attacks, bronchial spasm is the major feature. The common inflammatory chemicals involved are histamine, leukotrienes and prostaglandin E2 (PGE2).

Leukotrienes
These are chemicals made in the body as a result of eating too many meat and dairy products and not enough oily fish, raw seeds and nuts. The meat and dairy foods contain a fatty acid called arachidonic acid, and as you can see from the diagram, we make several other chemicals from it. However, asthmatics produce an excessive amount of those on the right of the diagram (leukotrienes) in preference to others. Tartrazine, non-steroid anti-inflammatory drugs and aspirin further exacerbate the problem by depressing the cycloxygenase pathway (on the left), and therefore allowing leukotrienes an unfettered run. The result is an excessive amount of very potent inflammatory leukotrienes increasing the symptoms of asthma.

Tartrazine is a yellow food colouring found in so many processed foods, drinks and sweets beloved by children. It is also found in some anti-asthmatic drugs. Read labels carefully in supermarkets and learn the 'E' numbers for all additives. In view of the fact that arachidonic acid is a major constituent of all animal protein, it is important to severely restrict these foods in an asthmatic diet, in order to solve much of the problem.

Allergy

Allergic reactions result in the release of histamine, which is another inflammatory chemical. Asthmatics are frequently allergic to colours and preservatives which are common throughout processed food. As many as 30% of asthmatics have been found to be allergic to sulphites (E221 to E227). Sulphites extend the shelf-life of food and get sprayed on salads displayed in restaurants. This keeps the food looking fresh and prevents oxidative changes

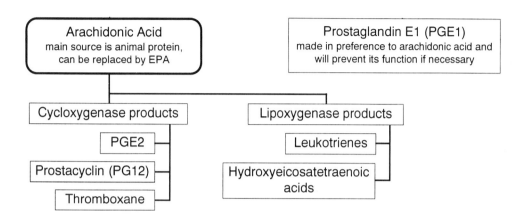

in avocados and fruit. Grapes are often coated with sulphites, and they are found in wine, beer, cider, gelatin, dressings and sauces, dips, vinegar, shellfish and potatoes, to name a few. An interesting theory is that the trace mineral molybdenum may block this type of allergic reaction, as the enzyme which neutralises sulphites is dependent on that mineral. Sulphites also lead to high levels of the inflammatory leukotrienes and PGE2.

Any number of foods may be causing an allergic reaction, but common ones are dairy products, eggs, citrus fruits, gluten grains, some nuts and pulses. Foods causing allergic reaction should be eliminated 100% until the immune system has strengthened, and then they may be incorporated into a rotation diet.

Histamine foods

In an individual who is releasing a lot of histamine as the result of an allergic reaction, foods with naturally high histamine content can exacerbate the problem. There is only so much natural anti-histamine which a liver can produce! However, once the offending al

lergens are removed, histamine foods usually cease to be a problem. Foods with very high levels are: shellfish, strawberries, tomatoes, chocolate, fermented cheese and drinks, sausages, sauerkraut, wine, baker's yeast and canned food.

Intestinal micro-flora

In the last ten years it has been clearly demonstrated that a lack of bifido bacteria in the intestinal tracts of very young children is a prime factor in the incidence of allergy. In the past, these bacteria were passed from mother to child through breast-milk. However this is no longer occurring, and it is believed to be due to contamination of breast-milk with pesticides and other environmental chemicals. In the 1950s it was found that breast-fed infants had a very low incidence of infections and allergies compared to bottle-fed children. Although this could have been partially attributed to immunity being passed from mother to child, it is now clear that bifido bacteria in milk played a major role in detox ifying chemicals in food and preventing allergic reactions. (These days, even breast-fed infants have a high incidence of allergy.) Any healthy bowel flora which do implant in the walls of the intestinal tract are very quickly destroyed by antibiotics that asthmatics are so often given. With a lack of bifido bacteria and acidophilus in children, allergies, fungal infections and deficiencies of vitamins, such as biotin and other Bs, occur.

Low hydrochloric acid (HCl) secretion

Several studies have shown that as many as 80% of asthmatic children are not producing sufficient HCl acid in the stomach, and some of them have severely low levels. This results in low absorption of vitamin B12, as well as the incomplete breakdown of protein foods. Protein should be reduced to individual amino acids before absorption, but if larger molecules reach the blood, the immune system recognises them as foreign and triggers an allergic reaction. This may lead to a release of histamine in the bronchi of an asthmatic.

A combination of low bifido bacteria and low HCl acid means that fungal infections such as candida readily occur. This fungus changes to a mycelial form, which means it grows roots that invade the bowel wall, and make it permeable to large food molecules. Another cause of fungal overgrowth in the bowel is the indiscriminate use of antibiotics.

Some doctors have discovered that replacing vitamin B12 rapidly improves asthmatic symptoms in children. However, the process involves injections once or twice weekly to maintain the status quo. The emotional trauma to the child may outweigh the benefits. It is surely better to replace the stomach acid and give high-assimilation vitamin B12 orally for a few months. Asthma caused by low HCl acid is the type which a child 'grows

out of' because he or she normally grows into producing adequate levels. Vitamin B12 treatment has been found to be particularly effective in sulphite allergy, as it blocks the effects.

When the intestinal environment is unhealthy in children, they may suffer any of the following: flatulence, bloating after meals, tummy aches after meals, burping, loss of appetite, picky eating, constipation, diarrhoeal tendencies or bad breath.

Vitamin B6 and magnesium deficiency

Some asthmatic children do not metabolise the amino acid tryptophan correctly, and the resulting high levels of the chemical serotonin causes bronchial constriction. Vitamin B6 corrects the fault, but it is also wise to reduce high-tryptophan foods in the diet such as meat, fish and dairy products. Bananas, avocado, plums and tomatoes are high in serotonin. Vitamin B6 is found in brewer's yeast, wholegrains, yeast extract and oily fish.

Magnesium and vitamin B6 work together, and asthmatics are frequently deficient in magnesium. This mineral has an anti-spasmodic effect on bronchial muscle and is also capable of blocking the broncho-spasm effect of the histamine released in allergic reactions. Magnesium is widely deficient in the food chain, due to the widespread use of artificial fertiliser.

From all of the above, it is clear that there are many possible causes of asthma, and often several aspects are present in one individual. However, most features are easily rebalanced with dietary changes alone. Asthma is one of the most rapidly increasing childhood diseases. The suggested culprits are many, but authorities generally agree that a common feature is that immune systems are being weakened by increased exposure to environmental toxins, which include pesticides on food, chemicals used in processing foods, as well as traffic and factory pollution. Weak immune function allows allergies to develop.

Drug medication deals only with reducing symptoms, that is, control of symptoms by inhibiting broncho-spasm and mucous membrane inflammation. It in no way addresses removing causes. If an asthmatic's life is to be returned to normal, the causes must be carefully investigated, and as far as possible eliminated. In the last ten years the death rate amongst asthmatics has doubled, but statistics indicate that it is anti-asthmatic drugs which are more often the culprits.

TREATMENTS

Diet

The aim of this is to strengthen the immune system, alter the fatty acid ratios in the body and keep the intestinal environment healthy, so that many of the causes of asthma are then eliminated.

- All foods should be natural and organically grown. A vegan diet is best, and studies have shown a dramatic improvement in symptoms by leaving out all animal protein. Care must be taken to combine vegetable protein correctly in order to ensure all the essential amino acids.
- An abundance of fresh vegetables and fruit – raw, lightly-steamed or stir-fried. This should form the main part of every meal, with other food treated as side dishes.
- Brown rice, millet, spelt, quinoa or yellow cornmeal are the best grains. Be sparing with wheat, oats, barley and rye, as they sensitise the airways.
- Raw nuts and seeds, but especially walnuts, almonds, sunflower, sesame, pumpkin seeds and flaxseeds in small amounts on a daily basis.
- Pulses – and be sure to vary the types of dried peas and beans eaten.

- Green tea and honey.
- Brewer's yeast or yeast extract, for vitamin B6.
- Cold-pressed flaxseed (linseed) oil for dressings. Do not heat this oil.
- Anti-leukotriene foods – garlic and onion, dill, asparagus, kale, lettuce, broccoli, cucumber, radish, red beet, artichokes, Brussels sprouts, peppers, pears, apples, berry fruits, fenugreek, tarragon, flaxseeds.
- Sautéed garlic releases a bronchial relaxant chemical.

Limit

- Meat, fish, eggs and dairy products to a minimum, as they are high in arachidonic acid and tryptophan.
- Oily fish for its EPA content is the best fish to eat.
- Soya products, as they are high in tryptophan.

Avoid

- All foods to which you are allergic.
- All packaged, processed and refined foods.
- High serotonin foods – bananas, avocados, red plums and tomatoes.
- All food additives, especially tartrazine and sulphite.
- Tap water, especially because of the chlorine content.
- Salt, because bronchial muscle becomes hypersensitive if the sodium/potassium balance is upset.
- Foods which feed intestinal fungus – sugar and white flour products.
- Known triggers, such as emotional upset.

Juices

- Lime, half an hour before breakfast.
- Any of the anti-leukotriene vegetables or fruits.

Supplements of value

Adult doses:
- ***Beta carotene*** – 15mg twice daily.

- *Vitamin C* – 1g three times daily.
- *Vitamin E* – 400iu daily.
- *Selenium* – 200mcg daily.
- *Zinc* – 25mg daily as citrate.
- High-potency *EPA* – 2-4g daily for one month, and then reduce to 1g daily, plus eating oily fish. EPA blocks some of the arachidonic acid production and lessens the effects of environmental allergens.
- *Vitamin C, zinc and EPA in combination* have been shown to prevent the asthmatic wheeze.
- All the above supplements have a marked effect on reducing inflammatory chemicals.
- *Bifido bacteria* for infants. *L acidophilus* and bifido bacteria for children. The product should guarantee potency, be acid-stable, require refrigeration and have an expiry date.
- *Magnesium* – 250mg twice daily, relaxes bronchial muscle.
- *Molybdenum* – 0.5mg twice daily to neutralise sulphites.
- *Vitamin B6* – 50-100mg twice daily, to correct tryptophan metabolism. The children's dose is 25mg twice daily.
- *B-complex* – once daily, or *brewer's yeast*, if taking extra B6 long-term.
- *Vitamin B12* – 1000mcg daily, if low stomach acid is a factor (children).
- *Betaine HCl acid* plus *pepsin* tablets – 1-3 with every meal for low stomach acid.

Molybdenum, B6, B12 and Betain HCl are to be taken only if necessary.

Children's doses are reduced according to age.

Herbs
Adult doses:
- *Cayenne* – 0.5ml tincture three times daily, desensitises airways but is a fiery remedy to swallow.
- *Ephedra* (*ma-huang*) – 1-4g dried stems, three times daily, or make a tea. This is a classic anti-asthmatic herb.

- Good mixtures for a daily tea are as follows:
Ephedra + grindelia + skunk cabbage.
Euphorbia + grindelia + senega.
Chamomile – inhalations of three drops of essential oil in boiling water, or use an infusion of the dried herb. It has an anti-inflammatory and anti-spasmodic effect.
Eucalyptus oil can also be used.

Homeopathy
Constitutional treatment is best, but the following remedies can be used for acute treatment. *Dose is every 15 minutes if necessary. Do not repeat a remedy while it is working.*
- *Aconite* 30c – attack comes on suddenly after exposure to cold dry wind, patient very anxious and fearful.
- *Arsenicum* 6c – attack occurs between midnight and 2am, the child is very restless, and is thirsty for sips only.
- *Carbo Veg* 30c – coughing, gagging, gasping for air, vomits mucous, needs to be cool. Worse talking, in humidity and at night.
- *Kali Carb* 6c – patient looks pale and lethargic and worse 2-4am. Better sitting and leaning forward. Better in a warm climate.
- *Nat Sulph* 6c – worse in damp weather and from 4-5am. Patient holds chest while coughing. Fluid retention and morning diarrhoea.
- *Pulsatilla* 6c – green phlegm coughed up, child weepy and craves fresh air.
- *Ipecac* 6c – lots of mucous coughed up, vomits mucous, feels sick.
- *Hepar Sulph* 6c – choking cough, asthma better in damp weather, worse in dry, cold weather.
- *Ant Tart* 30c – very loud wheezing, coughing and gasping consecutively.
- *Psorinum* 6c – if the asthma followed on from childhood eczema. Better lying down with legs outstretched.
- *Silicea* 6c – for asthma following a cold.

General
- Use an ioniser for clean air.
- Humidifiers help mucous expectoration.
- Exercise, and daily deep breathing.
- A stress-free environment.

In my experience, following a largely vegan diet with a little oily fish, avoiding allergic foods and taking anti-inflammatory vitamins and minerals leads to a dramatic improvement in adults. In children the same applies, although they may require healthy bowel flora and some of the optional supplements to correct deficiencies. The treatment as a whole strengthens the immune system, and thus the body's ability to heal itself. Constitutional homeopathy also strengthens the individual.

III: *24. RHEUMATOID ARTHRITIS*

This is the most common form of chronic inflammatory disease affecting joints. However it is really a systemic disease which produces local symptoms in the connective tissues of joints. Rheumatoid arthritis (R A) is an auto-immune disease, meaning that the body fails to recognise 'self' and destroys its own tissue.

There is often a familial association with other rheumatic disorders. Women are affected three times more often than men and some authorities believe the ratio to be 5:1. Onset is usually before 40 years, but the juvenile form occurs very young. The disease is not geographically-related and affects people world wide. However it is more common in temperate than tropical climates. Possibly this is because the easy-going attitudes of the races indigenous to tropical countries precludes a stress disease developing – or possibly it has much to do with their traditionally simple eating habits.

Extreme fatigue, vague muscle pain, loss of appetite and constipation are early warnings of the onset. Chronic catarrh is also one of the first symptoms – according to homeopathic principles, it is the body's way of trying to throw off the disease. It is the discarding of waste caused by excess food and the wrong type of foods. There is pain and swelling in the joints and the onset is usually insidious. The joints are warm, tender, swollen and painful on rising, and exercise is necessary to free them up. Swelling in the tissues of the hands causes increased sweating and muscle atrophy. The disease is usually bilateral, although it may start in one joint then spread to its opposite before affecting other joints. If unchecked it can cause severe destruction of the joints.

Exponents for natural healing view arthritis as essentially a disease of improper nutrition. Mental stress may precipitate it, and will certainly prolong the condition. It involves the dumping of waste products in the joints once the body loses the ability to cope with excretion via the normal channels of bowel, kidneys, skin and lungs. The acid-base balance is badly upset and the body is having to deal with a heavy excess of acid.

Causes

- *Over-eating* creates more acid than can be eliminated, and this leads to fermentation, flatulence and obesity, which increases the pressure on the joints.
- *Excessive meat and dairy intake* produces acid but no bulk for the large intestine. It also results in the formation of inflammatory chemicals, which may then be released in the joints. Studies have shown that vegetarians reduce their joint-inflammation quicker than meat-eaters.
- *Processed foods* which are de-vitalised and de-mineralised, and therefore contain few nutrients.
- *Incompatible food combinations*, leading to fermentation. When proteins and carbohydrates are ingested simultaneously, acid and alkali mediums are needed at the same time for the digestion. The end-result is that neither proteins nor carbohydrates get broken down fully, and go through the gut fermenting and putrefying, causing a toxic bowel.
- *Hypochlorhydria*, which means insufficient levels of stomach acid, is thought to be

responsible for 10-20% of rheumatoid arthritis cases. When hydrochloric acid secretion is reduced, it exacerbates the effects of poor food combining. In addition it may also inhibit the release of protein-digesting enzymes, so that these foods are not fully broken down into individual amino acids. The colon toxicity which develops as a result of poor digestion can lead to a leaky gut syndrome, whereby partial proteins pass into the bloodstream. Here they are perceived as foreign by the immune system and an allergic reaction is instigated. Non-steroid anti-inflammatory drugs have been shown to independently cause this increased intestinal permeability to undigested food.

• *An excess of acid-forming foods* such as meat, grains, tea, coffee, alcohol, and insufficient alkaline-forming foods like fruit and vegetables. It should be explained here that acid foods actually form an alkaline end-product once they have been metabolised, and alkaline foods are acid-forming.

• *Unsuitable fuel*, such as wheat and dairy products. These are relatively new foods in terms of human evolution, and many have not developed the means of coping with them properly. Anthropological studies have indicated that the bones of wheat-eaters in Egypt were riddled with arthritis whereas corn-eaters from further south in Africa were not. In a one-year study, where a group of rheumatoid arthritis sufferers were put on a gluten-free vegan diet, there was a significant improvement in symptoms. About half way through the study, dairy products were slowly reintroduced and left in the diets of those who did not experience an exacerbation of their symptoms. This is one of many studies which also highlights the advantage of avoiding meat.

• *Allergy*: there is evidence that food allergies often cause arthritis. A US study involving 20,000 arthritics indicated that when they avoided foods to which they were allergic, there was improvement in more than 50% of cases.

• *Chronic constipation* may cause the disease, as the poisons and toxins are reabsorbed, and if the system cannot cope, they will be dumped in joints. Faulty elimination of waste and toxins from the body and the resultant overloaded tissues, blood and lymph is characteristic of arthritis. Lack of exercise contributes to constipation. Additionally, bowel toxins directly affect the body's zinc/copper ratio by decreasing the absorption of zinc, and this is sometimes the only cause of arthritis.

• *Bacteria and parasites*: there has been a flurry of articles in the press concerning the relationship between proteus bacteria and rheumatoid arthritis. However, as far back as the mid-70s, researchers were reporting the benefits of anti- proteus treatment in arthritis. In Britain, a Dr Wyburn-Mason first found this bacteria in the tissues of people with active R A when he was conducting a study on 66 patients. They were given drug treatment and became completely free of symptoms within six months. In USA, the Indian herb yucca has been used with the same results. This herb is not absorbed, and acts as a cleansing agent which rids the bowel of infecting organisms like proteus. This demonstrates one of the reasons that naturopathic treatment works so well in arthritis. The diet cleanses the bowel of foreign bacteria and parasites, and increases the activity of healthy micro-flora. These prevent colonisation by foreign microbes.

A study involving 500 R A patients in Britain found that almost every one of them had antibodies to proteus in their blood. Klebsiella is another bacteria which has been implicated in R A, and amoeba is also a well-known cause. The reason that bacteria are implicated in the destruction of joints is that many people have the same tissue-type as the invading organism. When this occurs, the body mistakenly recognises its own tissue to be as foreign as the bacteria, and so sets up the destructive inflammatory process. Antibiotics may destroy the bacteria, but they will also destroy lactobacilli like acidophilus, which prevent the likes of proteus from making a home in the body. It is quite important to resist this line of treatment, and instead take acidophilus supplements, at the same time as a bowel cleanse, herbs, garlic, grapefruit seed extract and dietary change. Unless the bowel is detoxified and healthy habits instigated, arthritis will never be cured.

● *Histidine* is often lacking in arthritics. D D Gerber at the Downstate Medical Centre in New York discovered that they tend to have one quarter of the normal level. One test showed that joint-stiffness and the range of movement was improved after the amino acid was administered, at the rate of 1-6g daily.

● *Stress*, both mental and physical, is a major cause of rheumatoid arthritis. Dr Robert Bingham in USA states that almost all his patients could date the onset of their arthritis to a mentally-stressful situation, a single illness or a period of ill-health. That is, times when nutritional requirements were not adequately filled. I have found this to be a truth in most of my patients also. The condition often starts from an emotional upheaval like a major family upset, the death of a family member, redundancy or the shock of a cancer scare. It may also arise after longer-term lower-grade stress such as the constant emotional upheaval of caring for a retarded or very difficult child, continuous financial worries, an unhappy marriage, or a serious illness.

● Aside from stress acting as a trigger for the onset of the disease, attacks of pain often occur when an arthritic has been worrying or pushing himself too hard. This causes a release of inflammatory chemicals in the joints, and must be treated as a warning to stop and reassess the effectiveness of stress-control methods. If this happens to you, stop and ponder over whether you have got it right. Are you still absorbing emotional pain and pressure instead of pushing them aside? Are you absorbing worry instead of dealing with it objectively? Does your daily life involve periods of anxiety, tension or undue pressure? Small stressful events have been found to be positively related to an increase in anti-bodies and inflammatory chemicals, which is what occurs in an auto-immune disease. Major life events also have a profound effect on the ratio between the 'helpers' and 'suppressors', which control antibody formation. Helper T-cells raise antibodies, and arthritics produce an excess of these along with an excess of inflammatory chemicals.

● The anti-stress B vitamin known as pantothenic acid is very often significantly lowered in the blood of arthritics, and some studies indicate that the lower the level, the more severe the pain and inflammation.

TREATMENT

This involves some or all of the following:
● Dietary changes, improvements in elimination processes, supplements of vitamins and minerals, herbal and homeopathic treatment and dealing with stress. Heat, hydrotherapy, massage, poultices and exercise may also be necessary.
● The first step is to stop *causing* the disease, by attending to diet and elimination processes, as well as controlling stress.
● Acid-forming foods must be cut back, and alkaline-forming ones must be increased, until a ratio of 80:20 is achieved, in favour of alkaline-forming foods. Eating habits must be changed on a permanent basis, and the necessary supplements taken. Parallel treatment ensures the elimination of waste from the

bowel every day so that poisons cannot be reabsorbed.

● Acidic blood needs to be cleansed of all debris so that a healthy blood-supply reaches all tissues. Any anaemia must be treated, and exercise commenced to increase the supply of oxygen to the tissues.

● Stress must be dealt with, through the medium of yoga, meditation or relaxation techniques.

● A new approach involving total health is needed.

Food combining

Dr Hay, in his book *A New Health Era*, maintains that arthritis responds to nutritional treatment alone. In his view it is only necessary to correct the acid-base balance of the body for arthritis to disappear. That is, to increase the alkaline-forming foods to 80% of the diet, and to make sure that they are not erroneously converted to acid. With incorrect food-combinations, alkaline-forming foods may become acid. Disturbed emotions at mealtimes, and eating when tired or unwell produces acidity. Lactose in milk forms mucous and acid if not utilised properly. Insufficient alkalising minerals (sodium, potassium, calcium and magnesium) cause inefficient metabolism and an accumulation of acid. Kelp tablets contain minerals in proportions needed by humans, and this is an easy way of ensuring an improved level of alkali in the body. Dr Hay warns that starches and sugars are the chief dietary causes of arthritis, mainly because they are normally eaten with incompatible foods. Therefore proper digestion is prevented and fermentation occurs.

Many types of wholegrains, if properly combined, are fine in small amounts, and wheatgerm and kelp are necessary supplements. I know at least three crippled osteo-arthritics who did nothing more than correct their acid-alkali balance with diet, and now in their 70s, they mow the lawns and dig the garden.

Please see chapter II:1, 'the Essence of Food-Combining'.

Fasting

Initially the arthritic should start with a fast. There are a variety of types and lengths of fasts, but basically, you should stay on freshly made juices and whole fruit and vegetables until pain is considerably reduced. See chapter II:10 on Fasting, for making juices and potassium broth.

Fruit and vegetables should be fresh, raw and unprocessed. If you are unaccustomed to eating raw fruit and vegetables, the volume should be increased gradually, and skins removed initially. Use more in juice form and less as whole produce. You should try to find a source of organically-grown food, and do not use commercially-made fruit or vegetable juices – only home-made ones using a juicing machine.

● *Day 1*: water only, 6-8 glasses minimum.

● *Days 2-3*: fresh raw diluted fruit juice, but do not use citrus fruits. A glass every two hours with water in between.

● *Day 4-5*: add raw vegetable juices to the regime but don't combine them with fruit.

● *Days 6-7*: whole fruit and vegetables may be added, raw or steamed.

Once the pain has subsided, other foods are re-introduced, one per day, until a balanced diet is being eaten, but one which is mainly alkaline-forming. Foods must be fresh, whole and largely raw – lots of fruit, vegetables and salads, with small amounts of cheese, eggs, nuts, seeds, and sprouts, wholegrains (especially millet, buckwheat and corn), pulses, herbal teas, oily fish and organically-produced meat, if desired.

Diet

● 80% alkaline-forming, and as much raw as

possible. All fruit and vegetables fit this category except plums, cranberries, asparagus, peas, broad beans, Brussels sprouts and canned or sulphured fruits.
- Other alkaline-forming foods are millet, buckwheat, yoghurt, whey, fresh coconut, soya products and egg-white.
- Fruits and vegetables of special value are: all the berry fruits, blueberries, blackberries, cherries and hawthorn berries. These are flavonoid fruits which are powerful antioxidants to joints.
- Bananas, pineapples, apples and grapes.
- Carrots, celery, beetroot, parsley, cress, alfalfa, asparagus, yams, garlic, endive, mushrooms, avocado.
- Sprouted grains, seeds and nuts.
- Grains – millet, rice, spelt, quinoa and corn are the best. Use oatmeal and rye in moderation. Wheat causes major problems for many arthritics, so a slice of bread is to be reserved for treats unless it really does not increase stiffness.
- Nuts and seeds (raw and fresh), especially sunflower, sesame, walnuts, pumpkin seeds, almonds and flaxseeds for the essential polyunsaturated oils.
- Oily fish, twice weekly if desired – mackerel, herring, sardines, fresh salmon or trout. Some of this may be canned, but remove all surrounding oil.
- Dressings: use only extra-virgin olive oil or guaranteed cold-pressed polyunsaturated oils.
- Kelp and seaweeds, for rich sources of minerals.
- Spirulina and wheatgrass, as a potent source of vitamins, minerals, protein and plant pigments.
- Goats' milk or soya milk, eggs and cottage cheese (home-made) in moderation – twice weekly each.
- Cook with turmeric and ginger as often as possible.

- Herbal teas, freshly-pressed juices, mineral water, vegetable broth, rooibosch tea, grain coffee and naturally-brewed miso. Add powdered barley greens to juice daily.

Reduce
- All acid-forming foods, but especially meat and dairy products. Home-made cottage cheese is fine, or a low-salt goat cheese. Meat and dairy products increase the inflammatory prostaglandin E2 fatty acids, whereas oily fish in the diet instead, reduces inflammation.
- Pulses, to thrice weekly, except soya, which can be eaten more freely. Pulses as well as vegetables increase beneficial lactobacillus activity in the colon.
- Citrus fruits 2-3 times a week, and make sure that they are completely ripe. Arthritics sometimes do not metabolise these correctly, and an acid end-product results.

Avoid
- Foods to which you are allergic, as this is sometimes a major feature in arthritis. Allergy to the 'nightshade foods' is not uncommon: these are potatoes, tomatoes, capsicum peppers, aubergines, tamarillos, chili, cayenne and paprika. This food family has been shown to prevent the restoration of bone-cartilage.
- All wheat flour, and everything made from it – bread, pasta, cereal and cakes.
- All frozen and processed foods – cakes, crumpets, cereals, jams, sausages, bacon etc.
- Sugar and artificial sweeteners, and everything made from them.
- Coffee, tea, cocoa, alcohol and soft drinks.
- Added salt and hot spices.

Many arthritics have an inadequate mechanism for metabolising gluten carbohydrate, and feel a clogged-up sensation with increased joint-pain. The gluten grains are wheat, oats, barley and rye. Dried peas and beans may have the same effect on some. For people in this category, a simple diet of fish and cottage cheese with small amounts of nuts, seeds, rice, millet and corn dishes, along with an abundance of fruit and vegetables is more satisfactory. It is important to listen to your body and eat foods which suit it.

A note for the elderly

Many older folk are not accustomed to eating much raw food, and so cannot cope with the long chewing or the digestion. These people should gradually increase the vegetable content of the diet, and start by taking them cooked only. However, every day a selection of raw products like carrots, celery, cucumber and raw beetroot should be juiced and sipped slowly. In this way all the nutrients from the raw vegetables are taken in a very easily-digested form.

Do not confuse a juicer with a food-processor, as only the former separates the juice and fibre. A food-processor just turns food into a pulp, which still contains all the fibre. Seeds and nuts can be ground very finely and sprinkled on fresh fruit if they are too difficult to chew properly.

Juices

Raw fruit and vegetable juices are of enormous benefit to an arthritic, and whenever painful attacks occur it is wise to have a day or so on juices alone. These must be freshly-pressed and not canned or packaged. Do not store juice, as the living enzymes are destroyed quite soon after being released from the fibre. Juices especially good for arthritics are: carrots, celery, red beet, parsley, cress, wheatgrass and alfalfa; sour cherry, pineapple, blackcurrant and sour apple. Dilute the juices and drink them slowly. This is a good place to add your aloe vera juice, powdered wheatgrass and spirulina, for a nutrient-packed drink. They should not be added to hot liquids.

Daily menu suggestions
Breakfast choices
- On awakening, freshly-pressed fruit juice.
- Fresh fruit with a little plain yoghurt, chopped nuts and two tablespoons oatbran.
- Porridge oats, with soya or nut milk and raisins.
- Cooked mushrooms on rye bread.

Mid-morning
- Herbal tea, grain coffee or a fresh vegetable juice.
Lunch
- A large salad, with sprouted produce like alfalfa and mung beans.
- A side-dish of beans, lentils, tofu, black rye bread, brown rice, polenta, cottage cheese or a vege/nut paté or loaf.
- A thick vegetable soup in winter.
- Juice the vegetables, if you can't eat them whole.

See chapter II:13 on the Naturopathic Lifestyle for more ideas on what to eat with your vegetables – just avoid wheat and anything to which you are allergic.

Mid-afternoon
- Fresh fruit and herbal tea etc.
Dinner
- A large plate of vegetables, cooked or raw, or a small amount along with raw vegetable juice or cooked broth.
- A side-dish of oily fish, light meat, eggs or vegetarian protein as at lunch. Restrict the fish and eggs to twice a week of each, and meat to a small serving once a week.
Bedtime
- Rooibosch tea, miso or a herbal tea, like chamomile, fennel, peppermint or fenugreek.

See chapter II:13 for natural flavourings and sweeteners. Make biscuits or occasional desserts only with allowed grains and sweeteners.

Supplements of value

Adult doses:

It is a good idea to get professional advice on which of the following would best suit your individual requirements.

Antioxidants to repair the immune system and support the adrenal glands as well as inhibit joint destruction. Try to buy most of these as a single tablet:

- *Beta carotene* – 6mg daily.
- *Vitamin C* – 1g three times daily.
- *Vitamin E* – 400iu twice daily.
- *Selenium* – 200mcg daily.
- *B-complex* – 50mg daily – very important for all arthritics.
- *Pantothenic acid* – 500mg twice daily.
- *Zinc* – 25mg daily as citrate or picolinate, with *manganese* 5mg.

For the *auto-immune* aspect:

- *Calcium EAP2* – 80mg three times daily.
- *Evening primrose oil* – 500mg 3-4 times daily.
- *EPA* – 1-2g daily, or fish oil, three teaspoons, is the most effective oil for reducing pain and stiffness.

Anti-inflammatory products:

- *Boron* – 3mg 3 times daily. This is a mineral which has only been in use for five to ten years. Clinical studies have indicated excellent results in decreasing arthritic symptoms. Boron was recently reported to antagonise fluoride, and so it may have its greatest effect in those drinking fluoridated water, which is known to be harmful to the human body.
- *Quercetin + bromelain + pancreatin* – 250mg of each between meals, with vitamin C, is better than any drugs.

The antioxidants and auto-immune products are also anti-inflammatory.

Pain relief:

- *DLPA* 400mg – 3 times daily, half an hour before food, with juice.
- *Béres Drops Plus* – this also improves immune competence.
- *Shark cartilage* contains the same mucopolysaccharides (chondroitin sulphate) as green-lipped mussels and is therefore anti-inflammatory. Studies indicate that it has a quite remarkable and rapid healing effect with 60-70% of people experiencing astonishing improvement. This may have more to do with the product's ability to prevent the abnormal capillary growth that occurs in arthritic cartilage. Wear and tear and inflammation allow blood vessels to penetrate, and the resultant calcification destroys the cartilage in the joint.

Other products of note:

- *HCl acid* and *enzyme tablets* – with meals, if digestion is poor.
- *Glutathione* is a composite amino acid which is antioxidant and of use in inflammatory conditions.
- *Alfalfa* tablets are anti-inflammatory and rich in manganese, which arthritics are often deficient in.
- *Brewer's yeast* is a good food in arthritis, and an excellent source of natural B vitamins.
- *Methionine* and *cysteine* are amino acids that remove calcium plaque from joints.
- *Silica* 33mg – 3 times daily, removes bony spurs and repairs cartilage.
- *Histidine* is an amino-acid, often low in cases of rheumatoid arthritis. It balances the helper/suppressor ratio and is therefore useful in auto-immune disease and allergy.
- *Citricidal* (grapefruit seed extract) – to destroy proteus. *Garlic* is also effective.
- *L acidophilus* – a guaranteed potent lactobacillus supplement will maintain a healthy bowel environment and control proteus.
- *Celloids® PCIP* x1, and *Celloids® MP* x1 – 2 hourly, if necessary for pain and swelling.
- *Glucosamine sulphate* – 1-2g daily. This

substance is the precursor of joint lubricant and will restore the protective gelatinous consistency of this fluid. It is also the precursor of chondroitin sulphate, which is the anti-inflammatory substance in joints.

Herbs

Choose from the following to decrease pain, stiffness and swelling, by blocking the inflammation. Many companies sell capsules containing a mixture of arthritic herbs.

• *Curcumin* extract – 400mg three times daily. This is a turmeric extract, and is as powerfully anti-inflammatory as any drugs, and without side- effects.

• *Chinese Skullcap* (scutellaria) – 2-4g three times daily. This is a potent anti-oxidant and its anti-inflammatory effect is similar to some cortisone drugs.

• *Chinese thoroughwax* (bupleuri falcatum) – 2-4g, three times daily. This is a steroid type anti- inflammatory herb which also protects the adrenal glands and liver (in contrast to the drug forms of steroids).

• *Ginger* – 1-2g, three times daily, of powdered root, or make a tea from the fresh root, or cook with 1oz daily.

• *Devil's claw* – 1-2g of powder three times daily, or this can be bought as tablets. The herb also stimulates the lymphatic system.

• New Zealand *green-lipped mussel* – 350mg three times daily. This is very effective, but sometimes six weeks go by before the initial effect is felt. Hospital trials have indicated 70% improvement in rheumatoid arthritis and 40% in osteo-arthritis with this mussel extract. It is anti-inflammatory and contains mucopolysaccharides, which repair the collagen part of cartilage.

• *Guaiacum, celery seed, bogbean, wild yam, black cohosh, white poplar, prickly ash bark, willow bark, cramp bark* and *licorice*. These can be bought in various combinations in tablet form. Licorice is also

known to enhance the effect of Chinese thoroughwax and prevent the breakdown of adrenal hormones.

• *Yucca* – 2g, or *golden seal* – 1g, three times daily, are potent against proteus etc.

• *Flavonoid herbs*, which repair the cartilage destroyed by arthritis are: *blueberry* – 4g powdered berries twice daily; *hawthorn berries* – 1g powdered berries, three times daily.

A poultice for swollen painful joints: mix two tablespoons *mullein* + two tablespoons *slippery elm* + one teaspoon *cayenne* + one teaspoon *lobelia*.

Homeopathy

There are a great many remedies which may be applicable, depending on which joints are affected. Here are just a few general ones for acute symptom relief. *Dose 6c four-hourly, for a few days.*

• *Rhus Tox* – for joints which are worse in damp weather, and better after moving around a little. Also worse for excessive walking.

• *Bryonia* – hot swollen joints better for rest and worse for movement. Person is very irritable.

• *Ledum* – if a left upper and a right lower joint are affected, for instance left wrist and right knee. Better for cold. This is also of value after invasive injections have been given.

• *Pulsatilla* – hot swollen joints, pains flit from joint to joint, worse for heat and motion, better with pressure.

• *Dulcamara* – noticeably worse after cold or damp weather.

• *Apis* – if there is much swelling and redness.

Essential oils

Use these in a massage oil:
rosemary + *juniper* + *lavender*; *eucalyptus* or *camphor*. Put a total of 15 drops of essen-

tial oils to 30ml of a carrier oil, such as almond or avocado.

Elimination

- *Bowel* – It is important to have good daily function so as to not re-poison the system. If laxatives are necessary use flaxseeds or psyllium seeds. Buckthorn bark is a non-habit-forming herb which can safely be used long-term. A colon-cleansing blend of herbs and fibre may be necessary initially, or even daily enemas until the high fibre diet regulates bowel action. Exercise also improves any constipation. Natural unpasteurised aloe vera juice will detoxify and improve bowel function. A healthy bowel environment is essential to prevent arthritis and proteus infestations, so live acidophilus should be taken regularly.
- *Skin* – dry skin brushing daily with a loofah or natural fibre brush, until skin has a warm glow. Brush in circular motion all over the body. Shower for three minutes under very hot water and finish with thirty seconds of cold. Both these methods improve circulation and skin function.
- *Kidneys* – drink 4-6 glasses of allowed fluids daily (fruit and vegetables produce more liquid).
- *Lungs* – exercise and deep breathing to rid the body of acids.

Mealtimes

- Never over-eat, or eat too quickly.
- Chew everything very thoroughly.
- Mealtimes should be relaxed, so don't eat when anxious or stressed.

Exercise

Walking or swimming keeps the joints mobile and increases the sense of wellbeing.

De-stress

- Learn meditation or a relaxation technique, and practise it daily.
- Put aside time for yourself on a daily basis. Seek out situations which engender feelings of pleasure. Laughter, joy and positive thoughts are important, so make a point of actually counting your blessings, reading amusing books and enjoying social occasions.
- Examine past and present stresses and decide how to deal with them, so that the body will no longer be harmed each time. It is equally important to guard against self-pity, fear or a 'helpless victim' attitude, as these sentiments will damage your joints. Harmful emotions lead to a release of inflammatory chemicals in the joints.
- Stress can cause unimaginable havoc in the human body. The acid-alkali imbalance and the deposition of waste in joints may well be rooted in stress. Many arthritics suffer from suppressed resentments or anxiety, and are easily upset by situations not conforming to their own mode of behaviour. Perhaps these people have had more to be angry about than the average person, or perhaps they are over-sensitive. Often they are overly-giving types who always take care of others before themselves. This is a major stress on the body in the long-term, and has to be balanced with time for nurturing self on a daily basis. If you recognise any of this, then your arthritis will not disappear until you get to grips with healing your emotions. Every event which your mind perceives as a stress causes a release of inflammatory chemicals in the joints. It is very important to release harmful emotions and not bottle them up inside. Read chapter III:3 on Stress for useful guidelines.

Conclusion

It would seem that the important considera

tions in arthritis are to correct the acid-base balance of the body by means of diet, to correct all elimination channels and to learn how to cope with daily stress.

As to the type of foods or supplements which should be taken, this is a matter of biochemic individuality. Everyone is different and has his or her own biochemic requirements. Therefore one cannot lay down hard-and-fast rules but must experiment.

Some people find grains and pulses very 'clogging' and are better avoiding them. Gluten grains are to be totally banned in some, while others can happily eat a little whole cereal or wholewheat bread each day, as long as it is not mixed with protein. Milk is acid-forming unless raw and should be restricted – however, yoghurt, being alkaline-forming, is usually well tolerated. There are arthritics who remain completely well on daily small amounts of liver or white meat. Others experience pain on consuming meat because of a resulting cascade of inflammatory chemicals.

In my view, once pain has been alleviated by a juice fast, foods should be added back one at a time and assessed. If the pain returns, stop the food added, fast for another day on fruit and vegetables and then try another food. Continue until you have tried all wholefoods, and have come up with a healthy, mainly alkaline-forming diet which leaves you pain-free. Food-combining is obviously of paramount importance, and arthritics must be careful not to eat starches with protein or acid fruits. Milk, yoghurt and cheese, although protein foods, can be eaten in moderation at a starch meal.

As far as supplements are concerned, each person must be evaluated individually. It may be that, with the diet corrected and all the special foods incorporated, such as wheat-germ, brewer's yeast and sprouted seeds, very few extra vitamins are required. However, the antioxidants are very good insurance against all chronic illness.

III: *25. OSTEO-ARTHRITIS*

This is a wear-and-tear type of arthritis, with degeneration of the cartilage and bone ends. Bony spurs also form and restrict joint function. It occurs in men and women, and hereditary factors may be involved. Joints are painful, stiff and eventually deformed unless the condition is arrested. The wear-and-tear damage to the cartilage results in the release of enzymes which have a destructive effect on the joint.

The incidence increases with age, although 35% of sufferers have one knee affected by 30 years old. This type of arthritis is usually more painful after prolonged activity and is better for rest.

The aim of treatment is to restore the collagen matrix at the bone ends, and to this end it is important to avoid aspirin and non-steroid anti-inflammatory drugs. Experimental studies in 1982 clearly indicated that although these drugs suppress symptoms, they also increase the destruction of cartilage. Other anti-rheumatic drugs account for a very high percentage of drug deaths every year.

The nightshade family of vegetables mentioned in connection with rheumatoid arthritis (III:24) are thought to inhibit collagen repair in joints and even increase inflammatory reactions. It is important to be aware of whether this food family worsens symptoms.

Hormone imbalances influence osteo-arthritis, and experiments have shown that inhibiting oestrogen in women improves the condition – probably these people are not clearing oestrogen properly through the liver in the second half of the menstrual cycle. Attention to liver function could solve the problem, as it often does in those P M T sufferers who also don't remove this hormone from circulation. A poorly-functioning thyroid gland is thought to increase the risk of osteo-arthritis.

TREATMENT

Diet and juices
Follow the recommendations in chapter III:24 on Rheumatoid Arthritis. The diet is all-important and is often enough on its own to restore normal activity. An optimum weight is important, as obesity stresses joints.

Supplements of value
Adult doses:
- *Beta carotene* – 6mg daily.
- *Vitamin C* – 1g three times daily.
- *Vitamin E* – 600iu daily, to prevent cartilage destruction and promote its repair.
- *B-complex* – 50mg daily. Very high doses of niacinamide (B3) have been highly effective, but this must only be given under qualified supervision.
- *Zinc* – 30mg + *copper* 3mg.

All of the above are necessary for the proper synthesis of collagen at the bone ends.
- *Shark cartilage* – restores normal joint cartilage formation.
- *Methionine* – 500mg twice daily, clears oestrogen through the liver and is anti-inflammatory to cartilage. It removes calcium plaque from joints.
- *Silymarin* – 50mg three times daily, regenerates and is antioxidant to the liver.
- *Boron* – 3mg 3 times daily has caused complete remission in some and has a very good effect on all cases, according to very recent

studies.

• *Flavonoids* – 2g daily, especially extracts from berry fruits, as they have a remarkable effect on restoring collagen. They also act as antioxidants to cartilage and prevent its destruction.

• *Celloids® PCIP* x 1 + *Celloids® MP* x 1 – 2 hourly if necessary, for pain and swelling. *Celloids® SCF* x 1 – 3 times daily, to remove bony spurs and repair cartilage, or if you can't get Celloids®, take *silica*, 100mg daily (see Appendix 1).

Herbs and essential oils

• Deglycyrrhizinated *Licorice root* – 2g powdered root twice daily will bind to oestrogen receptors and prevent the accumulation of your own hormone. This is obviously not needed in men or menopausal women.

See III:24, Rheumatoid Arthritis, for arthritic herbs and essential oils.

Homeopathy

See III:24, Rheumatoid Arthritis for acute treatment.

III: *26. GOUT*

Gout is a type of arthritis associated with increased concentrations of uric acid in the body, which get deposited in joints and tendons, causing considerable inflammation and excruciating pain. The onset is usually sudden and acute in nature and normally affects a big toe. Fever and chills may follow.

Uric acid is formed from the breakdown of purines in foods such as meat, shellfish, dairy, eggs and beer. Usually there is no clear reason for the uric acid accumulation, but stress, lack of exercise and not enough rest are often associated. Alcohol is part of our vision of a typical middle-aged overweight gout sufferer, and the effect of imbibing is to prevent uric acid from being excreted through the kidneys. Some people simply produce an excessive amount of the acid and others with normal levels in the blood are unable to flush it from the system as they should.

TREATMENT

Hot epsom salt baths increase the elimination of uric acid through the skin. Use 1 cupful to a warm bath and soak for 20 minutes just before bedtime.

Diet

● Low protein. A vegetarian diet is of great value.
● Abundant vegetables. Garlic dissolves uric acid.
● Wholegrains such as brown rice, millet, corn, barley, oats and rye. Limit your wheat intake.
● Small amounts of nuts, seeds and pulses.
● High levels of water, juices and herbal teas to reduce the risk of kidney stones.

● Red sour cherries and all berry fruits are of special value. Cherries are best, as they very effectively neutralise uric acid and are antioxidant and anti-inflammatory to joints. Eat half a pound a day. Even canned cherries are beneficial, if fresh ones are out of season.
● Emphasise high potassium foods: dried fruit, avocado, banana, mango, nectarines, potato and tomato.
● The diet should be 80% alkaline-forming, as in the case of arthritis, which means largely fruit and vegetables.

Reduce

● Meat, dairy, eggs, poultry and fish to three times weekly. Avoid them totally in an attack. High protein diets increase uric acid synthesis in the body.
● Pulses – eat them only twice weekly as a protein source, as they do contain some purines.
● Mushrooms, spinach and asparagus.
● Fruit, as its sugar increases urate production.

Avoid

● All glandular meats, shellfish, mackerel, anchovies, sardines, herrings and yeast, as their purine levels are very high.
● Salt and spices.
● Gelatin, as it forms uric acid.
● Sugar and refined flour and everything made with them, as they increase uric acid production.
● Alcohol, coffee, tea and soft drinks. Beer is particularly high in purines.
● Fats.
● Added vitamin B3, as it competes with uric acid for excretion.

• Over-eating, and institute a weight-loss programme if necessary.

Juices
• Red sour cherry, fresh pineapple.
• Carrot, celery and parsley.

When in pain it is best to drink juices only.

Supplements of value
Adult doses:
• *Folic acid* – 20-40mg daily.
• *Vitamin C* – 500mg three times daily.

These reduce uric acid production by inhibiting the enzyme responsible.
• *Bromelain* and *quercetin* – 125-250mg of each, three times daily between meals. These inhibit uric acid as above, and have anti-inflammatory properties.
• *Vitamin E* – 400iu daily.
• *EPA* – 2g daily to inhibit inflammatory chemicals.
• The amino acids *alanine, aspartic, glutamic acid* and *glycine* all reduce uric acid.
• *L acidophilus* – 1 capsule twice daily digests uric acid.
• *Silica* – 100mg daily, dissolves uric acid crystals.

Herbs
• *Devil's claw* – 1-2g of powdered root three times daily.
• *Colchicum* – 10-15 drops of tincture hourly at first in an acute attack, and reduce to three times daily. This herb prevents inflammatory reaction.
• *Wild carrot, sassafras, germander, juniper, parsley, nettles, celery seed, buckbean, guaiacum* and *willow* are all specific to gout. Buy them as combination tablets, or make an infusion from two or three dried herbs.

Homeopathy
Dose 6c every 15-30 minutes until the pain reduces (10 doses maximum), and then 30c three times daily, if necessary.
• *Arnica* – if joints feel bruised or painful.
• *Urtica* – burning, itching pain.
• *Ledum* – slight swelling, but joints feel cold inside and are worse for movement.
• *Colchicum* – for chronic and acute forms of gout, tearing pain which is worse at night and worse for motion. This remedy is also for the effects of overwork or hard study. The person is depressed, irritable, peevish and feels nauseated from smells
• *Benzoic acid* – use this if colchicum fails and if highly-coloured or brown offensive urine is a feature. Worse for motion. Right foot is usually affected, pain moves from right to left foot. This is predominately a right-sided remedy, worse for motion or standing.
• *Bryonia* – right-sided tearing pain, worse for motion, better for rest. Person is lean and irritable.
• *Lycopodium* – right foot hot and left foot cold. Right side worse, and symptoms worsen from 4- 8pm, but it may not improve until much later in the evening. Better for motion. Person is overweight and has digestive problems.

Many gout sufferers fit lycopodium in a constitutional sense. If this is the case, a permanent cure may be effected with the remedy.

III: *27. HERPES SIMPLEX*

A highly infectious viral condition which can cause intense pain. There are two types: Simplex I affects the mouth and Simplex II affects the genitals. Once infected, the virus often lives in the roots of nerves and is reactivated whenever ideal conditions prevail. The herpes virus takes over nerve cells by actually reprogramming their DNA so that the nerves will then obey viral direction, should the immune defences drop low enough for it to emerge. Then multiplication occurs, and the characteristic blisters surface somewhere along the nerve pathway.

The herpes virus is initially transmitted by oral or genital contact or variations of both. After ten days of incubation it causes pearl-like blisters which then ulcerate. The condition may be excruciatingly painful in the first attack. Lucky people are over the problem in about two weeks, but in many the virus hides away in a nerve root.

It is believed that a calcium problem precedes a herpes flare-up because where low tissue levels of calcium occur, the cellular defences are reduced. One of the reasons that high levels of the acid form of vitamin C sometimes causes aggravation of herpes may be due to the vitamin's known effect of causing kidney excretion of calcium, when taken in high doses. It is the increased serum acidity which engenders the loss. Conversely, low levels of vitamin C can also trigger an outbreak, as this vitamin is needed to control the virus. Its acidity also increases calcium absorption from the gut. Clearly a balance is required, but the levels of vitamin C and calcium need to be high during a herpes attack.

Stress, overwork, a poor diet and inadequate sleep and relaxation all contribute to generally falling below par. This also reduces our defences against infection, and so a virus hiding out in a nerve root may surface time and time again.

Sun is another trigger, and this may also have something to do with low calcium levels. Vitamin D made in the skin as a result of sun exposure encourages the deposition of blood calcium into bone. Conversely, the heat of the sun gives rise to sweating and the consequent loss of minerals through the skin, calcium being one of them.

Treatments explained
Amino Acids
These are the fundamental constituents of all proteins. Two in particular play a central role in herpes: arginine stimulates growth of the virus and lysine suppresses it. The two amino acids are structurally very similar and yet have opposite effects. It is generally believed in scientific circles that the herpes virus doesn't recognise the difference between friend and foe and happily absorbs the enemy when it is offered. The two aminos actually compete for absorption from the intestines. L-lysine may be taken preventatively in small doses, which should be increased if an attack occurs. This treatment works like magic for some, but not for all by any means. It does not cure, it only prevents flare-ups. Manipulating arginine and lysine in a diet so that the lysine predominates is very helpful.

• *High lysine, low arginine foods* are as follows, in descending order: fish, chicken, beef, milk, lamb, cooked mung beans, pork, cheese, cooked beans, sprouted beans, brewer's yeast, shellfish, soya and egg.

• *High arginine foods* are as follows, in descending order: hazelnuts, Brazil nuts, peanuts, walnuts, almonds, cocoa, peanut butter, sesame seeds, cashew nuts, carob, coconut, pistachios, buckwheat, chickpeas, brown rice, pecans, wholewheat bread, oatmeal, raisins and sunflower seeds.

If you eat a high-arginine food be sure to balance it with a high lysine source. However, never eat hazelnuts, as their arginine content is more than twice the level of lysine in fish, serving for serving. For herpes sufferers, all high-arginine foods should be avoided, and a moderate-arginine food should be balanced by the intake of a high-lysine food. Basically, this means strict limitation of nuts, grains, chocolate and sugar, and eating of more fruit, vegetables, dried peas and beans and moderate amounts of fish, meat or dairy products. In addition, it is important to avoid getting sunburnt because besides the effects already discussed, it causes an adverse arginine-lysine balance. Added to the dietary changes, 1g of L-lysine may be taken daily so that its total intake will be at least 1500mg higher than the arginine intake. This should control the virus as long as stress-free health is maintained. Another amino acid, methionine, at the rate of 500mg daily is reported to be preventative.

Herbs

• *Echinacea* is a powerful anti-viral herb. It has an interferon-type action and is specific against the herpes virus. It also enhances the T-cell destruction of infected cells. If given in high dosage in the prodromal phase – when the tingling and tenderness is first felt – an attack may be aborted. An interesting case was recently reported, where a sufferer found that not only could he abort an attack but that the recurrence became less and less frequent.

One teaspoon of tincture hourly for a few doses, later reduced to two hourly, may abort an attack. If started when the lesions have already begun to erupt, the attack will be shorter and less severe.

• *Glycyrrhizin* is an extract from licorice root and inhibits viruses by deactivating their DNA and RNA. This occurs via the body's interferon production which licorice greatly enhances. The extract has been shown to irreversibly inhibit herpes simplex I.

• The South American herb *pau d'arco* is a powerful viral inhibitor, also having its effect by blocking viral DNA.

• *Kyolic*, an aged form of garlic, may block an attack if taken at first sign. The garlic can be consumed in large amounts, as it does not induce the side-effect of fresh garlic leading to stomach irritation, diarrhoea or headaches. Garlic's action against herpes is again the T-cell destruction of infected cells. Successful treatment has been reported with twelve capsules taken initially, and then three capsules four- hourly for three days.

TREATMENT
Outline

• Treat the symptoms.
• Shorten the attack.
• Prevent recurrence.
• Repair the immune system.

Diet

• Manipulate the lysine-arginine ration, as discussed above.
• Avoid all foods to which you are allergic, in order to strengthen your immune system.
• Good food sources of calcium are green vegetables and oily fish. Just one ounce of sardines contains 125mg of calcium.
• One tablespoon of flaxseed oil daily.

Supplements
Adult doses:
• *Calcium* – 1g daily.
• *Magnesium* – 1g daily, raises blood cal-

cium by its effect of putting more potassium into cells.

- *Vitamin C* – 1g two-hourly at first, and then reduce to 1g three times daily. Take it in the form of calcium or sodium ascorbate.
- *Bioflavonoids* – 1g daily.
- *Zinc* – 25mg daily as citrate or picolinate. This enhances immunity to prevent viral replication, and also regulates blood pH so that calcium is retained.
- *Evening primrose oil* – 500mg twice daily.
- *Vitamin B6* – 50mg daily, if outbreaks are related to menses. Take this vitamin for the ten days before a period begins.
- *Vitamins A, E* and *B-complex*, as well as *selenium* would enhance immune functions.
- *Lysine* – 1g daily as prevention. 2-3g daily in an attack. Take this half an hour before any protein food.

Herbs
- *Echinacea* tincture, 1 teaspoon two-hourly until improvement, and then reduce to 1 teaspoon four-hourly.
- *Licorice root*, 1 teaspoon of tincture three times daily, or 1g powdered root three times daily.

Celloids® minerals
- *Celloids® PCIP* x 1, two-hourly.
- *Celloids® PPMP* x 1, two-hourly.

Both are for pain and inflammation of nerves.

Topical treatment
See Herpes Zoster (III:28) for essential oils to use.

Homeopathy
Constitutional treatment is of benefit in preventing recurrence. The following remedies are for acute treatment, and the dosage is 30c, three times daily if necessary, for types I and II.
- *Nat Mur* – for pearl-like blisters on the lips that burn and itch. For large vesicles on the lower lip that are swollen or burn. A higher potency will often fizz away cold sores in a few hours, but only if a lower potency is already partially effective.
- *Rhus Tox* – works as well as Nat Mur. For red, itchy vesicles which are better for warmth and worse in bed and in cold or damp conditions.
- *Apis* – burning, stinging, red and swollen. Follows and precedes Nat Mur well.
- *Capsicum* – genitals burning or stinging, burning blisters on the tongue, ulcerative eruptions on the lips, and a red itchy rash on the face.

III: *28. HERPES ZOSTER (SHINGLES)*

This is caused by the same virus responsible for chickenpox. The condition is characterised by vesicles developing along a nerve pathway, usually on the face, head or trunk. The outbreak is preceded by severe pain, and some people suffer months of continual pain known as *post-herpetic neuralgia*, even after the rash has disappeared.

TREATMENT

Supplements
Adult doses:
- *Vitamin C* – 1g hourly as calcium ascorbate, dramatically reduces pain and healing time. The acid form may aggravate an attack.
- *Calcium* – 1g daily.
- *Magnesium* – 1g daily.
- *Zinc* – 50mg daily, as citrate or picolinate.
- *Vitamin A* – 25,000iu daily.
- *Brewer's yeast* tablets.
- *Bee pollen* tablets.
- *Vitamin B12* – 500mcg by intra-muscular injection, often causing dramatic relief within three days.
- *Vitamin E* – 1200iu daily. For those with hypertension, the dose needs to be started low and increased slowly.

Topical treatments of value
- Homeopathic *Hypericum* – 5 drops tincture in 1oz water.
- Homeopathic *Cantharis* – 5 drops tincture in 1oz water.
- *Tea tree oil* may stop it if applied early enough.
- *Peppermint oil* or *clove oil* are said to be effective.

Use the essential oils undiluted unless the skin is sensitive, in which case dilute with a few drops of oil, such as almond oil, before applying.
- *Betadine* solution.
- *Spinifex* sprayed on – this is an Australian Bush Flower remedy.
- *Vitamin E*, massaged into the root of the affected nerve for ten minutes, and then heat applied, is effective for post-herpetic neuralgia.
- *Zinc sulphate* solution – 0.025%.

Homeopathy
Dose 30c two–hourly and reduce frequency as symptoms improve.
- *Apis* – stinging and burning like a bee sting, better if using ice packs.
- *Arsenicum Alb* – restless, anxious and exhausted. Pain worse between midnight and 2am, better if using a hot flannel. Good for post-herpetic neuralgia as well.
- *Ranunculus B* – for herpes on the chest (intercostal neuralgia). The pain may be relieved in 20 minutes. Nerve pain and itching which is worse with the lightest touch or movement.
- *Mezereum* – severe pain, burning and itching. Worse when moving, in cold or at night.
- *Iris V* – for herpes zoster associated with gastric upsets. Worse during evening or night or rest, better for movement.
- *Rhus Tox* – blisters which are itchy. For herpes in the young. Better for warmth and movement.
- *Variolinum 30c* – three doses twelve hours apart as prevention, for those who have been in contact with chickenpox or shingles.

Post-herpetic neuralgia
- *Vitamin E* – 1200iu daily.
- *Calcium*, *Magnesium* and *Zinc* – as above.
- *B-complex* – 50mg twice daily.

Homeopathy
- *Gelsemium* or *Colocynthis* for post-herpetic neuralgia of the face or head.

III: *29. M E – Myalgic Encephalomyelitis*

This condition is known by a variety of names, such as post-viral fatigue syndrome, chronic fatigue syndrome, yuppie flu and chronic Epstein-Barr virus syndrome. Years back, the condition was called Royal Free disease because in the fifties M E struck down many of the staff at this London hospital and left them with the chronic symptoms for a long period.

The cause of M E is still disputed. A few still label sufferers as 'neurotic' but most now accept that there is an immune system association. The cause of the lowered immune response is hard to pin down at times. In some people there is evidence of previous infection, and it is assumed that the virus was not completely destroyed by the immune system, so that particles remained dormant in cells. When the host becomes weak, those viral components can re-awaken and start replicating, and the condition becomes active again. In some people a slight fever is present for a year or more and others never have any.

The *Epstein-Barr virus (EBV)*, which is part of the herpes group, is a prime suspect. Antibodies to EBV, coxsackie-B or cytomegalovirus are frequently found in people with M E. Viral particles are also often isolated from muscle tissue. By the time of adulthood, most people have been infected with EBV without ever knowing it happened. The virus hides in the salivary glands, and the B-lymphocytes of the immune system. EBV is highly infectious and is easily spread, since it is stored in the mouth. It is possible to pass it on for six months after an acute infection is over, and those who have been infected without experiencing symptoms will not know that they are infecting others.

Coxsackie-B viruses are entero-viruses which are found in the gastro-intestinal tract of a high percentage of M E patients. They are also the most common viral particles found in the muscles.

Cytomegalovirus infections produce similar symptoms to EBV, except that the throat and lymph glands in the neck are seldom affected, and an older age group is normally involved – 20-30 year olds.

Flu viruses may predispose to M E, and there is evidence that the rubella virus used in vaccinations lies dormant for years before being triggered and passed to others. American research indicates that it produces symptoms similar to EBV, and the severity of the symptoms relate to the number of rubella antibodies.

The immune system, stress and M E

There is a definite connection between the immune system function and the mind. We know that white blood cells have receptors for brain messages, and that the immune system can in turn communicate with the brain by means of hormone messages. This means that *distress or happiness in the mind are felt by the immune system, and have the effect of depressing or stimulating it.* In turn the immune system can complain to the brain if its function is reduced. Therefore our coping skills, attitudes and emotions can profoundly affect the cells of the immune system. Relaxed, stress-free individuals have an increased immune function, and the reverse occurs in those who do not mount an adequate response to life's problems. The emotions of the mind are transferred to the immune cells by endorphins, and in turn T-cells manufacture lymphokine messengers and endorphins that are believed to carry emotional messages to all parts of the body as well as the brain. If we are depressed or tense, every cell in the body will feel it.

M E people are usually high-achievers, in that they drive themselves hard and do not take adequate rest. At any level of society one can be a high-achiever and it is not only the highly ambitious over-worked executive who is at risk. Housewives with punishing schedules are just as likely to develop M E. Women who hold down a job at the same time as running a home and caring for children are often on overdrive, because there is no chance of relaxation in the evening, as the needs of the family cannot be put aside.

The key ingredients for stress-induced M E seem to be overtaxing the body and mind, a constant mental drive to keep going, and ignoring the body's demand for rest. It is the inappropriate response to stress which is at fault. Whenever we are working under pressure, a point is reached where the body demands rest. For those who consistently ignore this fatigue level and push themselves into overdrive, ill-health and the breakdown of adaptation systems will eventually occur. Where no viral connection is found in M E, a driven personality is usually a factor, and this alone can weaken immune response to the extent that extreme fatigue develops. When stress is present over a long period, the adrenal glands release corticosteroid hormones to produce extra energy. However, these same hormones also depress immunity because this function is not necessary in the stress-control process. When this happens, dormant viruses within the body can again become active and external ones can readily get a toe-hold and start breeding. It may be that a high percentage of M E cases have no viral association

until after their immune systems have been severely compromised by long-term over-achievement. Often these individuals fail to even recognise the difference between what they can safely achieve and what they intend doing.

Stress and/or viral activity can debilitate an individual for years once M E becomes a reality. Many of the classic symptoms of stress are a major feature of M E. For instance, a person close to the exhaustion stage of stress no longer conserves sodium. This leads to blood-vessel constriction in order to try to maintain normal blood pressure. Poor tissue oxygenation and a lactic acid accumulation follow. Lactic acid causes severe muscle pain, anxiety, tension, irritability and depression, all of which are major symptoms of M E. Treating the adrenal glands relieves many of the debilitating symptoms of this condition, including low blood pressure.

In addition to a viral or stress-induced immune suppression, one or two of the following are usually present before M E develops. A poor diet deficient in nutrients, heavy metal accumulation, candida or toxic bowel conditions, persistent upper respiratory tract infections, hormonal imbalances, allergies or emotional upsets. Any one of these conditions may be the direct result of over-taxing oneself and not taking time to eat nutritious meals. Good quality food is essential to help anyone through periods of high pressure.

Vitamin B12 and M E

Recent studies carried out in UK, Australia and USA have all indicated that M E is associated with increased levels of malformed red blood cells (RBC) in the blood. Vitamin B12 injections often reduce these, and the decreased levels are associated with a marked improvement in M E symptoms. In all the studies carried out, approximately 50% of the subjects experienced symptom and blood-picture improvements; the remaining people responded with neither red blood cell changes, nor symptom relief.

Vitamin B12 is vital for the proper formation of blood cells. Healthy red cells contain adequate amounts of haemoglobin, which carries oxygen to all parts of the body. Many seemingly healthy people get occasional B12 injections in order to boost their energy levels and it may be that the treatment works because their fatigue is due to an excess of faulty RBC.

Classic symptoms of M E

Fatigue which is not relieved by rest is the chief complaint and may be so severe that a person is totally bed-ridden and unable to even get up and dress, let alone prepare food or do any work. Others can work for part of the day and must rest frequently. The fatigue remains constant to a greater or lesser extent.

Muscle aches are associated with fatigue, and climbing a flight of stairs may cause severe muscle pain. It may also put a person to bed exhausted. Sometimes muscles only hurt at rest, and others feel pain whilst walking around, so that normal activity is made difficult. Joint pains may also be a feature.

Headaches are a common symptom which vary in severity, and the alteration of sleep patterns can be quite debilitating. Many cannot sleep at night and suffer nightmares and night sweats. Poor concentration, very poor memory, fuzzy-headedness, mood-changes, deep depression and anxiety are frequently present.

Low-grade infections are common, with sore throats and swollen glands being the most usual. Ringing in the ears, hearing that comes and goes, and poor sight may also develop.

Poor appetite is quite usual, and some complain of eating causing the whole body to become very cold. Pallor and poor thermo-regulation are a usual feature of M E, with marked coldness of hands and feet. Digestive upsets such as nausea, foul-smelling stools, diarrhoea or constipation are common. Digestion is reduced in stressed people, and if this is a constant feature over a long period, the colon becomes very toxic indeed. Many people with M E also have candida – this is partly due to lowered immune surveillance, which allows fungus to proliferate freely. Nervous disturbances like palpitations, twitches, dizziness and pins-and-needles often occur at various stages.

Those who have suffered long-term stress will recognise many of the above symptoms, albeit in less severe form. Not every M E person will suffer from all the classic conditions and some will be less severe that others. However, the diagnosis is often clear from symptoms alone, and blood tests just confirm the suppression of the immune system and the presence of viruses or antibodies.

The condition is curable but it usually takes a long time and certainly requires the taking of a lot of supplements. The diet has to be of excellent quality, with everything whole, organic and varied in content. Each person must be looked at as an individual, as not everyone requires the same treatment. We all have our own biochemic individualities so that the needs of one will be different from another. This must be catered for if treatment is to be successful. The body as a whole must be repaired, so that every organ functions optimally. A sluggish liver unable to detoxify adequately or a toxic bowel repoisoning the system would prevent a return to health.

The mind, emotions and coping skills need to be evaluated, and every area must be restored to normal. Relaxation techniques or meditation must be learned and practised frequently. M E sufferers need to realise the importance of pacing themselves when health is restored. They should never try to do more than 75% of what they feel capable of, or they will further strain the adrenal glands. The 25% of extra rest allows them to recover their normal function. Skills must be developed for coping with emotional problems and for releasing pent-up stresses. Additionally, those with M E need to work on their attitudes so that they feel in control of their own lives rather than driven by them. The work load should be viewed as a challenge rather than a burden, and to this end everyone needs to look at his or her own limits, strengths and weaknesses and work within them.

The body is a self-healing organism if it is given the ingredients to work with. To this end, all treatment is aimed at removing whatever is harmful and supplying the necessary ingredients, be they nutritional, spiritual or emotional. No two people will be treated in the same manner.

Professional assistance is *always* necessary for the treatment of M E, as many aspects need to be dealt with concurrently. Detoxification, liver support and candida treatment may be needed in addition to anti-viral and immune-enhancing nutrients.

TREATMENT
Outline
- Detoxify the body and support liver and adrenal function.
- Correct the diet.
- Support the immune system and use anti-viral medication if necessary.
- Treat any underlying infection or candida.
- Check for allergies to foods, as avoidance of allergens strengthens the immune system and improves wellbeing.
- Learn techniques for future stress-control.

Detoxification
A period of juice fasting may be necessary if the body is very toxic. The length of time is determined by the strength of the person, but usually the diet outlines will be adequate with occasional 2-3 day juice fasts.

Lymph drainage improves the body's ability to cleanse the tissues. Exercise achieves this by the movement of muscles against the lymph vessels. Those with M E cannot do aerobic exercise until well on the road to recovery, but as soon as possible they should take gentle daily walks and do passive muscle exercises for fifteen minutes every day. Postural drainage and remedial massage also help, as does dry skin brushing followed by hot and cold showering. The hot should be on for three minutes followed immediately by thirty seconds of cold water.

The blood and lymphs can be cleansed with a variety of herbs such as *echinacea*, *burdock root*, *red clover*, *yellow dock* and *devil's claw* (harpagophytum), and the blood-flow to the spleen is enhanced with *barberry* or *golden seal*. Improved splenic blood-flow increases the release of immune factors such as macrophages, and the golden seal increases their function.

Liver detoxification can be achieved with juices such as lemon, grapefruit, greens and beetroot. Dandelion, golden seal or artichoke tea increase liver function and the herbal extract silymarin protects and regenerates the liver. Coffee enemas have a rapid effect on the liver, by causing it to dump its toxic load into the intestines. A liver and gall bladder flush can also be achieved with three days of olive oil and lemon juice dosing, 2oz of each at bedtime, and an enema on the fourth morning, followed by a retention coffee enema. After this liver-detox juices or dandelion tea should be taken daily.

Bowel toxicity is dealt with in chapter III:7 on Bowel Toxaemia, but acidophilus, fibre, garlic and the herb sarsaparilla, golden seal and walnut all play their part in cleansing the colon. Enemas and colonic irrigations are valuable in detoxifying M E patients.

If heavy metal accumulation is confirmed by hair analysis, chelation with nutritional supplements should be carried out over several months.

Again I must stress that professional guidance is essential, as not everyone needs the same treatment.

Diet

If candida is deemed to be present, follow the candida diet outlined in chapter III:8, but if yeasts, moulds and ferments do not need to be avoided, the following is much less restrictive.

- Vegetables and fruit in abundance, and as much in the raw state as possible, especially garlic. Green vegetables contain natural sodium for those muscle aches.
- Sprouted seeds, nuts, grains and beans in abundance – raw.
- Fish, lamb, lamb's liver/kidneys.
- Vegetarian protein – pulses, wholegrains (wheat, spelt, quinoa, rice, oats, barley, rye), nuts and seeds. Combine these correctly to make whole protein.
- Low-fat yoghurt or cottage cheese in moderation.
- Olive oil or sesame oil for dressings.
- 2-3 pints liquid – spring water, herbal tea.
- Seaweeds for minerals.
- All food should be fresh and not tampered with by man or machine. It should also be organically-grown as far as possible.
- Eat as much food in its raw state as possible – high intake of raw vegetables and sprouted produce.

Avoid

- All sugar and all white flour and everything made from them – jam, biscuits, cakes, white bread, crackers, jellies, pickles, sauces, preserved fruit, frozen or canned vegetables.
- All canned or packaged or processed food.
- Tea, coffee, carbonated drinks, squashes, alcohol.

- All flavourings, preservatives, additives, artificial sweeteners.
- Breakfast cereals with sugar and all other processed cereals.
- All cured, smoked, preserved or pickled meats.
- Irradiated or microwaved food.
- Milk and cheese – use butter sparingly.
- All oils, except cold-pressed polyunsaturates, olive or sesame. No roasting or frying.
- Salt.
- Foods to which you are allergic.

Menu choices

Breakfast

- Oatmeal, rice or flaked millet as porridge.
- Home-made muesli – millet, rice, soya, wheat flakes, oatmeal and rye with nuts, seeds and dried fruits. Serve cereals with soya milk, yoghurt or nut milk. No sugar.
- Eggs and wholewheat toast.
- Wholewheat pancakes.
- Fruit, yoghurt, chopped nuts and wheatgerm.
- Dilute fruit juice – homemade.
- Herbal tea, spring water.

Snacks

- Seeds, nuts, yoghurt, fresh fruit, crudities.

Lunch

- Salad and cottage cheese, or an omelette.
- Salad and dishes made from pulses, tofu, rice, millet, barley, or soya.
- Baked potato and salad.
- Home-made soup, salad and home-made bread.
- Sprouted produce every day.
- Dress salads with olive oil and lemon juice, and use a very wide range of vegetables.

Dinner

- Fish, especially salmon, mackerel, sardines, trout.
- Free-range poultry with no skin.
- Lamb or lamb's liver/kidney.

- Vegetarian protein, by combining pulses and grains or nuts.

Serve these with lightly steamed vegetables and a side salad. Avoid potatoes and bread at the same meal as meat. No roasting or frying.

Immune system supplements
These also support the adrenal glands.
- *Beta carotene* – 6mg daily.
- *Vitamin C* to bowel-tolerance, for its anti-viral effect. 10g daily is the minimum.
- *Vitamin E* – 200-400iu daily.
- *Selenium* – 100-200mcg daily.
- *Zinc* – 15mg as citrate daily.
- *Manganese* – 5-10mg daily.
- *B-complex* – 50mg daily (B6 as P-5-P).
- *B12 injections* from your doctor or naturopath.
- *Calcium/Magnesium* – 250mg of each daily as citrate, aspartate, or amino acid chelate. Higher doses of magnesium as citrate or aspartate should be tried to see if fatigue and neurological and muscle symptoms improve.

Many companies make a multi-formula covering some of the above in similar dosage.
- *Evening primrose oil* – 500mg times three daily.
- *Béres Drops Plus* – stimulates immune function.

Other supplements
- *Celloids® SP* (see appendix 1) – if sodium loss has caused muscle pain and increased emotional disturbance. Low blood pressure in M E patients indicates a need for this form of sodium.
- *Celloids® PCIP* – 1 tablet three times daily if there is a viral involvement.
- *Lactobacillus acidophilus*, daily.
- *Oxyplex* or another antioxidant enzyme product daily.
- *Calcium EAP* (discussed in chapter III:37 on Multiple Sclerosis) improves cell membrane integrity, so that viruses cannot penetrate. In this way, they are prevented from infecting healthy cells and using their energy sources for replication. *Evening primrose oil* also maintains the correct fluidity of cell membranes, as do omega-3 fatty acids found in oily fish and flaxseeds.

Immune system and anti-viral herbs
- *Shitake mushrooms, echinacea, golden seal, licorice* and *astragalus*.
- *Myrrh* or *wild indigo* may be needed with echinacea, for sore throats and swollen glands.
- *Yarrow, chamomile* or *boneset* tea may be used freely as immune stimulants.

Energy enhancement
This is done by providing nutrients to encourage normal energy production.
- *Potassium* and *magnesium*, 1g each, for improved oxygen usage, reduced muscle pain and increased energy, demonstrated in one clinical study to benefit 90% of people taking part. Many also need added sodium. A specific feature of M E is a heavy loss of magnesium from cells, to the extent that cellular defences are broken down. Those who are given regular intravenous injections of magnesium have experienced marked improvement in symptoms. As yet, it is not known whether oral doses are as effective.
- *Ginkgo* herb has a similar effect. Some of my patients have experienced enormous relief from mental symptoms after only a short period on ginkgo herbal extract. Ginkgo improves the circulation to the brain, and this helps memory and concentration, and relieves depression and fuzzy-headed feeling.
- *Coenzyme Q10* (CoEQ10) oxygenates the body, and this has a beneficial effect on energy levels. 50mg daily is normally necessary and benefits are not felt for a few weeks. Anything which increases fat-burning increases energy, so the amino acid carnitine is also of value here.

• **L-glutamine**, another amino acid, is very useful for improving brain energy, alertness and moods. Its added benefits are that it decreases sugar and alcohol craving and heals wounds. L- glutamine has also been successful in treating jet-lag.

• **L-tyrosine** is important in supporting the adrenal glands, and low blood pressure indicates a need for this amino.

• **Sleep** is an important part of increasing energy, and in M E the pattern is often badly disrupted. The taking of sleeping tablets is to be avoided, as drugs worsen the symptoms of M E in the long-term. Use relaxation techniques and taped music at bedtime to assist falling asleep. Vitamin B6 is involved in the REM part of sleep, and as some people do not convert it to the active form of pyridoxine-5-phosphate any supplement should contain B6 as P-5-P. A sleep after lunch is important as well, because this prevents over- tiredness at bedtime, which can in itself prevent sleep.

Lifestyle

Because people who develop M E tend to put themselves under pressure, it is important that they learn to pace their lives. Of course the illness slows them down to a snail's pace, but an eventual return to full energy levels may tempt some to go back to former driven habits.

Learn a relaxation technique such as autogenics, which can be taught in its simplified form in 15 minutes. A reflective measure such as meditation is also of great value. Usually the relaxation precedes the meditation, which should be done daily for 15 minutes or more. Autogenics involves some meditation, in that one focuses the mind gently on a particular physical reaction. The other advantage of this therapy is that it doesn't involve tensing and relaxing muscles. For many people the latter type of technique doesn't work, and for an M E sufferer with weak muscles it is a painful process.

Visualisation techniques can follow on from relaxation. Here you mentally travel to a sanctuary – a place where you feel safe, happy and at peace with yourself. Time in the sanctuary should be used for self-healing on all levels. There are many books on the market teaching these techniques, and some of my favourites are in the appendix section.

Exercise is very important, and in the first stages this will need to take the form of passive stretching or yoga exercises. Tight muscles must be relaxed, and the lactic acid build-up, which causes the pain, needs to be freed. As soon as possible, start going for short walks and build up to eventual aerobic exercise several times weekly when feeling well enough.

Deep breathing exercises daily are valuable for increasing the body's oxygen supply, which brings multiple benefits. Yoga breathing utilises a quick deep inhalation and a slow exhalation, whereby breathing out takes four times longer than breathing in. This is a very good way of calming feelings of stress, anxiety or anger.

For those who do not cope with life's ups and downs very well, certain skills need to be learnt. It is important to be able to view changes in life as an interesting challenge rather than a threat and it is vital that we feel in charge of our lives. Those who feel as though events or other people control their destiny have poor coping skills. All this can be changed by first accepting responsibility for oneself. In this way we become totally involved and passivity is not possible. A positive outlook equates with happiness and with being able to look forward to each day for bringing something new, exciting or rewarding. Counselling can help develop a changed outlook, as can meditation and visualisation.

Homeopathy

Constitutional treatment always helps, and should be combined with nutritional therapy. Homeopathy will assist the person's coping skills, and raise energy levels by assisting the vital force.

See chapter III:5 on Fatigue for some useful remedies to try, before seeing a homeopath.

Finally, M E is a multi-faceted illness, and a return to good health requires an initial acceptance of responsibility for one's own recovery. All the aspects outlined above need to be dealt with, and a supportive family is of great value here, because in the initial stages assistance is necessary on every level.

III: *30. CARDIO-VASCULAR DISEASE (CVD)*

Earlier in the century it was discovered that cholesterol clogged up blood vessels and led to CVD. For this reason it was assumed that cholesterol *per se* caused the problem, and so processed oils and margarine came into vogue. However, in the past two decades it has become clear that our cholesterol intake is not the cause of atherosclerosis (degeneration of arteries), as our consumption has not changed since the beginning of the century. Other things in the diet have changed markedly, and it is these which are responsible for causing cholesterol to stick onto the linings of blood vessels. The prime changes have occurred as follows.

• *Sugar* consumption has increased phenomenally, and that is readily converted to cholesterol and triglycerides.

• *Grains* are processed so that the vitamins and minerals are stripped out and only the white starch is eaten. Refined flour causes an imbalance in the protective essential polyunsaturated oils and is also converted to cholesterol and fatty acids.

• *Total fats* have increased dramatically because large amounts of processed oils and margarine are used. These are hidden everywhere in processed and fast foods, as is sugar. The statistics indicate that during the twentieth century, milk and butter consumption has been reduced by approximately 60%, meat and cheese raised by 300%, but the cholesterol intake has experienced a 0% change. The downside is that margarine use is up 900%, shortening 200% and oils a whopping 1200%. Most of those oils are bought processed because the public doesn't know the danger. We have been lulled into a false sense of security by the word *polyunsaturated*. These oils are essential to the body but only if *unprocessed*, otherwise we convert them, as well as excess sugar and processed grain, to cholesterol and triglycerides for storage.

• *Stress* levels are higher, and this raises serum cholesterol as well as interfering with oxygen supplies to the heart. Alcohol consumption has also risen a lot and an excess certainly increases cholesterol levels independently of food intake.

• *Chlorination of water* has become widespread, and it causes the destruction of vitamin E which is cardio-protective.

It has been said that the rate of CVD is climbing at the same rate as the increase in sales of processed oils and margarine and the spread of water chlorination. In Asia, where the traditional diet protected against CVD, the incidence is climbing dramatically as western fast foods and processed convenience products are introduced. Additionally, many Asians have moved towards a Western breakfast, eating either fried bacon, eggs and sausages, or sweet white bread and soft drinks instead of the traditional rice congee and Chinese tea.

Western diets are associated with CVD, with high levels of meat, dairy products and omega-6 fatty acids (from margarine and processed oils). Traditional Northern Asian diets have high levels of omega-3 fatty acids (oily fish) which protects against CVD.

Causes of CVD

Modern medicine has targeted the following:
• Cigarettes, alcohol and caffeine, overeating and over-weight, lack of exercise,

stress and hypertension, high cholesterol, fat and salt levels in the diet.

Naturopaths add the following to this list:

• Sugar, white flour, processed cereal, processed oils and margarine, fried cholesterol foods and low fibre intake.
• Constipation.
• Toxic bodies with low levels of oxygen circulating.
• Exposure to toxic substances like lead and chlorine.

Water chlorination

In the 1960s a Dr J M Price in USA attributed the dramatic upward trend of CVD in the West to the introduction of water chlorination several decades earlier. He also noted that Japanese who moved to Hawaii, where the water was chlorinated, soon developed this 'Western disease' while their compatriots at home did not. Dr Price decided to test his theory by adding chlorine to the water given to one group of young chickens while another identical group acted as controls with clean water. Within a few months 95% of the chlorinated group had developed advanced atherosclerosis while the controls had no sign of the disease. Other studies have corroborated these findings – this is one of the compelling reasons for avoiding tap water. Governments now almost universally add chlorine, along with a cocktail of other dubious chemicals like aluminium and sodium fluoride, instead of cleaning the water with a natural substance. The householder then has to invest in expensive filters, distilled or mineral water if he wants to maintain his health.

Stress

Without doubt a primary cause of CVD is stress, which leads to a series of hormonal and chemical releases in the body. These constrict blood vessels, increase fat and cholesterol lev-

els in the blood, cause damaged blood vessel walls, atherosclerosis and thromboses – all of which directly result in CVD.

Studies which have investigated lifestyles in relation to heart attacks clearly show that where life is difficult, the death rate is highest. For instance, Eastern Europeans have a higher incidence of CVD than their Western counterparts. Happy, outgoing people who feel secure do not die of heart attacks or cancer. Another aspect is that these people also tend to lead healthy lifestyles, as they have smaller need for comfort-eating, drinking or smoking. Because they feel good about themselves, they also tend to exercise more readily and set aside time for relaxation.

A study involving rabbits and a high cholesterol diet highlighted the fact that only those who were picked up and stroked before being fed remained healthy. The rest developed atherosclerosis. This shows that the contented rabbits released 'happy' chemicals which sent out all the necessary messages to ensure that cholesterol was either not absorbed or was rapidly cleared through the gall bladder from the bloodstream. They did not release 'unhappy' stress hormones like adrenalin and cortisole.

Another study run by a Dr Dean Ornish in San Francisco involved 41 people with serious CVD. Half followed the standard orthodox advice and half changed their lifestyles and attitudes, at the same time as reducing total fats to 10% of calories. The individuals outside the experimental programme experienced a definite worsening of symptoms, whereas the rest not only dramatically lowered their cholesterol and decreased their angina attacks by 91%, but 82% of the group actually stripped the plaque off their blood vessel walls. These results were confirmed by scans and angiograms after just one year. No supplements were used but the diet was extremely restrictive, in that animal protein was reduced to one glass of non-fat milk or yoghurt, and oils and margarine were forbidden. The participants took part in meditation, breathing exercises, yoga and moderate daily exercise as well as discussing problems in a twice-weekly support group.

Dr Ornish believes that, as much as anything, the plaque reduced as a result of resolving emotional deprivations and imbalances, such as hostility, selfishness and cynicism. Many individuals reported feeling emotionally lighter and learning to love themselves and those around them. This study indicates that happiness resulted in chemical messages that instructed the blood vessel cells to release layers of cholesterol plaque. Remember that stress hormones have the opposite effect, damaging blood vessels and increasing cholesterol. Clearly, a happy heart can turn itself into a healthy heart.

Cholesterol

Only 10% of our daily requirement comes from food. 90% is made in the liver and intestines, from fat, sugar and protein, as we need a steady supply to be used as part of the wall of every cell in the body. The sex and adrenal hormones and vitamin D are also made from cholesterol and the skin is protected from cracking by a layer of it. In fact an adult may synthesise as much as 2000mg of cholesterol daily, depending on the food intake. The more that is eaten, the less the body makes. At any one time it contains 150,000mg of cholesterol.

Cholesterol sticks to blood vessels only if they are unhealthy, or if this fat is oxidised or not cleared from the blood as it should be. The oxidation of cholesterol in food occurs if it is overheated, as in frying meat, eggs or butter, or if antioxidants are lacking. So where does all that cholesterol come from, which is circulating in the bloodstream of those with high counts? Some quite obviously

eat too much saturated fat and others are heavily into processed foods, using margarine, shortening and oils. A diet containing these oils, sugar and white flour produces an excess of acetates, and this forces the body to form cholesterol in order to reduce the acetate level. So those 'cholesterol free' oils are converted to cholesterol in the body because they are of no biological use.

The essential polyunsaturated oils from *un*processed sources of oils are saved for vital function and are never converted to cholesterol. In fact, these oils actually *reduce* blood cholesterol levels. Studies indicate that avocados and walnuts lower cholesterol much faster than a low-fat diet. Oily fish and seeds do the same, and this is why evening primrose oil and EPA capsules are taken, to reduce cholesterol and triglycerides quickly and safely. A clinical trial reported in the *New England Medical Journal* (1993) indicated that when obvious fats were replaced with 3oz of walnuts, LDL cholesterol was reduced by 16.5%, and the HDL/LDL ratio markedly improved within a month. A different report stated that a group who had eaten avocados lowered their cholesterol by 9% in an equally short time, whilst those on a low-fat diet reduced cholesterol by only 2.6%. In 1993 the *British Journal of Nutrition* published the results of a four-week trial which proved that 50g daily of ground flaxseeds or 20g of the oil lowered total cholesterol by 9% and LDL by 18%, thus significantly improving the HDL/LDL ratio.

While some studies indicate that polyunsaturated oils will lower cholesterol independently, others have shown that the total fats must remain constant when polys are added, which means that the saturates must be correspondingly reduced. To be healthy always, aim for 50% fats in polyunsaturated form, and only 15-20% of total calories as fat.

Stressed people also have high blood levels

of cholesterol. This is because our response to stress is the secretion of hormones from the adrenal glands, which in turn release fats and cholesterol into the bloodstream for energy production. Unless these fats are burnt up in energy production for 'fight or flight' exercise, the excess remain in the blood. Unfortunately, most stress occurs in sedentary situations. A certain amount of extra cholesterol is needed for the production of adrenal hormones during long-term stress.

There have been a great many clinical trials reported where weight, alcohol, smoking and cholesterol intake have been reduced, and exercise raised, along with substituting fats with margarine and processed oils. These have failed spectacularly to reduce the incidence of CVD: in fact, most have reported an increased rate of death from heart attacks. The respected American medical publication *Journal of the American Medical Association* reported a fifteen-year study of 1,200 Swedish businessmen at risk of CVD. Half of them continued with their harmful diets and lifestyles. The other half lost weight, exercised, lowered their cholesterol and substituted margarine and oils for animal fat. Five years later it was noted that the second group was dying of CVD at twice the rate of the so-called 'unhealthy' group!

High-density lipoproteins (HDL), low-density lipoproteins (LDL) and triglycerides

Triglycerides form at least 90% of the fats we eat and most of the stored fat in cells. They are chains of saturates, monounsaturates and essential polyunsaturates in various proportions. Meat triglycerides, for instance, carry very few polyunsaturates, whereas flax-seed oil triglycerides are entirely composed of them. Triglycerides are our stores of all types of fats but an excess is associated with CVD. Sugar and refined carbohydrate are also partially converted to triglycerides if not used immediately.

Fats are carried in the blood by lipoproteins. If they were not anchored to protein, they would all float to the top and our brains would be full of fat! Triglycerides are transported by VLDL and HDL, and cholesterol by either LDL or HDL. LDL carries cholesterol towards cells such as muscle cells and those lining blood vessels, whilst the HDL carries cholesterol away from the cells to the liver and gall bladder for excretion. Therefore the HDL are the good guys and the ratio between HDL and LDL is very important – the higher HDL, the less the risk of CVD.

Studies indicate that if total cholesterol is high, there is less risk of CVD if the HDL is also raised because this indicates that the system for excreting cholesterol is working well. On the other hand a moderate total of cholesterol with high LDL is bad news, as it means that cholesterol is not being cleared to the liver. The more LDL in the blood, the more likely it is to be oxidised, and then cause atherosclerosis. LDL must be protected by antioxidants, otherwise free radicals turn it into the destructive type, which can then initiate damage to arterial walls and cause blood clots to form.

To raise HDL, exercise is important, as well as low alcohol, and a high fibre intake from whole grains (not wheatbran), vegetables and pulses. Studies indicate the following are also effective: EPA, olive oil, garlic, ginger, vitamin B6, vitamin B3, magnesium, selenium, chromium, and vitamin C and vitamin E.

As more and more nutritional research is published, it is becoming clear that the amount of cholesterol in the blood is not as important a factor as is the efficiency in controlling its dynamics. Where sterols (in beans and oatbran) and antioxidants are abundant in the diet, excessive cholesterol will be cleared from the blood quickly and that which remains will be protected from free radical attack. Consequently LDL is less likely to damage the linings of blood vessels.

Plaque formation

This is initiated by damage to the walls of blood vessels from free radicals, whose activity is promoted by such things as drugs, pesticides, radiation, excessive alcohol, tobacco, rancidity and oxidised LDL cholesterol. Free radicals are produced by the body's energy-production system but they escape to cause harm only if antioxidant minerals and vitamins are deficient. A quick feed of glucose to the blood as a result of a meal containing sugar and white flour will cause an insulin response, and this hormone also severely irritates blood vessel linings.

Once the blood vessel walls are damaged a fatty layer develops underneath the surface layer of cells lining the blood vessels. Oxidised LDL cholesterol from the bloodstream is the usual cause of this. Eventually, these layers are dislodged, and the platelets adhere to the damaged surface. These red blood cells then start sticking together in clumps, and release substances which trigger the formation of a rough fibrous layer of cells.

Cholesterol can now stick to a coarse roughened surface very easily. In time this becomes hardened with a layer of calcium, and atherosclerosis is a reality. The final step in CVD is that sticky platelets form a thrombosis, and completely block an essential blood vessel in the heart (coronary thrombosis), in the brain (stroke) or an artery supplying the legs. The process is insidious and even one year-old children show some lesions. Autopsies performed on seemingly fit

young men in the Vietnam war indicated heavy plaque deposition in 18-21 year-olds. Is it any wonder that half the world now dies of CVD?

The role of alcohol in this process is still not clear-cut. It is known that it can cause the initial oxidation of LDL cholesterol but on the other hand moderate levels appear to encourage formation of the HDL cholesterol that removes fats from arterial walls. Before cracking open another bottle, you should wait for the scientists to do more research in this area.

Homocysteine

This is converted to the amino acid methionine during protein metabolism and it is known to instigate damage to blood vessel linings (endothelium) if it accumulates. Where sufficient vitamin B6, vitamin B12 and folic acid are present in the diet, the homocysteine immediately goes through another conversion and no harm is done to the endothelium. Atherosclerosis will occur in those with circulating homocysteine even if cholesterol levels are normal. One study where autopsies where performed on 194 people with low cholesterol (and no diabetes or hypertension), indicated that 187 of them had died from atherosclerosis. Homocysteine damages the elastin in the walls of blood vessels.

Clearly it is important to maintain healthy blood vessels by avoiding poor quality food and being sure to eat food which supplies antioxidants and all other nutrients. Vegans have a low incidence of CVD, but vegetarians have the same risk as meat-eaters, because they tend to increase dairy products and not use nuts, seeds and pulses.

Sugar, flour, calcium, sodium, alcohol and coffee

Sugar, white flour and pretty packaged *processed cereals* break down into glucose very quickly and cause a rapid rise in blood sugar. Since the body maintains serum glucose within a very narrow range, any excess results in an outpouring of insulin from the pancreas and blood vessel damage occurs. Where there is an excess of sugar to be burned for energy, the energy-producing Krebs cycle in every cell overheats, so that acetates are formed. This situation forces the body to convert them to cholesterol and triglycerides, which are then stored in fat cells, blood vessel walls, the heart, kidneys and liver. These processed foods also cause the sticky platelets, which lead to more blood vessel damage and thrombosis. We are inclined to think of these foods as being just of no value, whereas they are actually extremely *harmful* in several different ways.

Calcium from poor quality sources, like pasteurised cow's milk, is most likely to harden cholesterol plaques. This milk also contains small amounts of xanthine oxidase, which once in the blood, initiates atherosclerosis. Better sources of calcium are oily fish, green vegetables, nuts and seeds. Raw untreated milk, because it is not heated, is a health product and still contains lipase for breaking down its fat content. Research has shown that people with heart disease have low levels of lipase in their blood because they use pasteurised dairy products and heated processed oils that have no lipase left intact.

Calcium will be leached from the blood in any situation which leads to an excess of phosphorus in the blood. It then circulates while waiting for transport through the kidney tubules and may stick to cholesterol plaques. Processed food, all meat and carbo-

nated drinks are sources of very high phosphorus.

Sodium in the form of sodium chloride (salt) added to food during cooking and processing depletes the vital organic sodium in the body. When this occurs, all parts of the body become acid and cannot function properly. At this stage body calcium comes out of solution and is deposited in joints and kidneys, and cholesterol is hardened onto blood vessel walls. Once the liver stores of organic sodium are depressed, the blood cannot be cleansed adequately, and there may even be insufficient quantities for bile salts, so that the bile becomes an irritant to the intestinal walls.

Organic sodium is abundant in a variety of fruits and vegetables, but it must be taken raw if this mineral is to remove acidity from the body and strip cholesterol off blood vessel walls, leaving them supple and healthy again. *Do not confuse vital raw organic sodium with the poisonous sodium chloride in your kitchen.*

Alcohol causes the body to make more cholesterol, because when several drinks are taken it causes the walls of cells to become too fluid and so extra cholesterol has to be inserted to maintain the norm. Once the alcohol intake ceases, the cell membranes become too stiff and so cholesterol is removed and put into circulation. Another down-side of alcohol is that it raises triglycerides. One glass of red wine at lunch and dinner is said to be protective, because it raises healthy HDL cholesterol levels. HDL clears cholesterol from the blood, and is also believed to strip free cholesterol from blood vessel walls. Furthermore, very moderate levels of alcohol are thought to enhance the process.

Coffee also raises cholesterol if more than three cups a day are consumed and it may be that the two go together. Even decaffeinated coffee has been shown to raise cholesterol and LDL – but not tea. In fact a French study of

Chinese tea discovered that *oolong* and *pu erh* teas could lower total blood fats by 25% in one month. In a study of coffees, 818 healthy men were divided into three groups, and for two months given either caffeinated coffee, decaffeinated, or none at all. Only those drinking the caffeine-free coffee experienced blood cholesterol changes – LDL levels rose, which means that something in the decaffeinated coffee is harmful.

Eggs

Eggs have high cholesterol! Let's put this in perspective. One egg has 250mg of cholesterol, whereas we synthesise about 1500mg a day within our bodies. Free-range eggs actually contain lecithin to emulsify fats, but battery-farmed ones don't, because the manufacturers of chicken-feed remove the polyunsaturated oils in order to prolong shelf-life. Fried eggs, though, are dangerous because the sizzling fat alters the structure of the cholesterol to a type that stimulates plaque formation. This is called oxy-cholesterol and it is the only type which stimulates atherosclerosis. The frying of meat or butter will also change their cholesterol content to the oxy- form.

One test involving 25 men with high cholesterol being given two egg yolks daily did not result in any rise of total cholesterol or LDL. In another test, where half a cup of egg yolks was given daily, there was an increase in cholesterol levels of only 9%. A third study of interest involved a group of people on a high-fat diet, who were given three eggs weekly for two months, and then divided into three sub-groups. The first continued as before, but for another five months, the second lot increased their intake to seven eggs a week, and the third group ate 14 eggs weekly. At the end of the five months, tests indicated that the blood cholesterol variations were slight, but identical in all three groups. Additionally, there

were no changes in the helpful HDL, or unfriendly LDL levels, and blood-clotting factors had remained constant. This very clearly shows that even two eggs every day have little effect on cholesterol levels and nor does it in any way increase the risk of CVD.

Another fascinating case was highlighted concerning an 80 year-old man who ate 25 eggs a day for 15 years and maintained normal serum cholesterol levels, along with no significant evidence of atherosclerosis. This case beautifully illustrates the body's adaptive ability, as the man was found to have increased bile synthesis and excretion, thereby quickly clearing blood cholesterol. He also had reduced cholesterol absorption rates from the gut. A diet high in sterols (beans and oatbran) will facilitate both these functions. It is also possible that this man was a contented stress-free person, and this alone caused his body to clear the unwanted cholesterol.

Some people carry a unique gene which enables them to devour large quantities of eggs with no serum lipid increase. However, the individuals taking part in tests are not in this category, as they are volunteers, or are chosen at random, and the uniform results indicate clearly that a modest intake of eggs does no harm. It should also be remembered that eggs are a near-perfect form of protein – but don't fry them!

Sticky platelets

This subject is mentioned under cancer (chapter III:38), but sticky platelets are equally destructive in CVD. Their aggregation is a part of the clotting process, which otherwise should not happen. In the case of CVD it does occur if the blood vessel walls have been damaged. Other causes are stress, lack of natural polyunsaturates, the presence of sugar and white flour, smoking and disease.

Substances found in good diets are preventative – garlic, oily fish, vitamin E and vitamin C, and evening primrose oil. The prostaglandin hormones made from EPA, fish and flaxseeds (PGE3) prevents sticky platelets and the constriction of blood vessels by one chemical path. The prostaglandins made from evening primrose oil and seeds (PGE1) has the same action via a different pathway. Evening primrose oil is said to be less effective alone, and should be combined with EPA. PGE2 made from the arachidonic acid in meat and dairy fat makes platelets more sticky, so you can see the importance of a balanced intake of these foods.

Sterols and fibre

Sterols are constituents of vegetable protein, and by competing for cholesterol-binding sites in the gut, they decrease food cholesterol absorption. Sterols are found in all dried peas, beans, and lentils, but especially in soya and alfalfa. Rice, oats, sunflower and sesame seeds, garlic, leeks, asparagus, beets, aubergine, blackberries and many herbs also have very good levels. Alfalfa has been found to actually shrink atherosclerotic plaque and reduce circulating cholesterol levels. Shellfish have high cholesterol levels, but some also have high sterols to ensure the cholesterol is not absorbed – these are clams, crabs and mussels. Lobster and prawns do not have this protection.

Another advantage of vegetable protein is that it lowers the ratio of lysine to arginine, which, in turn, reduces the body's synthesis of cholesterol. If the amino acid lysine is high, synthesis is increased. The soluble fibre found in oatbran and ryebran, pectin and guar gum removes cholesterol from the bloodstream to the liver and gall bladder. Whilst other fibre like psyllium seeds cannot do this, they have another beneficial effect of increasing the excretion of bile. In this way the cholesterol waiting in line can be more

quickly converted to bile for removal by the gall bladder and bowel.

Essential polyunsaturated oils

This means only those not processed with heat or affected by exposure to light and oxygen. They are very hard to buy in oil form, but easy to find in the food chain. It is only unprocessed oils and their food sources which have beneficial effects on the heart and circulatory system. Fish oils tend to be best for lowering triglycerides and the omega-6 oils have their greatest effect on reducing cholesterol. A veritable cascade of studies involving manipulation of fatty acids in the body have been published in the last few years. Here are the conclusions of some interesting studies.

- High-fat diets which include olive oil and garlic are found in countries with low CVD risk. The French fit into this category.
- High-fat diets with high levels of fish have very low levels of CVD. Eskimos on a traditional diet eat vast amounts of fat and very little fibre, and yet are free of most chronic diseases because of the extremely high omega-3 oil content in their fish. They ingest 14-15g of EPA daily and have low triglycerides, cholesterol and LDL levels.
- Meat increases blood cholesterol dramatically. Half a pound added to vegetarian diets increased serum cholesterol by 20%.
- Olive oil and garlic lower cholesterol and LDL in a diet with 30% of calories from fats. A high complex carbohydrate diet with 20% of calories from fat also lowered cholesterol and LDL. The Greeks have a low incidence of CVD and use garlic and olive oil daily.
- If the fat content is low, olive oil alone lowers cholesterol by 5%, and almond oil by 11%. Olive oil had no effect on triglycerides in this test.
- Trans-fatty acids (in margarine and pro-

cessed oils) raise LDL and lower the valuable HDL even more profoundly than does saturated fat. This is because the essential polys are blocked, and also because the trans-fatty acids adversely alter the competition between omega-3 and omega-6 oils.

• Boiled coffee raises cholesterol LDL and triglyceride, whereas changing to drip coffee lowers them. This was a study carried out in Finland. It is thought that filtering removes 80% of the cholesterol-raising substance in the coffee.

• 2,000 men who had a coronary were divided into three groups for a two-year study and the results were compared with those in a control group. Group A did no more than lower their fats to 30% of calories and experienced no change in mortality rate. Group B only increased fibre to 18g and had a slight increase in mortality rate. Group C ate oily fish twice-weekly and experienced a 29% decrease in mortality rate compared with the control group.

• Diets which contain food sources of omega-6 oils (*eg* sunflower seeds) reduce cholesterol and LDL, even though saturated fats are not reduced. HDL is raised at the same time. *If saturated fat is simultaneously lowered, the reduction of cholesterol and LDL is even greater*.

• A diet of salmon as a protein source reduced triglycerides by 75%, LDL by 26% and cholesterol by 27%. A diet of pollock also reduced triglycerides by 78%, but the LDL did not change, and the cholesterol was actually raised 19%. The interesting part of this study is that although both fish are high in EPA, salmon (like all EPA supplements) also contains DHA whereas pollock does not. Therefore the DHA may be more important than the EPA content of fish oils.

• Further studies indicate that monounsaturated oils (olive and almond) may raise HDL more effectively than polyunsaturates, and are as good at reducing the susceptibility of LDL to oxidation. It is also clear that olive oil is better than a low-fat diet in regulating cholesterol and reducing the risk of CVD, according to Dr M Werbach of UCLA in the USA, who has examined a wide range of clinical studies.

The results of more studies are as follows:

• Oatbran fibre, 7 tablespoons daily, reduce cholesterol levels by 13%. 6 tablespoons is ideal in the diet as maintenance but 12 tablespoons are needed to reduce cholesterol markedly. Those prone to gall-stones should not eat this much.

• With the correct diet, plus 200mg of nicotinic acid daily, blood cholesterol and LDL was lowered 50%. Even long-term plaque regressed.

• Low-fat plus exercise and stress-release led to plaque regression. This test used no food supplements.

• Vitamin C is the best antioxidant to blood vessels, and completely prevents oxidation of fat. It converts LDL to HDL and strips plaque from walls. In an earlier test vitamin C was thought to raise cholesterol, but it was soon recognised that serum levels rose, because plaque was being stripped off the walls of blood vessels!

• Vitamin E, 500iu daily, over three months, raised HDL 13.6%.

• Over the past ten years, scientists have been studying the French diet, because of the paradoxical association between high saturated fat levels and a low incidence of CVD. In fact, the French are second to the Japanese for the lowest rate of CVD in the world.

There are many aspects of the French diet which in naturopathic terms are cardio-protective. The quality of raw ingredients is always high – no bottled, packaged sauces, no fast foods, canned or frozen vegetables. Garlic is used liberally, butter in place of margarine, extra-virgin olive oil is the only one in a French kitchen – no trans-fatty acids from margarine and processed oils. Meat and vegetables are fresh and fruit and vegetables are eaten seasonally. Milk, with its plaque-stimulating ingredients, is not part of the diet even though cheese is eaten daily and butter used liberally. Of prime importance is the fact that, to the French, a good meal is to be savoured, which means that it is a social occasion, eaten in a relaxed manner and ample time is set aside. Additionally they eat only three meals a day with nothing in between and the main meal is eaten in the middle of the day.

The alcohol content of this nation's diet is what most puzzles scientists, but it is a fact that, like the Italians, the French tend to drink only with a meal – and this means wine of good quality. None of those chemical-laden varieties drunk by other nationalities from sun-up to bed-time. Red wine in moderation is known to prevent sticky platelets and to raise the healthy HDL cholesterol. Because it contains phenolic compounds, which are powerfully antioxidant, it also prevents the oxidation of LDL cholesterol, which means that the fat in the meal cannot damage the linings of blood vessels. 1-2 glasses with the main meal of the day is a moderate amount. The reason we steer clear of recommending alcohol is the fear that moderation will very easily become excess – and don't we all know it!

People who eat processed foods, drink milk and soft drinks, snack all day like cows, drink coffee, spirits and beer between meals, avoid garlic and use margarine and processed poly-unsaturated oils, rush their meals and eat a heavy meal only three hours before bed-time, would not be protected against CVD even if they did add wine to lunch. It is interesting to note that where people drink milk regularly, there is a higher than average incidence of

CVD, osteoporosis and arthritis.

Very low cholesterol

Because cholesterol is essential in so many ways, it follows that very low levels carry a down-side. A detailed examination of some of the largest clinical prevention trials indicated that lowering cholesterol did not improve survival. True, the incidence of heart attacks was reduced but total mortality rose due to deaths from cancer, accidents and suicide in the test groups.

The death rate from cancer was especially high in those using cholesterol-reducing drugs. A huge World Health Organisation study in the 1970s revealed that those using drugs to lower cholesterol actually had an increased death rate from cancer, rather than CVD. In fact the death rate in the treated group was 25% higher than in the control group receiving no treatment. The reason for this is that very low cholesterol levels lead to aggression and other mental disturbances, as well as an increased risk of accidents. It must be remembered that every cell membrane requires cholesterol, and if cells can't function correctly all manner of things go wrong. Very low cholesterol levels are found in criminals and those with a history of violence or suicide. One test showed that monkeys on a low cholesterol diet become very aggressive. Clearly moderation is important. Science is now warning doctors of the danger of lowering cholesterol with drugs.

Daily requirements of fat

26% of total calories as fat is considered to be the top level in prevention, but regression of plaque requires a level of 10%. Of this percentage, at least half should be natural poly-unsaturated oils (oily fish, seeds and pulses) and the remainder a mixture of saturated (coconut, meat and dairy) and monounsaturated (olive oil). In the 1800s, 40% of the fatty acids in our diet came from omega-3 oil (oily fish, flaxseeds, pumpkin seeds and walnuts). Now we take in a mere 3%.

A 2,000 calorie diet would have a fat content of 200 calories for a 10% fat level. Since 1g of fat yields 9 calories, only 23g of total fat is allowed. Of that, at least 12g in the form of EFA should come from oily fish, flaxseeds, sunflower seeds, sesame and pumpkin seeds or walnuts. A quarter pound of fresh salmon yields 5g of saturated and 5g unsaturated fat. A quarter cup of seeds yields 17-20g of oil, 14g of which is unsaturated, and one tablespoon of their oil contains 10-12g of unsaturated fat. One teaspoon of oil is found in any of the following: 3 pecans, 6 almonds, 1 walnut, 2 teaspoons of sunflower seeds or 2 tablespoons of wheat germ. Olive, peanut, macadamia, cashew, pecan and almond oils are 70 to 92% monounsaturated. They contain very little polyunsaturated oil. Sesame seeds and walnuts are 50% oil, of which nearly half is unsaturated. Pumpkin seeds contain 50% oil and 60% of that is unsaturated. Sunflower seeds are also 50% oil but 65% is unsaturated, and flaxseeds are 35% oil of which 75% is unsaturated. On the other side of the coin 1oz of camembert cheese contains 4.5g of saturated fat, 1 cup of low-fat cottage cheese 3g and one egg 2g.

TREATMENT
Supplements in treatment

• *Vitamin C* has a powerful antioxidant effect on blood vessels, and strips cholesterol from the walls.

• *Vitamin A* should be taken as its pro-vitamin, *beta carotene*, because it reduces fats in the blood more effectively. Beta carotene lowers the total cholesterol count, which means that VLDL, LDL and HDL are all reduced.

• *Vitamin E* suppresses arachidonic acid from meat and dairy products, and therefore a series of chemical reactions which cause atherosclerosis, thrombosis and hypertension. Daily doses over 250iu have been found to dramatically lower the incidence of CVD. Vitamin E will prevent the oxidation of LDL cholesterol so that it cannot attack blood vessel walls. In a US study involving 10 men taking 400-600iu of vitamin E daily, Dr J Balla and his colleagues discovered that, after only a few days, the LDL was no longer able to initiate a free radical attack on blood vessels. However, a reversal occurred if the vitamin was discontinued. Other studies have also shown that vitamin E penetrates LDL cholesterol and inhibits its oxidation.

• *Selenium* is needed as part of the antioxidant chain reaction.

• *Magnesium* is always deficient in CVD, and many a life has been saved by massive injections of the mineral at the time of a heart attack. Magnesium is necessary for the proper function of heart muscle and blood. In high doses it dilates blood vessels and therefore increases the flow of blood and oxygen to heart muscle. This mineral also reduces platelet stickiness and calms down any arrhythmia of the heart beat.

The famous German physician Dr Hans Neiper conducted a study with more than 150 cardiac patients. It showed that those with very severe CVD could recover their health and prevent all further heart attacks with high-dose magnesium combined with moderate levels of bromelain and potassium.

A Dr Gerhard Schumann in Germany repeated the study with 150 of his patients who were on the verge of heart attacks and not one person succumbed. At the same time in California, a Dr Garry F Gordon treated 700 patients over a two-year period with the same dose of magnesium and potassium and reported that less than 1% later suffered a heart attack. He described Dr Neiper as a medical genius. Where magnesium levels are high, more cholesterol is tolerated because this mineral helps control its dynamics. When we used to eat only whole foods which were grown on compost and animal manure, our magnesium levels enabled us to eat a lot more fat with no ill-effects. Artificial fertilisers have changed all that for the worse.

• *Calcium* reduces cholesterol by preventing its absorption. *Zinc* deficiency is associated with atherosclerosis.

• *Chromium* lowers cholesterol, triglycerides and raises HDL.

• *Garlic* and *onion* prevent sticky platelets, lower triglycerides and cholesterol, and raise the healthy HDL. The equivalent of 25g (6 cloves) daily has a powerful effect. Studies have shown a remarkable reduction in mortality in people who have had heart attacks and then started on regular garlic. Even 1g daily used in clinical studies has reduced the death rate by half, compared to controls using no garlic.

• *Silica* both prevents and reverses atherosclerosis. In a study where rats were fed a high-cholesterol diet and developed atherosclerosis, dosing with silica then stripped off the plaque lining the blood vessels. The rats given silica along with the cholesterol diet did not develop atherosclerosis. Silica is the most common mineral in the earth's crust but it is removed along with the fibre in food-processing. This mineral is an important cross-linking agent in connective tissue and is therefore important in blood vessel walls, where it also provides protection against free radicals. The daily requirement of silica is unknown but a good diet averages 200mg daily. No toxicity has been noted, even at 750mg daily.

• *Bromelain*, found in pineapple, is an enzyme which acts like a pipe-cleaner on blood vessels, thus removing cholesterol. It also prevents sticky platelets.

• *Lecithin* is made in the body from the B vitamin choline, the amino acid methionine, vitamin B6, folic acid, magnesium, potassium and polyunsaturates. It emulsifies fats and assists in removing cholesterol plaque.

• *Niacin* (nicotinic acid) inhibits cholesterol synthesis and reduces it markedly. The HDL/LDL ratio is improved dramatically. Triglycerides are lowered as well and the blood-clotting mechanism is normalised. 200mg daily is sufficient, and if more than 1g daily is taken long-term, liver enzymes need regular checking.

• *Vitamin B6* metabolises cholesterol and inhibits platelet aggregation. If it is plentiful, fat metabolism takes care of itself. If it is deficient, homocysteine prevails, and damage to the linings of blood vessels occurs.

• *Carnitine* is an amino acid which carries fat to be burnt as fuel. In this way it lowers cholesterol and triglycerides, and clears fat from the heart. This amino is normally stored in the heart, but when the oxygenation is poor, carnitine is lost.

• *Ginger* inhibits sticky platelets better than garlic and also lowers cholesterol.

• *Co-enzyme Q10* (CoE Q10) is necessary for energy-release and preventing free radical formation in the process. It also reduces the side-effects of beta blockers. Results will be noticed only after 6-8 weeks of supplementation. Scientists have found CoE Q10 in LDL (the undesirable type of cholesterol), and its function is to prevent the LDL from being damaged and then in turn harm blood vessel walls. For this reason, the ratio between CoE Q10 and LDL is maybe more important than the ratio between LDL and HDL in preventing CVD.

• Other substances which oxygenate the blood and tissues are *pangamic acid*, which is also known as *vitamin B15*, and the herb *pau d'arco*. Pangamic acid reduces hypoxia and athletes using it report greatly increased stamina.

• *Taurine* excretes cholesterol from the gall-bladder. It improves the heart status by transporting calcium, magnesium, potassium and sodium. Taurine is used to control angina spasm and prevent strokes.

The basic cardiac diet
Largely vegetarian.

Protein:
• Vegetable protein from soya and other dried beans and peas, nuts and seeds, lentils and grains (especially rice, oats, millet, corn, spelt and quinoa).
• Oily fish in small servings of mackerel, sardines, salmon, trout, or other fish caught in very cold water areas, three times weekly.
• Low-fat meat and eggs, in small servings infrequently.
• Low-fat dairy products occasionally, but not milk.

Extra fibre:
• Fibre from flaxseeds or psyllium seeds.
• Fibre from pectin foods: sunflower seeds, lemons, apples and bananas.
• Fibre from oatbran or ricebran – 1oz daily is enough.
• All the fibre can be added to breakfast fruit or muesli.

Carbohydrate:
• Two plates of vegetables daily, one cooked and one raw – use garlic and onions liberally. Red peppers lower cholesterol significantly.
• Whole grains and beans.
• Fruit for breakfast and between meals.

Essential fats:
• Nuts and seeds, especially walnuts, pumpkin, sesame, sunflower and flax seeds.
• Dressing of extra-virgin olive oil, lemon and garlic.

Wonder foods:
• Kelp tablets and seaweeds, for organic minerals.

• Spirulina powder for a potent blend of protein, vitamins, minerals, carotenoids, chlorophyll and vitamin B12.
• Sprouted nuts and pulses, especially alfalfa, supply mega-nutrients.
• Lecithin granules to emulsify fats.

Drinks:
• Herbal tea, ginger tea, grain coffee, mineral water or fresh pressed vegetable/fruit juice. Chinese *oolong* and *pu erh* teas. Fenugreek tea.

This diet is high in essential vitamins, minerals and enzymes. Keep fat to 15 to 20% of calories. 1g fat equals 9 calories.

Some natural sources
Vitamin B foods: nuts, seeds, whole grains, soya, brewer's yeast, wheat germ, fish, cantaloupe, banana, avocado, carrot, cabbage, tomato and green pepper.
Calcium foods: all green vegetables, fish, almonds and other nuts, seeds and seaweed.
Magnesium foods: soya beans, almonds and other nuts, brewer's yeast, whole grains, tofu, spinach, fish and seaweed.
Potassium foods: dried fruit, mango, banana, nectarines, pumpkin, avocado, potato, spinach, mushrooms, Brussels sprouts, carrots, broccoli, brewer's yeast. salmon and seaweed.
Sodium foods: kelp, seaweed, raw fish, celery, asparagus, Brussels sprouts, cauliflower, onions, beans, peas, courgettes, romaine lettuce, sage, water chestnuts, soya, coconut, watermelon, papaya, apple, lemon, banana, pineapple, peaches, strawberries, cherries, unpasteurised whey and yoghurt. These help clean up blood vessel walls and remove acidity, but they must be eaten raw to gain benefit.

See chapter III:34 on hypertension for the milligram values of these minerals in food.

Avoid

- Stress, over-eating and over-weight, alcohol (except for a glass of wine with the main meal), smoking and coffee.
- Sugar and white flour, and everything made from them. A very small serving occasionally is alright - binges and repentance are definitely not.
- Salt and high-protein meals.
- All processed foods.
- All margarine and oils that are processed using heat.
- High-cholesterol foods are to be strictly limited to low-fat varieties, or very small amounts – cream, butter, cheese, milk, meat or eggs – do not fry them! Even skimmed milk has been found to raise cholesterol synthesis via the casein component, not by fat. This does not happen with cheese.
- Shrimp, lobster and offal.
- Chlorinated water, as it destroys vitamin E and stimulates atherosclerosis.
- Soft water, as it lacks minerals.
- Heavy metals, aluminium pans, lead-glazed ceramics, tap water if the plumbing is copper or lead.

Juices

- Carrots, celery, red beets, asparagus, garlic, onion.
- Red grapes, black currants, rosehips, blueberries, pineapple, lemon, apple.

Supplements of value

The following are cardio-protective, and most can be found in a single tablet. Antioxidants A, C, E and selenium, with B vitamins, manganese and zinc as follows:

- Beta carotene – 6 to 15mg daily.
- *Vitamin C* – 1g twice daily.
- *Vitamin E* – 400iu daily. Start on 100iu and increase slowly if hypertension exists.
- *Selenium* – 100-200mcg daily.
- *Zinc* – 15mg daily, with *manganese* 5mg.

- *B-complex* – 25-50mg daily, to include B2, B3, B6 folic acid and B12 (the latter two in microgram dosage).
- *Calcium* and *magnesium* – 500mg each at bedtime, as citrates, aspartates or amino acid chelates. A daily juice supplies adequate potassium.
- *Flaxseed (linseed) oil* – 2 teaspoons daily.
- *EPA* – 1g three times daily, if not eating fish.
- *Lecithin* – 1 tablespoon daily.
- *Brewer's yeast* – 1-2 tablespoons daily for chromium and all B vitamins.

Herbs

- Hawthorn berry tea, as a heart tonic.
- Fenugreek and turmeric reduce cholesterol and triglycerides.

Exercise

This is most important for those who have suffered a heart attack or angina. It is the best means of prolonging life. Brisk walks should be gradually increased in length as a person becomes more fit. Swimming and cycling are very good forms of exercise. The exercise must be aerobic, which means that the pulse rate is kept at a constant level throughout. This increases oxygen in the blood and tissues.

Everyone has their own safe level of aerobic exercise and the way to determine it is as follows: take the maximum rate of 220, deduct your age, then deduct your resting pulse rate, taken over a one-minute period after sitting quietly for 15 minutes. Finally multiply this figure by 0.60, and then add the resting pulse rate, to arrive at a safe pulse rate which is also aerobic. This is in fact 60% of maximum, which also happens to be better than 80% of maximum when trying to lose weight. As you become more fit, the exercise of your choice will have to be done more quickly to maintain the 60% figure. The minimum time for exercise is 30 minutes three times weekly.

Stress release

Learn to meditate, do yoga or practise some other relaxation technique. Breathing exercises have significant value in halving the incidence of angina and heart attack. Take holidays frequently and make time for fun on a regular basis. Emotional problems and imbalances must be resolved in order to prevent insidious damage to the heart and blood vessels. Read chapter III:3 on Stress for guidelines in this area. Happiness equates with health and studies have proven that dietary indiscretions can be overcome by a body in which the cells are all sending and receiving messages of contentment. We are self-healing organisms but even this ability breaks down if the cells of the body are receiving anxious or depressed messages from the mind.

III: *31. ATHEROSCLEROSIS*

A disease of the arteries in which cholesterol plaque has developed on the inside of blood vessels. The process is insidious, and there are often no symptoms until a very narrowed opening is suddenly completely occluded by a thrombosis. This is most common in the small coronary vessels which carry nutrients to the heart muscle. As the deposits increase and harden, blood vessels lose their elasticity. Eventually the plaque may cause a blood vessel to burst as in a stroke or a ruptured aneurysm.

TREATMENT

Diet

Follow the basic cardiac diet and lifestyle recommendations (chapter III:30) with the following aspects emphasised:

● To remove cholesterol plaque, take lecithin, silica, zinc, sulphur, soya, sesame, iron foods, alfalfa, vitamin C, nicotinic acid, exercise and practise stress-release.
● To dissolve calcium deposits, take beetroot and grapefruit juice, apple cider vinegar and vitamin C.
● Natural sodium foods remove calcium deposits and keep them in solution: kelp, seaweed, raw fish, celery, asparagus, courgettes, Brussels sprouts, cauliflower, onions, peas and beans, romaine lettuce, sage, water chestnuts, soya, coconut, water melons, papaya, apple, lemon, banana, pineapple, peaches, strawberries, cherries, whey and yoghurt.
● Brewer's yeast, garlic, oatbran, ginger and lecithin.

Supplements of value

Take the same as for CVD, with the following additions if necessary – and use higher doses where a range is indicated under CVD. Try to find combinations of supplements to reduce the number of tablets taken. Not everyone requires all of the following: it depends on the severity of the condition. You could perhaps see how you get on with adding just silica and increasing vitamin C, EPA and garlic for a start.

● Increase *vitamin C* to 1g, 6-10 times daily, as sodium or calcium ascorbate – make up a solution to sip throughout the day.
● Increase *EPA* to 2g, three times daily.
● *Silica* – 100mg daily. This mineral is high in the lining of healthy blood vessels and absent in atherosclerosis.
● *Niacin* (nicotinic acid) – 100mg once or twice daily with food.
● *Chromium polynicotinate* – 100mcg, twice daily.
● *Bromelain* – 200mg, three times daily.
● *Garlic* – 1-2g three times daily, or a powdered equivalent.
● *Amino acids* – to chelate cholesterol plaque and clear it from blood vessels. *Methionine* – 500mg, *carnitine* – 250mg, *cysteine* – 500mg, *glycine* – 500mg, *glutamic acid* – 500mg. Take all of these twice daily half an hour before food with fruit juice.

Herbs
● *Hawthorn berries* – 0.5-1g, three times daily, dilates coronary vessels and improves heart function.
● *Ginseng* – 200mg three times daily, as a

tea.

• *Ginkgo* – 500mg three times daily, or 40mg of extract three times daily. This dilates peripheral blood vessels, increases serum oxygen levels, is a powerful antioxidant, prevents sticky platelets, is powerfully anti-inflammatory, contains high levels of flavonoids, speeds up the storage of information in the memory and increases concentration and mental ability – Wow!

Homeopathy

• *Baryta Carb* – 6c twice daily, for progressive senile confused state with high blood pressure or palpitations.

• *Glonoinum* – 6c, for pounding in the arteries and a congested headache.

III: *32. ANGINA*

This often occurs where atherosclerosis already exists to a marked extent and the heart cannot cope with extra demands, such as unaccustomed exercise. Usually a major artery is already at least 50% blocked. However it also occurs independently if there is cholesterol coating or as a result of spasm in the coronary arteries. The attack wears off as soon as the extra exertion ceases, whereas in the case of a myocardial infarction (heart attack) the pain continues. Cold weather, stress or over-eating can also trigger an attack.

Angina is characterised by a dull pain in the chest which radiates to the jaw and often down the left arm as well. Difficulty in breathing and a feeling of faintness is common. Treatment involves dealing with the atherosclerosis or coronary spasm as well as relieving the symptoms. It is vital to avoid encouraging sticky platelets, and to increase the oxygen supply to the heart muscle.

There is a wealth of evidence pointing to the fact that a heart attack is due to a lack of oxygen in the heart muscle. This can be the result of a clot forming in furred up blood vessels, which reduces the blood flow to the heart muscle. However, many reports in medical literature point out that clots have often not been found during autopsies on those who died of heart attacks. It is also true that many patients who have been referred to surgeons for by-pass surgery have been found to have no cholesterol build-up in their coronary vessels.

So what is causing the lack of oxygen in the hearts of these people? Again we come back to stress. When we are stressed the adrenal glands and nervous system constrict blood vessel walls, thus narrowing the opening. Additional to this is the fact that a stressful incident causes the release of many chemicals and hormones which can trigger a spasm of the coronary arteries. This shuts off the oxygen supply to the heart muscle and results in angina pain. Conversely hyperventilation in stress results in low levels of carbon dioxide in the blood, which then becomes excessively alkaline. This is another cause of coronary spasm because the oxygen in the blood cannot be used when carbon dioxide levels are reduced. When oxygen levels are low, the heart muscle has to use an anaerobic source of energy and this causes an acid build-up so that muscle cells cannot function and therefore die. This is thought to directly cause a heart attack.

A Dr B Keen, working from this angle, used an oral extract of the herb strophanthus on 15,000 of his patients over a 20-year period, and although many had already had heart attacks only 20 subsequently suffered another attack. Amazingly, not even one of the 15,000 had a fatal infarction. The herb restores the proper alkaline/acid balance in the heart muscle, which indicates that the tissues are being correctly oxygenated. This is probably why coenzyme Q10 and other oxygenators work so well in improving heart function.

Clearly it is very important to improve coping skills, so that responses to stress do not lead to coronary spasm. It is equally important to not feel like an invalid fearing another attack, as this emotion is stressful. People who are shown how to take charge of their lives through guidance on diet, exercise and stress management react positively. Those who undergo by-pass surgery don't, because the surgery is very traumatic and acts as a constant reminder of their mortality. By-pass surgery carries serious risks, is horrendously expensive and does not increase life expectancy.

TREATMENT
• Follow the cardiac diet and atherosclerosis dietary recommendations.
• Take regular exercise and practise stress-release techniques.

Supplements of value
Treat any atherosclerosis from the supplements suggested in chapter III:29. Choose from the following, which are especially recommended for angina, in addition to *antioxidants A*, *C*, *E* and *selenium* with co-factors *B-complex*, *zinc* and *manganese*:

• *Taurine* – 1,000mg twice daily.
• *Carnitine* – 250mg three times daily, to clear fat from the heart muscle. Take both of these half an hour before food, with juice.
• *CoEQ10* – 30mg three times daily, oxygenates and prevents attacks. It is deficient in 70% of angina patients.
• *Bromelain* – 200-400mg three times daily, to prevent clots.
• *Magnesium citrate* – 250mg, three times daily.
• *Potassium* – 2g, as 8oz of freshly-pressed vegetable juice.
• *EPA* – 2g, three times daily.
• *Garlic* – 1-2g, three times daily.

Herbs
• *Hawthornberriesubstitutesforcallingyour*
• *Black cohosh* tincture – 15-60 drops.
• *Bach Flower Rescue Remedy* – 4 drops in

a cup of water and sip frequently.

Emergency Homeopathy
Dose 30c every two minutes for 4-5 doses.
• *Cactus Grandiflora* – for an 'iron band' feeling around the chest, and pain which may also travel down the left arm. Cold sweats and low blood pressure. Worse lying on the left side.
• *Lactrodectus Mactans* – for severe chest pain radiating down the arm, rapid pulse, numbness in arms, body is cold.
• *Aconite* – fear of death and great anxiety. Rapid onset of stitching pains.
• *Arsenicum* – anxious and worried, with burning constriction in the chest, intense chilliness and thirst for sips only.
• *Lilium Tig* – a vice-like pain, the heart feels as though it is being alternately squeezed and relaxed. Pain in the right arm.
• *Glonoinum* – throbbing sensations, feels faint and has a fluttering heart.
• *Spigelia* – strong palpitations that can be seen by an observer; breathing is easier if lying on the right side.
• *Naha* – pains extend to the neck, left shoulder and down the left arm. An inordinate fear of death. Irregular pulse and low blood pressure. Pain in the forehead and the heart feels heavy.
• *Spongia* – bursting, swelling feeling in the heart. Can't lie down for fear of choking, rapid violent palpitations, numbness in the left arm.
• A mixture of *arnica* 30c, one dose, and *Bach Flower Rescue Remedy*, for shock, plus the appropriate remedy from above,

doctor, but will save a life while waiting for him to arrive.

III: *33. CHOLESTEROL REDUCTION*

TREATMENT

Follow the recommended lifestyle for avoiding cardio-vascular disease, paying particular attention to exercise, stress-management and dietary dos and don'ts. It is possible that supplements will then be unnecessary.

Diet

Follow the basic cardiac diet, and bear in mind that the following foods reduce cholesterol:

- Walnuts and pumpkin seeds.
- Pectin foods: sunflower seeds, lemon, apples and bananas.
- Fibre from flaxseeds or psyllium seeds.
- Oatbran or ricebran – 5 tablespoons daily, cooked or raw.
- Alfalfa sprouts.
- Dried peas and beans, especially soya.
- Onions, garlic and brewer's yeast.
- Oily fish.
- Corn, broccoli, beets, okra, carrots, red peppers, avocado, spirulina and seaweeds.
- Grains, soya, garlic and beets also reduce any excess cholesterol production in the body.
- Chinese *oolong* and *pu erh*, and fenugreek teas.
- Note that coffee, alcohol and diuretics *prevent* the lowering of cholesterol.

Supplements which lower cholesterol

- *Vitamin C* – 1g, three times daily, or more often.
- *Niacin* – 100mg, twice daily with food.
- *Vitamin B6* – 50mg, twice daily.

- *Chromium polynicotinate* – 100mcg, twice daily.
- *Selenium* – 150mcg daily.
- *Calcium* and *magnesium* – 500mg each daily, as citrate or aspartate.
- *Lecithin* – 1-2 tablespoons daily.
- *Zinc* – 15mg daily, plus *copper* 3mg (if low).
- *Evening primrose oil* – 500mg x four daily.
- Organic *iodine* – 300mcg daily.
- *EPA* – 1g daily is enough, if eating oily fish. This oil has a much more dramatic effect on triglycerides than cholesterol, although it markedly raises the healthy HDL.
- *Arginine* inhibits synthesis of cholesterol, along with niacin, iron, evening primrose oil and sulphur (sesame and wholegrains).
- *L acidophilus* daily, increases bile synthesis, thereby increasing cholesterol excretion.

Many of the above can be bought in a single supplement.

III: *34. HYPERTENSION*

90% of all cases of high blood pressure are described as essential hypertension because there is no single apparent cause. Only 10% of cases have an easily recognisable cause. Blood pressure is expressed in terms of the systolic pressure over the diastolic, *eg* 100/80. The top figure represents the contraction force of the left ventricle in the heart as it pushes blood into the arteries, and the diastolic pressure is that which remains in the arteries when the left ventricle is at rest.

The condition is rare outside developed countries, and is almost entirely associated with western diets. There is a rising incidence of the condition in Asia, as countries there adopt the worst of western eating habits, associated with increased salt, sugar, refined carbohydrate and fat. There is also a definite association between hypertension and low fibre intake, low levels of potassium, magnesium and calcium, and a lack of the essential polyunsaturated oils. Many people just accept raised blood pressure levels because they feel fine but this is foolish. It is always possible to feel well, up until the moment of a heart attack or stroke.

Blood pressure is controlled by the brain, the kidneys and adrenal glands and the autonomic nervous system. The brain secretes hormones from the pituitary gland, such as the anti-diuretic hormone (ADH), which prevents water loss through the kidneys, in order to maintain a high blood volume and so raise pressure if it drops. When the kidneys register a low blood pressure, they secrete a hormone which leads to constricted blood vessels and stimulation of an adrenal hormone which then increases sodium and water retention, in order to raise pressure. This also happens during stressful periods. Problems arise only in those who live under constant stress, as they produce these hormones continuously and so maintain an abnormally elevated blood pressure.

The autonomic nervous system has its effect on blood pressure by increasing or decreasing heart action and the tone of the blood vessel walls. Where the sympathetic and parasympathetic sides of this system are balanced, blood pressure remains constant. However, in the A-type personality, the sympathetic nervous control predominates so that blood vessels become constantly constricted and hypertension develops.

Blood pressure can alter through the day by as much as 30 points, and will always rise when a person is pressured, nervous, anxious or rushing for an appointment. It is often higher on awakening in the morning as well. Never accept a single reading as being an accurate reflection of your average blood pressure.

Consistently high blood pressure is of considerable concern because of the insidious damage it does to the brain, heart and kidneys. The arteries in the brain are particularly vulnerable to increased pressure, as they are not protected by surrounding muscle tissue and can therefore rupture easily, causing a stroke. The kidneys too are very vulnerable, as a constant high pressure of blood in the vessels supplying them causes thickening of the small arteries. This narrows the blood vessels, and in response the kidneys further raise the blood pressure in an effort to increase the supply of blood.

A persistent systolic pressure over 160 or a diastolic pressure over 95 is classified as dangerous in relation to long term health, and must be lowered. Where the diastolic pressure is high, fluid in the tissues cannot return to the venous end of the circulatory system, and so fluid retention occurs. Taking diuretics only relieves the symptoms, which will return when the diuretic drug or herb is stopped. The best way to permanently relieve the symptom is to lower blood pressure through diet, exercise and stress-release techniques.

Fats
See chapter II:6 on Fats versus Oils.

High levels of fats, processed oils and margarine inhibit the essential polyunsaturated oils from controlling tissue hormones called prostaglandins (PGs), which in turn regulate blood pressure. A balance between the various types is very important, and in the case of hypertension the PGE1 and PGE3 series are too low. Formation of these prostaglandins is blocked more by processed oils and margarines than by saturated fats. Although the latter must be used very sparingly, processed oils and margarines should be totally avoided. Instead, olive oil can be used for dressings and cooking. It should be noted that aspirin has been shown to prevent dietary control of prostaglandins and, by extension, prevent the control of blood pressure by natural means.

PGE3 is provided from flaxseed oil or oily fish (omega-3 oil), and *PGE1* is made from most seeds, walnuts and evening primrose oil (omega-6 oils). Many studies have indicated that omega-3 oils will not only lower high blood pressure but even lower normal pressure. However, quite high amounts are needed. Tests indicate that 10g daily of the fish oil extract EPA is necessary for any appreciable lowering of the blood pressure, if it

is the sole method used. Prevention is provided by a small serving of oily fish three times weekly.

PGE2, which is made in the body from meat and dairy products, causes sodium and water retention and constricts blood vessel walls to raise blood pressure. Conversely a diet rich in oily fish increases urinary output by 10%, as it acts like a low-sodium diet. This is a very good reason for following a largely vegan diet, with oily fish being the only animal protein.

Sugar and refined carbohydrate

Sugar, white flour and other processed grains and cereals are intimately involved in hypertension and have also been shown to cause an unhealthy reversal of the cholesterol HDL/LDL ratio. Certainly hypertensive individuals often display a refined carbohydrate intolerance, which can be picked up by Kraft's glucose-insulin test – this is at least 50% more accurate than the more commonly-employed glucose tolerance evaluation, so make sure that you get the best available test done.

Studies have indicated that hypertensive patients have high levels of insulin in their blood, which indicates a blood sugar problem. This usually only occurs in diabetics and obese individuals. Insulin initiates damage to blood vessel linings so that cholesterol can then stick to them. In one group of hypertensive men, studied alongside a healthy control group, there was found to be a significant correlation between high blood pressure and the body's insulin response to oral glucose. The higher the sugar and insulin response, the higher the systolic and diastolic blood pressure and the higher the dangerous LDL cholesterol. Sugar also increases adrenalin which in turn stimulates the sodium retention mechanism, so it increases blood pressure from two different angles. Treating these people, by dietary restriction of sugar and processed grains alone reduces blood pressure but the B vitamin niacin with EPA speeds the process.

High diastolic pressure and minerals

This may be related to fluid retention as a result of food allergies, or because of a dietary sodium/potassium imbalance. Where sodium levels are too high, fluid levels surrounding the cells rise, which causes the blood pressure regulatory mechanism to malfunction. Hypertension does not occur unless there is firstly a low level generalised fluid retention. However, a high diastolic pressure can in turn cause further water retention in the tissues because the high pressure prevents the return of fluid from the tissues to the circulatory system. Lowering the salt content of the diet may not correct the problem on its own, as potassium intake must be increased at the same time. Those who have high blood pressure usually consume more salt than normal, and it is an interesting fact that this further increases the desire for salt, so that a vicious cycle exists. It can only be broken by a long period of salt restriction combined with high potassium intake. Increasing potassium foods in the diet as well as avoiding salt may alone correct faulty diastolic pressure.

It must be emphasised that processed foods have very high levels of sodium chloride, so home-preparation of meals is important – even salt substitutes often contain a lot of sodium chloride. Potassium dilates blood vessels, causes a sodium and water loss and suppresses the sodium retention mechanism in the adrenal glands. It is of prime importance in preventing high blood pressure. In one study reported in *British Medical Journal* 37, mildly-hypertensive people, given potassium

for 32 weeks, experienced an average reduction in systolic pressure from 158 to 143 and diastolic from 101 down to 85. Another study indicated that anti-hypersensitive drug dosage could be reduced by 50% in those increasing their potassium intake. Various supplements will reduce a diastolic pressure involving tissue fluid retention, notably *Celloids® SS* and *Celloids® PC*, homeopathic *Nat Mur*, the herb yarrow, or a mixture of the B vitamin niacin, vitamin C, zinc and a multi-vitamin/mineral supplement. Although Celloids® SS is sodium sulphate, this tissue salt removes fluid from the tissues, in contrast to the retentive effect of common salt. It is only when chloride is combined with sodium that hypertension results.

It should be noted that if magnesium is low, a low potassium level will follow, which cannot be rebalanced until the magnesium is returned to normal. There is an increased need for magnesium in diets high in fat, salt, calcium and phosphorus, and it is also thought that faulty magnesium metabolism may be involved, where the hypertension is hereditary. Certainly magnesium, when given alone, will lower blood pressure in those who are sensitive to this mineral. Calcium is frequently deficient in hypertensive subjects and supplementation has improved the condition significantly in clinical trials.

Vegetarians generally have lower blood pressure because the potassium levels are higher and the fatty acid balance is better. Additionally they have more fibre, calcium, magnesium, vitamins C and A in their diets.

Coffee, cigarettes and alcohol

The relationship between these and all heart disease is well-known. Alcohol raises cholesterol and increases blood pressure by causing the release of adrenalin, which in turn constricts blood vessels and leads to increased sodium retention. Caffeine raises blood pressure if several cups of coffee a day are drunk. However this may be due to the diuretic effect of flushing out essential minerals like potassium, magnesium and calcium. Cigarettes also use up essential nutrients, particularly vitamin C, which is used at the rate of 25mg per stick. Nicotine, like alcohol, stimulates adrenalin, so that the two together are a dangerously potent mixture.

Stress

Everyone knows that stress raises blood pressure, but a recent report indicated that job stress even causes enlargement of the left ventricle of the heart, which means it has to work harder. Clearly the heart and blood vessels feel the emotions and for this reason it is very important to practise stress-release techniques. It is true that if our emotional responses are balanced and salt intake is low, blood pressure will remain level. However, when we are constantly stressed, all the systems involved in blood pressure control become overworked. Eventually blood vessel walls thicken and the heart and adrenal glands enlarge so that they become less receptive to messages from the nervous system. This causes the fine control over blood pressure to disappear. Eventually, small fissures appear in blood vessels and ruptures occur.

Stress causes sodium retention and adrenalin release, which directly raise blood pressure. However the adrenalin also causes a loss of magnesium and then calcium – two minerals vital to normal pressures along with potassium. A combination of stress, a type-A personality and a moderately high salt intake is a major reason for the type of hypertension which is resistant to treatment and eventually results in a heart attack or a stroke.

Weight

The need to reduce excess weight in order to lower blood pressure is widely recognised, but it will also work with those only moderately over-weight. Obese people usually commit all the dietary faults associated with hypertension and these must be corrected as part of the weight-loss programme.

Herbs

- **Hawthorn berries** are wonderful in all cardio-vascular disease. They lower blood pressure, dilate coronary vessels, strengthen heart action and improve circulation. They also protect calcium levels and have a sedative effect on the central nervous system.
- **Mistletoe** reduces blood pressure when combined with other herbs. It affects the capillaries and arterioles (small arteries) and reduces the heart rate.
- **Cactus Grandiflora** is a cardiac herb with diuretic action as well. Cactus + hawthorn + garlic reduce blood pressure and cholesterol markedly within three months.
- **Yarrow** dilates and tones arterioles and increases the peripheral blood flow by 50%. This herb is of value in high diastolic pressure and all types of thromboses.
- **Valerian** works with chamomile and reduces blood pressure in stressed and anxious people.
- **Chamomile** relaxes blood vessel walls. It also prevents sticky platelets and thus the risk of thrombosis.
- **Lavender** is an anti-spasmodic herb with hypotensive properties, and is of great value in anxiety and stress. Use the essential oil, 1 drop on each temple twice daily.
- **Lime flowers** are for nervous tension as well as high blood pressure.
- **Linden** has an anti-spasmodic effect and is of value in the type of hypertension causing a dull congested headache. This can be used as a tea three times daily if appropriate.

TREATMENT

Diet

- Eat a largely vegetarian diet.
- *Juice fasting* reduces blood pressure quickly, so one day a week on juices only would be of value. One cup of freshly-made mixed vegetable juice contains 2g potassium.
- *Garlic* is of special value in reducing blood pressure, and numerous studies have indicated average reductions in systolic and diastolic pressure of 20mmHg (*eg* 150 down to 130). 15g a day of garlic is said to prevent heart disease. This amount represents between one and four cloves. In one study only 9g of fresh garlic was used daily, and after four weeks blood pressures had been lowered by six points. In all cardio- vascular disease, garlic may be taken fresh, powdered or in the form of oil capsules.
- Eat plenty of *potassium foods* (6g daily), especially bananas, dried fruit, nectarines, mango, avocados and melons. The high potassium vegetables are: jacket potatoes, tomatoes, spinach, broccoli, pumpkin, Brussels sprouts and celery.
- Eat plenty of *calcium foods* (1g daily) – oily fish, green vegetables, raw nuts and seeds, pulses and a little low-fat goat's milk and cottage cheese.
- Eat plenty of *magnesium foods* (1g daily) – soya beans, nuts, brewer's yeast, wholegrains and dried peas and beans.
- Eat a high-fibre diet – fruit and vegetables, whole grains, pulses, raw nuts and seeds including sunflower and flaxseeds. Millet, oats,spelt and rice are the preferred grains, and oatbran makes an ideal breakfast. These foods are also a rich source of minerals and vitamins. Buckwheat lowers blood pressure by its beneficial effect on blood vessel walls.
- Oily fish, as the EPA has a powerful blood pressure lowering effect.
- Seeds and walnuts for the other essential oil.
- Dressings made from extra-virgin olive oil or genuine cold-pressed polyunsaturates. Olive oil for cooking.

Mineral food values

Potassium food values

1 cup fresh vegetable juice	2g
3oz salad vegetables	200-1000mg
3oz broccoli, spinach, chard *etc*	400-600mg
3oz dried fruit	700-1800mg
½ cup of pulses	500-1000mg
¼ cup sunflower seeds	350mg
3oz grains	300-500mg
1 avocado	1200mg
1 banana	500mg
1 mango	400mg
1 jacket potato	700mg
½lb fish	600-800mg

Magnesium food values

3oz soya beans	310mg
1oz nuts	80mg
3oz brown rice	120mg
3oz wholewheat bread	90mg
3oz banana or dried fruit	80mg

Green vegetables also contain reasonable levels.

Calcium food values

1 cup of green vegetables	200-300mg
3oz sardines	375mg
3oz pulses	150mg
1oz nuts	80mg

Eggs, grain and fruit also contain reasonable levels.

Spirulina is a very good source of all three minerals.

Avoid

- Any food to which you are allergic.
- Sugar and refined carbohydrate (white flour, white rice, cornstarch) and everything made from them.
- All processed foods – they are high in salt and low in other minerals.
- All processed oils and margarines.
- Added salt and strong spices.
- Caffeine, alcohol and cigarettes.
- Aspirin, as it upsets the fatty acid balance.
- Stress, as it raises blood pressure, cholesterol and damages blood vessel walls.
- Animal protein from meat and dairy products should be heavily restricted.
- Hypotensive drugs – because the long-term side-effects are unacceptable.

Juices

- Carrots, spinach, red beet, parsley and pumpkin.
- Blackcurrants, grapes, cranberries, citrus and the potassium foods above.

Supplements of value

- *EPA* – 6g daily lowers blood pressure. If eating oily fish three times weekly, 2g daily is sufficient.
- *Evening primrose oil* – 1g daily.
- *Lecithin* – 2 tablespoons daily.
- *Potassium*, *magnesium* and *calcium*, if not getting enough in food. Most people need extra magnesium.
- *Spirulina*, for its natural B vitamins, beta-carotene, minerals and protein.
- *Garlic* – one clove three times daily, or the equivalent in tablets or oil capsules.
- *Vitamin B-complex* – 50mg daily.
- *Celloids® SS* and *Celloids® PC* (see Appendix 1) – 1 tablet each three times daily, if fluid retention is involved.
- Other supplements which have been used successfully are *bromelain*, the herb *ginkgo* and the amino acid *histidine*.

Herbs

Many of these can be bought in various combination tablets with garlic.

- *Hawthorn berries* – 1g three times daily.
- *Mistletoe* – 2-4g three times daily.
- *Yarrow* – 2-4g three times daily.
- *Lime flowers* – 2-4g three times daily.
- *Valerian* – 0.3-1g, three times daily.
- *Cactus Grandiflora* – 0.5g three times daily.

Exercise

Work up to a one hour brisk walk three times weekly, or forty five minutes of more strenuous aerobic exercise such as swimming.

Stress release

Learn to meditate or use some other stress-release technique, and practise it daily, as the mind has a powerful effect on lowering blood pressure.

Change your lifestyle if necessary so that your emotional responses to stress become balanced. Resolve any emotional feelings which may be preventing you from feeling good about yourself and your lifestyle.

Acupressure

Pressure the top of the middle finger for 30 seconds, four to six times daily. Press under the ears until tender, several times daily.

III: *35. HYPOGLYCAEMIA (Low Blood Sugar)*

Hypoglycaemic symptoms can be caused by many other conditions besides diabetes. Poor eating habits, with diets composed of refined carbohydrates like white flour and sugar products, can lower blood glucose levels dramatically. The reason for this is that they are rapidly converted to glucose, and then they flood the bloodstream with sugar. In response, the pancreas secretes insulin, which removes the sugar to storage and leaves you with hypoglycaemia. Alcohol and coffee have the same effect. It is possible to find yourself in a vicious cycle of fluctuating blood sugar levels, because every time you appease the symptoms of hypoglycaemia with chocolate or a bowl of processed cereal, there is a period of feeling good before cravings and uncomfortable sensations return. If the sugar craving is subdued instead, with such things as wholegrain foods or fruit, this type of carbohydrate breaks down into glucose slowly, thus maintaining a stable level of blood sugar. It is the fibre in the food which prevents the quick release of simple sugar from carbohydrate.

Allergic reactions to foods other than sugar are a frequent cause of hypoglycaemia, as is persistent stress. Where allergy is involved, the problem clears with avoidance of the specific food. However, persistent stress alters the function of the adrenal glands. This means that they are consistently pumping out hormones designed to raise blood sugar for energy. Eventually the process of changing stored sugar into energy happens too slowly, because the adrenal glands are tired. This also causes sugar craving, and when you succumb, there is an answering insulin release

and a return to hypoglycaemia.

Less common causes of low blood sugar are thyroid and pancreatic dysfunction. Even the contraceptive pill will create the problem in some women.

The symptoms of low blood sugar are hunger, sweating, tremor, a fast heartbeat and anxiety. If the onset of the condition is gradual then these symptoms are not so obvious. Instead, central nervous system responses occur – emotional instability such as irritability, anger or weepiness, headaches, poor concentration, dizziness and a confused mind. Twitches, cramps and numb feet and hands may also be a feature. In a few cases, hypoglycaemic symptoms occur without blood sugar levels altering. Allergy, very long-term stress or heavy coffee drinking may be the cause in these instances.

TREATMENT
Outline
- Allergy test.
- Correct the diet.
- Support the adrenal glands, if over-stressed.
- Practise stress-release techniques and exercise daily.
- Add supplements according to individual need.

Diet
- Pulses and wholegrains, such as oats, millet, spelt, quinoa, barley and rye.
- Seeds and nuts.
- A large serving of vegetables twice daily.
- High fibre fruit.
- Moderate levels of meat, fish or dairy

products.

• Brewer's yeast for chromium. Foods and herbs rich in this mineral are wholegrains, egg yolk, cheese, beef, mushrooms, lettuce, tomato, beans, onions, caraway, cinnamon, coriander, nutmeg, mace, poppy seeds, cumin, cloves and bay leaves.

In the initial stages, always eat an allowed snack between meals and at bedtime. Never skip a meal.

Make sure that breakfast and lunch always contain a good serving of unprocessed grains or pulses, as the carbohydrate content breaks down slowly over several hours.

Breakfast choices
• Oatmeal porridge, and cow's or soya milk.
• Wholegrain, sugar-free muesli with chopped nuts and nut milk.
• Fruit (especially berries) with low-fat live yoghurt, nuts and two tablespoons of oatbran.
• Wholegrain rye bread and poached eggs, mushrooms or tomatoes.
• Buckwheat pancakes and berry fruits.

Lunch and dinner choices
• Salads or steamed vegetables with vegetarian protein, such as bean dishes, tofu, lentil paté, buckwheat, brown rice salad, millet or buckwheat pasta.
• Steamed vegetables with fish or organic meat.
• Salad and a mushroom or tomato and onion omelette.
• Salad and a wholegrain pasta dish containing cheese.
• Salad and rye bread with a nut spread or vegetable paté.

Desserts
• Fresh or baked fruit and live plain yoghurt.

Between meals and bedtime snacks
• A few raw nuts or seeds, an oatbran snack

bar, a wholegrain crispbread, fruit and yoghurt, or a vegetable juice. These may be very important in preventing hypoglycaemic symptoms in the early hours of the morning, and in the hour or so before regular mealtimes. Do not succumb to anything containing sugar, white flour, caffeine or alcohol.

Avoid
• All processed and refined foods, such as sugar, white flour products and processed cereals (pizza, white pasta, cakes, biscuits).
• Fruit juice and these low-fibre fruits – melon, grapes, lychees, nectarines, peaches, pineapple and pomegranates.
• Honey, molasses *etc*.
• Glycaemic foods, until the hypoglycaemia is under control, and then reintroduce them as part of the diet – wheat, corn, yams, beets, potato, banana, sweet grapes, dried fruit.
• Coffee, alcohol, soft drinks and flavoured milk.

Supplements of value
Adult doses:
• **Chromium polynicotinate** – 200mcg daily, improves proper insulin activity by 85%, in people with slight glucose intolerance.
• **Pectin** and **guar gum** fibre – 5g each at every meal, slows the blood sugar response after eating.
• **Vitamin C** – 500mg four times daily, for sugar craving.
• **B-complex** – 50mg once daily.
• **Pantothenic acid** – 100mg daily.
• **Vitamin E** – 400iu daily.
• **Zinc** 15mg + **manganese** 5mg – daily at night on an empty stomach.
• **L-glutamine** – 500mg three times daily, in juice, half an hour before meals, for sugar or alcohol craving.

The above also support the adrenal glands in stress, as do the herbs *licorice* and *ginseng*.

III: *36. DIABETES MELLITUS*

Diabetes is a serious metabolic disease associated with western diets. There exists a disordered metabolism of fats, carbohydrate and protein because of a malfunction in the insulin-producing beta cells of the pancreas. Where insulin secretion is too low, cells cannot use glucose and so this sugar circulates in the blood until the kidneys excrete it along with a lot of water. The major signs of diabetes are sugar in the urine, unusually high thirst levels and the passing of a lot of urine. Without sugar for energy, the body has to burn protein and fat instead, and so fatigue and weight-loss are also key factors.

Type-1 diabetes begins in childhood and occurs because the pancreas is unable to produce adequate levels of insulin. There are many known reasons for this and it is a tragedy that children are automatically put on insulin for life instead of looking for the cause and possibly completely overcoming the problem.

Some children develop an allergy to cow's milk protein, which is similar in structure to a protein inside the pancreatic beta cells. If this protein surfaces in an infection, the immune system then destroys it (along with the beta cells themselves) because it recognises it as being as foreign as the cow's milk allergen. Allergic reactions to other foods can also cause serious blood sugar disturbances, so this is a facet which should always be considered in a new diabetic.

Low levels of vitamin B6 also lead to insulin deficiency because a substance called xanthine acid then collects in the blood and destroys beta cells. A supplement of B6 with magnesium and zinc would solve this type of diabetes if started early enough. Toxic intestinal conditions which are very common in children because of low levels of healthy bowel flora is another possible cause of diabetes. This leads to a low-grade pancreatitis.

Type-2 diabetes is the maturity-onset form which occurs in 50-70-year old individuals whose pancreatic function is either diminished or just unable to cope with dietary excesses and overweight. These people can control the condition through diet and natural supplements. Those who are overweight should shed excess fat and avoid alcohol, white flour products and white rice, as these make insulin less sensitive. The orthodox medical approach is to use glucose-reducing drugs given orally.

Stress

Emotional trauma can cause any part of the body to malfunction – so why not the pancreas as well? When we are stressed, adrenal hormones cause the release of sugar and fats into the blood so that they can be used for energy. The brain must switch off the insulin response to this, so that the increased fuel can stay in the blood while the alarm stage of stress response is in operation. For those who live with constant stress, blood sugar remains high and pancreatic release of insulin is depressed. Could it be that type-2 diabetes is brought about by years of stress? Certainly those who take stock of their total lifestyle return closer-to-normal pancreatic function than those who only change their diets.

In the case of type-1 diabetes, some have the condition because of permanently damaged beta cells in the pancreas but others can definitely link the onset of the disease with an emotional trauma. It seems a tragedy to leave these people on insulin for life, when the pancreas may have returned to normal function. Unfortunately, when insulin is given long-term it causes a feedback situation whereby the pancreas eventually stops producing its own. The same happens in the adrenal glands when cortisone is administered long-term. In fact the whole body works on feedback systems.

Another aspect of stress is that the immune system becomes disordered, to the extent that auto-immune diseases (self-destruction) become a possibility. Many diabetics do have antibodies to pancreatic cells, which suggests an auto-immune attack as a possible cause.

Diabetic complications

These are caused by insulin damage to blood vessel linings (endothelium), which is common in the eyes, causing diabetic retinopathy, and in the kidneys. Peripheral blood vessel damage and subsequent poor circulation can cause ulcers in the lower legs and feet. Diabetic neuropathy is another complication, whereby peripheral nerves are damaged by sorbitol (a product of glucose metabolism), causing a variety of symptoms from pins and needles to gross muscle weakness. The diabetic is also very prone to infections and high cholesterol levels. Cataracts may develop because of an accumulation of sorbitol in the lens.

TREATMENT
Explained

Since diabetes is associated with a diet high in refined carbohydrate, animal protein and fat and low in fibre, a diabetic diet is geared to reversing this. Hence a high complex carbohydrate diet, which is high in fibre and low in protein and fat, is far superior to the old dietary recommendations of a low carbohydrate/high protein combination. The latter only increases the tendency to atherosclerosis in diabetics. Where carbohydrate is provided in complex form, it breaks down slowly into simple sugar, so that blood levels remain constant, and insulin requirements are lowered. The presence of fibre prevents glucose from being released quickly, and a low-protein diet automatically reduces saturated fat levels. The excess of sugar in the blood of a diabetic is often due to a lack of insulin receptors on cells rather than a lack of insulin itself. Complex carbohydrate increases these receptors.

70-75% of calories should come from complex carbohydrate, 15% from protein and 10-15% from fats or oils. This ensures a very high fibre content, which will prevent high cholesterol levels, atherosclerosis and damage to blood vessels. The carbohydrate is derived from whole grains (millet, rice, oats, spelt, corn, barley and very little wheat), pulses (dried peas and beans), fruit and vegetables. The diet should be very high in vegetables and high fibre fruits. Fruit juice and highly glycaemic foods like wheat, banana, potato chips and sweet grapes should be strictly limited. The glycaemic rating of food indicates the rate at which it is converted to simple sugar, and even some high fibre foods have a high glycaemic rating, and so need to be avoided. For instance, a grain of wholewheat becomes glycaemic the moment it is crushed, so that the wholegrain is as glycaemic as white flour.

Protein is derived from pulses, grains, nuts, seeds, vegetables, fish and lean meat. The major portion should be eaten as beans and vegetables, and in fact, a vegan diet is best.

Fat is derived from nuts, seeds, fish, vegetables, grains and beans. The nuts and seeds are important, but must be in moderate amounts. In 1988 a study of 21 patients suffering diabetic neuropathy indicated that a vegan diet plus regular exercise completely alleviated the intense pain within two weeks in 17 of the patients, whilst the remaining four experienced noticeable relief. Insulin requirements in this group also decreased.

Chromium increases glucose tolerance and its level in the blood determines the degree of insulin sensitivity. Where circulating levels of insulin are high, the body's ability to mobilise chromium is reduced. Simple starches like white flour increase chromium excretion, as do all glycaemic foods. This mineral is best taken as brewer's yeast or as chromium poly-nicotinate supplements. A side-benefit of taking chromium is that it lowers cholesterol and triglycerides, as well as raising the healthy HDL levels. Many spices and herbs have very high levels of chromium, and they have been found to increase the activity of insulin three-fold!

Inositol and *biotin*. These two B vitamins, with B12 and B6, are known to prevent diabetic neuropathy, and biotin works with insulin to maintain normal blood sugar levels. A study reported in 1990 gave 400mcg of biotin daily to severe cases, and after just 4-8 weeks, symptoms were markedly improved. Where biotin is low, nervous system metabolism is adversely affected. Inositol is needed at the rate of 1000mg daily, and this can be obtained from the diabetic diet. Two tablespoons of lecithin contains 450mg, and a 3oz serving of brown rice or oatflakes contains 300mg. Add an orange, and the day's allowance is covered. Nuts, pulses and green vegetables are very good sources. Biotin is high in brewer's yeast, eggs, oats and wheatgerm and substantial amounts are made by the intestinal bacteria.

Fish oils have been used in studies recently in an effort to reduce serum cholesterol and triglycerides in type-2 diabetes. In one study 10g of MAXEPA was given, with marked improvement in serum cholesterol and triglycerides. However, blood glucose levels increased and peripheral insulin sensitivity decreased. Another study showed some degree of blood cell destruction, and even after vitamin E was added this tendency remained. More research is needed, but for the moment it would appear that fish oil supplements should be avoided by diabetics, and the control of fats should be through diet alone. However, evening primrose oil significantly improves neuropathy.

Vitamin C reverses the sorbitol accumulation, which leads to cataracts, kidney and nerve damage. Vitamin C at 2000mg daily in one study reduced sorbitol by 44.5% in diabetics. When blood sugar is high, sorbitol collects and is driven by osmotic pressure into nerves, blood vessels and kidney tissue. To lessen the kidney damage, protein levels need to be kept low – 0.5g per kilo of weight is believed to be ideal. This means that protein, as a fraction of total calories in the diet, would be below 15%.

Total phosphorus and sodium levels also have to be kept down, which means largely avoiding meat as a protein source. The flavonoid *quercetin* has a vitamin C sparing effect and is a powerful antioxidant in its own right. *Pignaginol* is another flavonoid and is better absorbed than most. It is 100 times more powerful than vitamin E as an antioxidant, and protects capillaries and the retina. Both flavonoids prevent diabetic retinopathy. All the nutrients protecting against damage to blood vessel linings are very important, and these include vitamins A, C, E, and selenium, B vitamins, zinc and manganese. The latter two minerals are normally deficient in diabetics, and are necessary for sugar and insulin metabolism.

Vitamin E reduces insulin requirement, increases the fatty acid which protects blood vessel walls (prostacyclin), inhibits sticky platelets which damage blood vessel walls and raises healthy HDL levels so that cholesterol is cleared from the blood quickly. The free radical scavenger enzymes, SOD and catalase are also increased by vitamin E, and this is another weapon against atherosclerosis. *Selenium* is always given with this vitamin, as they function together in their antioxidant activity. Diabetics must protect their circulatory system and maintain low cholesterol levels, if they are to be healthy in middle and old age.

Magnesium is low in diabetics, and poorly controlled patients have the most depleted levels as well as an excessive loss of the mineral in urine. It is considered that low magnesium may be an actual cause of diabetes, and certainly supplementation with this mineral reduces insulin requirement and improves all neuromuscular symptoms, as well as playing a role in insulin secretion and effect. Magnesium is involved in controlling blood factors like cholesterol and sticky platelets and is thought to prevent retinopathy.

Niacinamide (B3) alleviates pancreatic beta cell defects and protects against further damage. This vitamin also lowers insulin requirements. Many additives found in processed foods, such as colours, directly causes vitamin B3 and B6 deficiency. 'The pill' leaches several B vitamins and many other essential nutrients. Vitamin B6 inhibits sticky platelets, and is a component of GTF chromium (in brewer's yeast) – it helps lower cholesterol and triglycerides and inhibits the formation of xanthine acid which creates high serum glucose levels and a consequent beta cell destruction.

Supplements which have been found to be of value in increasing insulin production and activity are niacinamide 400mg, chromium polynicotinate 200mcg, vitamin C 2g, vitamin E 400iu, flaxseed oil and the following herbs.

Herbs

• *Fenugreek seeds* benefit diabetics. In a study where 100g were taken daily, 24 hour sugar-excretion went down by 54%, and serum levels remained steady. This indicates that fenugreek increases the body's sensitivity to insulin and improves glycaemic control. This may be due to the guar gum fibre which is so beneficial to diabetics. The test individuals also lowered their triglycerides and cholesterol with fenugreek seeds.

• *Red gum bark* from Australia or India, has been shown to regenerate beta pancreatic cells, something no other herb is known for. Dosage is one teaspoon of tincture three times daily.

• *Nettles* and *goat's rue* stimulate the pancreas and increase its insulin output. Goat's rue is an effective antioxidant which slowly reduces the insulin requirement. It is often used with jambul, another hypoglycaemic herb, and the dose is half a teaspoon of the tincture, three times daily.

• *Blueberries* contain powerful antioxidant flavonoids, and myrtillin extract from the berries has an insulin effect which, although weaker, is much less toxic than the drug. A single 1g dose of extract has been found to be effective for several weeks. Its value is in reducing insulin requirement, and retarding the sorbitol build up. The dosage is 4g of dried powdered berries daily.

• *Bitter melon* stimulates beta cells to produce insulin. It is also known as balsam pear, and has a strong hypoglycaemic action. The melon contains natural steroids more potent than the tolbutamide given to type-2 diabetics. 2oz daily of the juice is an optimal dose.

• *Onion* and *garlic* lower blood sugar and increase insulin secretion. Clinical evidence points to a chemical in these foods competing with insulin for binding sites, and this frees the hormone in the bloodstream to reduce glucose. Onion and garlic have the same effect if cooked or eaten raw.

- *Green tea*, *black catechu* and *red gum* contain epicatechin, which regulates pancreatic beta cells.
- *Dandelion*, *salsify*, *artichoke* and *green beans* are insulin herbs.
- *Juniper berries* regulate the pancreas, *golden seal* and *licorice* stimulate it.
- *Wild yam* has been shown to lower blood sugar by 10% within thirty minutes.

Diet

- Pulses, for protein and their very low glycaemic index rating – soya and other dried peas, beans and lentils.
- Grains, such as oats, millet, spelt, quinoa, barley and rye. These must be whole grains and fresh. Iraqis use barley as a means of improving glucose tolerance.
- Seeds and nuts, especially buckwheat, pumpkin, flax, sesame and sunflower seeds, coconut, cashew nuts, almonds and walnuts. A little each day is excellent, but too much raises the total fats in the diet.
- Vegetables, at the rate of two large plates daily – especially garlic, onion, cucumber, beans, artichokes, turnip and swede.
- Avocado, in moderation, is high in fibre but also high in unsaturated oils.
- Vitamin B3 and vitamin B6 foods: nuts, seeds, wholegrains, soya beans, brewer's yeast, wheatgerm, fish, cantaloupe, banana, avocado, carrot, cabbage, tomato and green pepper.
- Fruit, especially apples, lemons, all berry fruits, guava, mango, papaya, pears, prunes and figs.
- Oily fish, three times weekly in a small serving, or flaxseed oil one tablespoon daily.
- Brewer's yeast, two tablespoons daily. Other chromium-rich foods are, whole

grains, egg yolk, cheese, mushrooms, lettuce, tomatoes, beans and onions. Chromium-rich herbs are caraway, cinnamon, coriander, nutmeg, mace, poppy seeds, cumin, cloves and bay leaves.

- Fibre supplements from guar gum and pectin reduce insulin requirement. The dose is 5g of each per meal.

The diet must be highly alkaline-producing and as much raw as possible. High potassium levels are also necessary, as insulin reduces this mineral. The above diet covers these requirements.

Avoid

- Over-eating and over-weight.
- Fruit juice, and these low fibre fruits: melon, cherries, passion fruit, grapes, lychees, nectarines, peaches, pineapple and pomegranates. Glucose and fructose are highly insulinogenic.
- Skimmed milk, as the casein (protein) part raises cholesterol, and cow's milk protein triggers diabetes in some children.
- Margarine and processed oils.
- All processed and refined foods, such as sugar, white flour, corn starch, white rice, processed cereals and everything made from them, including white pasta and pizza.
- Fish oil extracts.
- Tea, coffee, alcohol and smoking.
- Honey, fructose, dextrose, molasses.

Reduce

- Glycaemic foods: wheat in any form, banana, corn, sweet grapes, potatoes, yams, peas, carrots, beetroot, white rice and any other processed grains, dried fruit, fruit juice and honey.
- Meat and dairy products.
- Total fats.

Juices
• String beans (which contain insulin), cucumber, artichoke, watercress, lettuce, parsley, carrot, celery and bitter melon, for potassium and other nutrients.
• Juniper berries regulate the pancreas, as does green tea.
• Bitter melon juice, 2oz daily.

Others
• Exercise improves circulation, reduces the need for insulin, improves cholesterol levels, and maintains weight, by increasing metabolism. It also increases chromium levels in the tissues and glucose tolerance.
• Dry skin brushing improves circulation, as do hot showers followed by thirty seconds of very cold water.

Supplements of value
Adult doses:
• *Vitamin C* – 500mg four times daily.
• *Pignaginol* – 200mg daily, a flavonoid which is antioxidant to the eye tissue, and retards sorbitol build-up.
• *Vitamin A* – 10,000iu daily, as diabetics don't convert beta carotene very well.
• *Vitamin E* – 400iu daily.
• *Selenium* – 200mcg daily.
• *Magnesium* – 400mg daily, as aspartate or citrate.
• *B-complex* – 50mg daily, to also contain inositol, biotin and B12.
• *Zinc* – 15mg daily.
• *Manganese* – 5-10mg daily.
• *Evening primrose oil* – 500mg three times daily.
• *Vanadium* – 1000-2000mcg daily, increases the activity of pancreatic beta cells, the insulin producing part.
• *Chromium polynicotinate* – 200mcg daily.
• *Lecithin* granules – 1-2 tablespoons daily.

The above nutrients assist insulin production, protect blood vessels and nerves against damage, and strengthen the immune system. Cholesterol and triglyceride levels will remain within acceptable levels with the above nutrients, and adherence to the diet. Some components of the B complex, such as nicotinic acid may need to be added in higher dosage.

Herbs
Adult doses:
• *Fenugreek seeds*, freely, as well as the high chromium spices.
• *Dandelion root* – one teaspoon to a cup, and make a tea.
• *Goat's rue* – half a teaspoon of tincture three times daily, or 1-2g three times daily of the dried herb.
• *Blueberries* – 4g three times daily of the dried berries.
• *Red gum bark* – half to one teaspoon of tincture three times daily.

Stress management
Take stock of your lifestyle and make any necessary changes, so that emotional responses to stress can normalise. Learn a stress-release technique and practise it daily. Seek help if necessary to become a whole person mentally and spiritually.

III: *37. MULTIPLE SCLEROSIS*

This is a condition where the myelin sheath which covers nerves comes away – demyelination. It occurs in patches at different times and in different locations of the central nervous system. The result is dysfunction of any muscles within the body, be they major or minor in size. For instance, if the eye muscles are affected, rapid loss of vision may suddenly occur, and then weeks later spontaneously improve. If the spinal column is involved a limb may suddenly begin to lose function, but again this may be resolved over a period of weeks or months. A common feature is for all symptoms to disappear after an initial attack and not return for several years. In some patients there is a slow progressive deterioration without any let up, but others may have wide fluctuations of attacks and remissions. The onset is usually between twenty and forty years and is rare beyond fifty years old.

An interesting fact is that the disease is more common in temperate climates and rare in the tropics. The further from the equator, the higher the incidence, except in Japan where it is rare as a whole. This is perhaps because the traditional Japanese diet has an excellent fatty acid balance and is high in minerals.

The cause is not known, but there is evidence that the myelin sheath in M S is different from that of normal people. It is possible that M S may have many interlinked causes.

Viruses

Some scientists favour a viral cause, on the basis that studies have indicated that other demyelinating diseases have viral implications. Viruses are thought to interfere with the body's ability to use the essential fatty acids which are so vital in stabilising M S. On the other side of the coin, GLA (from Omega-6 fatty acid) is necessary for the body to make its own anti-viral weapon, interferon.

A viral infection can alter the ratio between helper and suppressor T-cells and so instigate an auto-immune disease. If the helpers are too high, an excessive number of antibodies are produced and then the body may start recognising a part of itself as foreign and destroy that part. Studies indicate that suppressor T-cells often fall just prior to an attack. To date science has not managed to isolate an individual myelin protein to which the antibodies may be reacting. Given the fact that M S myelin is different, and given the fact that an auto-immune factor may be present, it makes sense to strengthen the immune system as a part of treatment.

Stress

It is widely accepted that all auto-immune diseases have an emotional basis which triggers the immune system to misfire and start making antibodies against its own tissue. Major stressful events have a profound effect, but even small daily stresses lead to an increase in antibodies.

Many M S patients can relate the onset of their disease to a major emotional disturbance, such as the loss of a loved one, or long-term unhappiness, anger or low self-esteem. Those who recover best are the ones who do not accept the orthodox prognosis of inevitable deterioration. These people are fighters, who view M S as a challenge to alter their lives and become whole on physical, mental and spiritual levels. A great many sufferers have, in this way, recovered full mobility, and although not 'cured', they have a fully-functioning body which remains so throughout life. Healing the emotions is as important as altering the diet; probably more so because if you are genetically prone to this illness, it will strike whenever stresses are mishandled.

Fatty acids

Most research is in the direction of dietary fats, because the myelin sheath is a mixture of protein and fat. It is becoming increasingly clear that dietary omega-3 oil (from oily fish and flaxseeds) is deficient in areas where M S is most prevalent. In addition, saturated fats in meat and dairy products and processed omega-6 oils (sunflower, corn, peanut *etc*) are widely used in the same countries. In a study where 144 people had to restrict their saturated fats to 180 calories per day over a 34-year period, 95% not only survived but remained physically active.

The Japanese, who are rarely affected by M S, eat a lot of fish and very little meat or dairy products, and therefore consume high levels of omega-3 oils. Too much processed oil and saturated fat in western diets prevents any small amounts of fish or flaxseed oil in the diet from being used. Deficiencies of these omega-3 oils are thought to cause the formation of faulty myelin. Clearly, manipulating fatty acids in the diet is of great benefit.

Another advantage of increased fish oil is its beneficial effect in preventing blood platelets from clumping together. This is a normal function in clotting but should not occur otherwise. M S patients do have sticky platelets, and this may be the reason for their damaged blood brain barrier (BBB) and more porous blood vessels. The BBB is a membrane designed to prevent anything toxic from reaching the brain via the circulatory system. When it is damaged, toxins can enter the cerebro-spinal fluid, which acts as a shock absorber and protector of the brain. Sticky platelets are known to be capable of damaging any blood vessels in the body, including the BBB. Eating oily fish three times a week will prevent this from occurring.

Omega-6 oils (genuinely cold-pressed) from sunflower, safflower, pumpkin and sesame seeds, walnuts, corn and soya are also essential to humans. For this reason, evening primrose oil has long been given for M S. Yet, studies have shown that normal doses of it have no effect. On the other hand, one study reported in 1978 that just 23g daily of omega-6 oil from sunflower seeds resulted in reduced severity and frequency of relapses. This same study also concluded that evening primrose oil had no effect. Omega-6 oils are low in the blood of some M S patients, and it has been noted that during a relapse of the disease the levels may fall even further. This may be due to a virus reducing the fatty acids. For evening primrose oil to be of benefit, it seems that at least 4g should be taken daily. It is believed that omega-6 oils have their main effect by normalising the suppressor T-cells and so decreasing the auto-immune reaction. These oils also lead to the strengthening of blood vessel walls and to improving the conduction of nerve-messages – an essential part of reducing M S symptoms, though it would seem that omega-3 oils are even more important. However, do remember that the conversion of omega-6 oils to GLA requires vitamin C, B1, B2, zinc and magnesium as co-factors.

Free radical attack as a cause of demyelination has a valid basis also, in that reduced antioxidant activity has been observed in the blood cells of M S patients. Because they have low levels of the free-radical scavenger glutathione peroxidase in their red and white blood cells, aggressive antioxidant treatment also makes sense.

Two studies in UK have reported that M S patients are frequently deficient in the mineral molybdenum and vitamin B2. Both studies determined that the molybdenum had to be given in homeopathic form to be effective. Some doctors use weekly vitamin B12 injections successfully, and a deficiency of this vitamin produces symptoms very similar to M S. The late Dr Carl Pfeiffer discovered the need for another B vitamin, pyridoxine with zinc, when he found that his M S patients were spilling these nutrients into their urine.

Dr Hans Neiper, who has vast experience in treating M S, firmly believes that it is a generalised membrane disease, which means that the walls of all cells do not function properly. There is defective porosity because the electrical-charging mechanism is faulty. Like a battery, if the cell wall can not be charged, it ceases to function as it ought. In the case of M S, the lack of charge means that the cells of the myelin sheath cannot defend themselves against immune aggression, and so an auto-immune attack destroys the sheath in patches.

Where cell membrane disease exists, it has other effects, all of which are quite common to M S – calcium loss from bones occurs, small blood vessels become fragile, kidney infections are possible, red blood cells become fragile, and absorption is poor through the cells of the small intestine. The oxygen/carbon dioxide exchange is faulty in the lungs, and in the case of M S this worsens parallel to the progression of the paralysis. If the electrical discharge from the cell walls of the urinary tract is inadequate, then infections can be frequent, and this also often occurs in M S. In the 1950s, an American biochemist first discovered that a substance called EAP (2-amino-ethanol-phosphate) was especially important for loading electrical charge to cell walls. Dr Neiper has since determined that M S patients apparently do not produce enough EAP, and that this may also be hereditary. M S does have hereditary tendencies.

Dr Neiper says that if treatment with EAP is started early, there is remarkable improvement in all muscle and sphincter function, as well as in vertigo and ataxia (shaky, unsteady gait). A group of his patients treated with EAP since 1968 has not deteriorated in the last 23 years. Those with osteoporosis have improved bone density, and have not had any more fractures.

One interesting side investigation by Dr Neiper found that squalene also appears to increase cell wall electrical charge. M S people suffer chills, but 1-2 teaspoons daily of squalene increased body warmth markedly in his patients. The absence of cancer in sharks is thought to be due to their squalene, which converts field energy for body use. Insects also get 90% of their energy from the universe, and this protects them against cancer and viruses, as they have no immune system. From these fascinating snippets it is clear that if the cell wall electrical charge functions correctly, the cell is protected from attack by viruses or a disordered immune system. Additionally, EAP would appear to be a missing ingredient in M S individuals.

TREATMENT

Diet

• Eat a largely vegan diet, plus oily fish, like mackerel, herring, salmon, trout and sardines, three to four times weekly.

• Eat heavily reduce dairy products, and avoid all meat, as saturated fat must be no more than 10g daily.

• 40-50g of polyunsaturated oils in total, from oily fish, flaxseed, sunflower seeds, walnuts and soya, or by using the oil in genuinely cold-pressed form. Half the oil should be

omega-3 oil (fish and flaxseed predominantly).
- The above combination will increase the essential fatty acids in the central nervous system, reduce any auto-immune activity and prevent sticky platelets.
- On the days that fish is not eaten, get protein from a mixture of dried peas, beans and soya, with whole grains.
- Fruit and vegetables in abundance.
- All foods should be home-prepared – especially dressings, sauces, mayonnaises *etc*, where oils are featured.
- Proper food-combining is essential, as M S people often suffer from malabsorption. A report in *The Lancet* highlighted various studies that showed abnormal stool fat and meat fibres, as well as the malabsorption of vitamin B12. In fact the 1970s produced a series of M S studies, some of which noted the presence of the measles viral protein and abnormal immunoglobin ratios in the small intestines of M S patients, which indicates some functional disorder.

Avoid
- All margarine, shortening and processed oils (if in doubt, don't buy). This includes mayonnaise, peanut butter, dressings *etc*.
- All processed foods, because oils are usually involved.
- All meat and animal fat.
- Foods to which you are allergic, in order to strengthen the immune system.

Supplements of value
Adult doses:
- *Flaxseed oil* – 1 tablespoon daily.
- *Cod liver oil* – 1 tablespoon daily.
- *Sunflower seed oil* – 1 tablespoon daily.

The doses above are to be adjusted according to the food intake of the two essential fatty acids. Any oils used must be genuinely cold-pressed, and fish oil must be fresh. For this reason it is better encapsulated, where it is protected against rancidity.

- *EPA* – 1g twice daily.
- *DHA* – 700mg twice daily – this occurs in EPA supplements.
- *Antioxidants*: *beta carotene* – 15-30mg daily; *vitamin C* – 1g twice daily; *vitamin E* – 600-1000iu daily; *selenium* – 200-400mcg daily; *glutathione* – 1g twice daily with wheatgrass juice.
- *B-complex* – 50mg once daily.
- *Zinc* – 25mg once daily as citrate or picolinate, with *manganese*, 10mg.
- *CaEAP2* (calcium ethanoleamine phosphate ester) – 600mg three times daily. This product has a powerful effect against auto-immunity, and is a natural precursor to the formation of lecithin which emulsifies fats. It also increases the body's natural production of essential fats required by the nervous system. The anti-viral effect is via the restored electrical charge mechanism in the cell wall.
- *Magnesium* – 400mg daily, or 600mg as MgEAP2.
- *HCl acid* and *digestive enzymes* – to improve absorption of nutrients.
- *Lecithin* granules – 2 tablespoons daily.

The antioxidants are vital in view of the fact that high levels of natural polyunsaturated oils are being ingested. Without antioxidants, free radical damage would occur. It is wise to see a naturopath initially, as everyone has different nutrient requirements.

Homeopathy
- *Molybdenum* – 200c twice daily for ten days, has reportedly improved all M S symptoms, on a long-term basis.
- Constitutional treatment.

Exercise

Frequent moderate levels of exercise is important to strengthen muscles and maintain mobility.

Stress management

Use daily self-healing meditation and imagery, at the same time as altering the biochemic ingredients of your body. Instruct your loving inner self to heal your physical body.

Examine and resolve any emotional blocks to healing. Viewing the mind, body and spirit as one is an essential first step in the healing process, because only the holistic approach will bring optimum results.

III: *38. CANCER*

There is overwhelming evidence that the majority of cancers have their causes rooted in a poor lifestyle. This may be an inadequate diet, poor handling of emotions, polluted air, water and food, or drugs. Figures show that 82% of all cancers are related to diet, tobacco, pollution, alcohol, occupational hazards, abnormal sexual behaviour, chlorination of already-polluted water, and chlorinated hydrocarbons in pesticides.

Cancer of the stomach and oesophagus has been linked to cured, smoked and pickled food, low zinc and selenium, vitamins A, C and E, folic acid and B2. The nitrites and nitrates in cured meat like bacon, ham and salami combine in the stomach with naturally-occurring 'amines' (in all food) to form a carcinogen product (nitrosamines). These nitrites are also a major part of chemical fertilisers, so our natural foods contain them unless organically grown. Unfortunately, nitrates in the soil find their way into water systems, so that even the water in the tap is contaminated. Organic foods and filtered water are essential to health, but one can guard against nitrosamines by taking extra vitamin C. Linus Pauling, the Nobel Laureate, takes 13g vitamin C every day as preventative medicine.

Low zinc occurs in those who eat a lot of cereals, because these foods contain chemicals called phytates that cling to minerals and carry them out of the body. Anyone eating grains in any amount should either soak, ferment or sprout them in order to be rid of the phytates. Studies in China have lead to the conclusion that excessive calcium also reduces zinc absorption. In areas where high calcium/low zinc diets predominate, the incidence of oesophageal cancer is five times higher than in areas where diets are low in calcium and high in zinc.

Cancer of the oesophagus has also been attributed to low vitamin C and selenium levels. In fact, studies indicate that selenium is the most important antioxidant against this and stomach cancer. It is of little use to list the foods containing the mineral selenium, because vast areas of the world have serious soil depletion of it. China, Australia, New Zealand, wide areas of USA and Europe are known to contain almost no selenium. Even within UK some areas are rich, and others contain only traces. East Anglia has very high levels of this mineral, which is a known protection against all cancers.

In China, where the rate of oesophageal cancer is high, researchers have discovered that the risk factor is greatly enhanced by smoking, alcohol consumption and low levels of fruits and vegetables. The risk is also increased by insufficient protein and vitamin C. Those who eat dried salt fish and little fruit have very low stocks of vitamin C, and where protein intake is low, zinc levels drop.

In a study of 21 communes in China where oesophageal cancer was prevalent, animal protein was found to form only 1% of the diet. Vegetables constituted a major part, but zinc is poorly absorbed from them. In addition, those communes where wheat and corn were part of the diet had even lower zinc levels because of the phytates present in the grains. Another probable factor involved in the zinc loss was the high level of folic acid in the largely vegetable diet. Where imbalances remain on a long-term basis, disease will inevitably follow.

Bowel cancer has been clearly linked to high-fat, high-protein and low-fibre diets. Alcohol (especially beer) and sugar also play a role. Fats damage the cells lining the colon, so that they divide more rapidly and become cancerous. In addition, bowel cancer is often associated with low levels of the fatty acid butyrate, which is increased in the intestines by high fibre and lactobacillus micro-flora such as acidophilus. A simple stool test can evaluate butyrate levels. Researchers have concluded that the incidence of bowel cancer is reduced when the pH of the gut is lowered. It is known that when certain types of fibre are converted to butyrate, the pH is improved. Oatbran fibre is of great value here, but wheatbran, pectin and guar gum fibres are not converted to this fatty acid.

A very interesting recent study indicated that vitamin D at 400iu daily reduced colon cancer incidence by 50%, and calcium at the rate of 1200mg daily reduced the incidence by 75%. The calcium is believed to inhibit the colonic cell damage caused by dietary fat and it also improves the pH of the bowel. Researchers believe that the vitamin D and the calcium have a beneficial hand-and-glove effect. Raw vegetables, whole grains and essential polyunsaturated oils protect against bowel cancer, as does vitamin A found in orange-coloured fruit and vegetables. One study indicated that a low-fat diet plus vitamin A results in a low incidence of bowel cancer, and even a high-fat diet plus vitamin A gave rise to some protection.

Bladder cancer is fairly clearly associated with saccharine intake, and in the case of prostate cancer there are normally low levels of vitamin A and zinc. From these few examples, it is already clear that deficiencies of basic nutrients like vitamins A, C, B and D do precipitate cancer, and if organically-grown nutritious food is rejected in favour of quick processed varieties, vitamin and mineral levels will certainly be too low to prevent cancer.

Breast cancer is associated with a high level of oestrogen prior to ovulation. Unbalanced hormones are directly linked to dietary faults such as high fats or poor liver function. One method of reducing oestrogen levels is to spend a half hour each day in the sun with no glasses or contact lenses. In this way the sun reaches the pineal gland in the brain which secretes the hormone melatonin. This hormone blocks over-production of oestrogen in the body.

Oestrogen is continually cleared from the blood by the liver, and this action will be reduced with a subsequent accumulation of the hormone, if the liver is overloaded by toxic body conditions. It appears that tumours have oestrogen receptors, and this is why oestrogen increases breast cancer. However, plant oestrogen found in soya beans and herbs actually blocks these receptors, so that the body's oestrogen cannot attach itself. It is a bit like musical chairs, but the herbal ones win every time. Cruciferous vegetables such as broccoli, cauliflower, Brussels sprouts, cabbage, and Chinese *bak choi* have the ability to convert body oestrogen to an inactive harmless form. Large quantities of vegetables are important in the diet for cancer prevention.

High levels of another female hormone called prolactin have been shown to effect a two-fold increase in breast cancer risk. Here again, high fat diets are implicated, as fats increase hormone concentrations. Vegetarian diets have been shown to reduce prolactin secretion, whereas stimulants of this hormone are found in meat.

A Dr Jonathan Wright has discovered that of the three types of oestrogen in a woman's body, only two are likely to be procarcinogenic (oestradiol and oestrone) whereas the third (oestriol) is probably anti-carcinogenic. 'Oestrogen Quotient' laboratory testing will determine your balance, and therefore your risk factor. Oestriol is the type of oestrogen formed in the liver from the oestradiol and oestrone that is being cleared from the bloodstream. Automatically blocking all oestrogen with drugs is like throwing a brick at an ant, and will surely lead to other problems in time. Dr Wright has noted that in six out of seven cases in his clinic, 100-300mg of potassium iodide daily significantly improved the balance between the three types of oestrogen, so that no drugs were needed to suppress body sources. The iodine is used to form the thyroid hormone thyroxine, which in turn prevents a build-up of oestrogen in the blood. A medical study in USA has clearly shown that breast cancer is much more prevalent in areas of the world where iodine levels are low. Fresh seafood, seaweed, kelp or iodised sea salt are excellent sources of this mineral. Frozen fish loses its iodine content as it thaws. Breast cancer is more rare in Japan than almost every other country – the Japanese eat more fish than most other races.

At a conference held in Washington DC, over fifty leading garlic researchers converged to highlight some new scientific investigations. Dr John Milner reported that a 4% aged garlic extract (Kyolic) inhibited breast cancer by 72%. It was most effective in the early stages, and appeared to work in tandem with selenium and vitamin C. Selenium is consistently low in those with breast cancer, as is vitamin E, with which it works hand in glove. Undoubtedly, garlic is one of nature's wonder foods. At the same conference a Dr Hoow, of UCLA Medical Centre, reported that Kyolic garlic significantly inhibited the growth of melanoma cells, which is good news for foolish sun-worshippers. Garlic can-

not be 'aged' at home – it must be bought as a 'kyolic' supplement.

Whilst on the subject of skin cancer, Dr Ian White has discovered that his Australian flower remedy mulla mulla will remove some cancers if it is used topically as well as taken internally.

Intestinal tract health

If vital nutrients are consistently low or missing, the body slowly seizes up and loses the ability to destroy rogue cancer cells. This will occur if you eat devitalised processed foods, junk, or food polluted with fertiliser, pesticides, colourings and preservatives.

The gastro-intestinal tract will be hit early on with inadequate nutrients to form stomach acid and enzymes. Pancreatic enzymes, besides digesting food, break down cancer cell walls so that the immune system can then destroy them. Enzymes in raw fruit and vegetables also do this to a certain extent, notably bromelain from pineapples, and enzymes in papaya leaves.

Modern research in the USA supports the empirical evidence in Australia that an extract of papaya leaves has a very powerful effect against cancer. The fresh leaves and stems should be chopped finely and boiled gently for two hours to make a decoction which is drunk daily until the tumour disappears.

In 1987, a Dr Richards wrote a very interesting paper in *The Lancet*, outlining the value of using enzyme therapy to destroy cancer cells. Large doses were necessary, which means that treatment must be supervised and not self-administered. The paper highlighted the fact that low enzymes were indicative of poor pancreatic function, impaired gut wall transmission of nutrients and impaired liver function. Without adequate enzymes, even food is not properly broken down, and goes through the gut fermenting and putrefying. Gas and bloating are the results. When nutrients are low, the gut wall loses a degree of its muscle power, and bowel action slows down. In a situation of optimum health, the bowel functions after every meal. Today this happens only in professional athletes, babies and animals.

Poor bowel function results in the accumulation of toxins, a high pH level, the destruction of healthy indigenous micro-organisms and reduced synthesis of B vitamins in the colon. Fungus, which inhabits the bowel of everyone, can then flourish and bacteria, parasites and pesticides will no longer be destroyed. This includes the cancer-causing nitrites in processed meats and water. The next thing to happen is that the bowel wall becomes more porous. Toxins then pass from the bowel, back into the circulatory system, and the body is in effect hit from behind by waste it has already disposed of once. It must seem like a final insult to a body coping with detoxifying and storing chemicals from junk food, colourings, preservatives, margarine and processed oils, white flour, sugar, polluted water and air. At the same time, a beleaguered system is endeavouring to keep organs, muscles, blood cells, the lymphatic system and skin functioning correctly and repair and make new cells; all on a diet deficient in vital nutrients. The stress becomes so great that the cancer surveillance system breaks down. The importance of bowel flora cannot be over-emphasised, as a lack of these is an important factor in the cause of all chronic illnesses.

Fatty acids - constituents of all fats and oils

See chapter II:6 on Fats versus Oils.

When cells accumulate fat they are effectively suffocated, so that oxygen consumption is reduced. Without oxygen for energy production, toxic waste accumulates in the cell and it then develops abnormally. Only if the immune system is strong will that diseased cell be destroyed – otherwise it may become cancerous. As in most chronic illnesses, fatty acid imbalance is a major factor in the disease process. Saturated animal fats must be reduced and processed oils and margarines totally avoided, even if these are made from polyunsaturated oils. The natural essential fatty acids (omega-3 fatty acids and omega-6 fatty acids) should predominate in the fat allowance of the diet; omega-6 oils are found in nuts and seeds, as well as reduced amounts in soya and some grains. Omega-3 fatty acids come from flaxseeds, pumpkin seeds, purslane, walnuts, soya and oily fish predominantly.

A great many studies have been done with flaxseeds and the EPA from fish oil, and all indicate tumour regression, especially of breast and colon cancers. Research is also increasingly indicating that if omega-6 oil is used alone it may actually promote tumour growth, whereas this propensity is inhibited if omega-3 oils are a part of the diet. This probably only applies to processed omega-6 oil.

Because of the heavy use of both animal fat and processed oil, coupled with the very low consumption of oily fish and raw seeds, a fatty acid imbalance must exist in at least 75% of the population. Dangerous processed omega-6 oils are present in all commercial crackers, biscuits, cake mixes, pastries, crisps and other snacks. The Japanese, who have the lowest level of breast cancer in the industrialised world, eat fish daily, and use cold-pressed sesame oil.

One final thing to remember about essential fatty acids is that they are a natural oil which will go rancid easily. Rancid oil produces free radicals in the body, which are extremely harmful. So always use nuts and seeds that are fresh and raw.

Cellular oxygen

Two scientists famous in the field of cancer research and treatment, Dr Johanna Budwig and Dr Max Gerson, both believe that cancer is cured by restoring cellular oxygen, increasing tissue pH levels and balancing the positive and negative polarity of the body. Dr Budwig produced research proving that this could be done with a mixture of flaxseed oil and sulphur protein, from a ferment of unpasteurised skim-milk called kwark (or quark). Dr Gerson proved that manipulating the mineral content of the diet also had the same effect.

When the body is laden with toxic waste and the nutrient levels are low, the cells are suffocated so that their normal oxygen intake and metabolism is disturbed, and energy release is reduced. Once the respiratory chain inside a cell is damaged, cells can very rapidly become cancerous because cancer cells are the only type capable of surviving low oxygen levels. Only they can produce energy from glucose without oxygen. When the cell burns glucose to produce energy, it does so in the presence of oxygen, which reaches the cell from the blood and surrounding fluids. This whole process is carried out in the mitochondria (power generator) of the cell, which includes what is known as the respiratory chain. An essential part of this chain requires the activity of an oxygen-dependent enzyme, and if the oxygen levels are low, the respiratory chain is then destroyed.

In Germany, a cancer researcher, Dr P Seeger, demonstrated that cancer begins as a result of interruption in the respiratory chain inside cells, and that this is the direct result of a lack of an oxygen-dependent enzyme. Furthermore, Seeger discovered that the degree of lost oxygen in cells is directly related to the virulence of a cancer.

About 50 years ago, Dr Otto Warburg won the Nobel prize for his work on cellular oxygen utilisation, when he proved that cells become malignant only after oxygen intake is reduced. Energy production inside the mitochondria of all cells uses almost all the oxygen absorbed by a cell, and therefore any reduction means that this important function is damaged. In practical terms this means that the final oxidation of nutrients does not occur, and so a fermentation process begins. In addition, the electrical charge on the cell wall is altered. Dr Warburg states that cancer begins when the activity of the respiratory chain is replaced by fermentation. Cancer cells thrive on low oxygen, on fermentation in an acid medium, and have a negative electrical charge. They also contain more sodium and less potassium than normal cells because when cells are damaged, sodium invades at will, and this causes a loss of potassium and a change in electrical charge.

The essence of Dr Gerson's cancer diet is fresh fruit and vegetable juices with the juice of raw liver, all of which alkalise the tissues and supply mega-doses of minerals and enzymes to normalise cell oxidation. Sprouted foods and grass juices like wheat or barley are also very high in the minerals and enzymes which restore the respiratory chain. Any product which acts as a hydrogen acceptor has the same restorative effect, and the best of these are beta carotene, beetroot, flavonoids and propolis. The squalene mentioned in chapter III:37 on Multiple Sclerosis restores cellular electrical potential, as does potassium. Once oxygen is restored, fermentation ceases and cells function normally.

Linus Pauling states that vitamin C increases cellular oxygen, and Dr Budwig's research with polyunsaturates led her to the conclusion that cold-pressed flaxseed oil and the sulphur amino acid cysteine would produce the same effect. She went on to prove her theory by successfully treating a great many patients. She has stated that cellular oxygen can be restored in a matter of months, with a diet of flaxseed oil at 20% of calories, plus 250g of unpasteurised skim-milk kwark. The latter provides high levels of the sulphur protein called cysteine. The remainder of Dr Budwig's diet consists of fresh raw fruit, vegetables, seeds and nuts, along with very small amounts of wholegrains and freshwater trout. No other protein, fats or oils are allowed until the tumour has shrunk considerably. Antioxidants are necessary with this diet to protect the natural oil and cysteine from destruction. Cysteine is found in eggs, pulses, and especially in sprouted forms of beans and lentils.

In her research, Dr Budwig also found that trans-fatty acids found in margarine and chemically-processed oils accumulate in cancer cells before healthy ones. Through publishing this information Budwig lost her government research job. Margarine manufacturers have a powerful influence on governments, as do sugar and cereal processing companies. Both Dr Budwig and Dr Gerson have documented a wealth of case histories where terminal cancers have been reversed with their respective diets.

An old therapy for raising cellular oxygen relies on the internal use of hydrogen peroxide. This is very toxic when undiluted, but when taken in therapeutic dosages, it is completely non-toxic and highly germicidal. It kills viruses and other organisms by oxidation as it spreads through the tissues.

Scores of physicians are on record for using hydrogen peroxide therapy to cure a wide variety of diseases, including AIDS. Most disease-causing organisms, including those found in cancer tissue, cannot tolerate high levels of oxygen and are destroyed by it. Several AIDS victims are known to have been cured by an oxygenation therapy. Because hydrogen peroxide is anti-viral, it is also useful against the Epstein Barre virus and herpes, as well as against bacteria, parasites and fungus including candida albicans.

Hydrogen peroxide occurs naturally in rain, snow and any rushing water. It is a constituent of all raw fruit and vegetables, and is produced by our immune system in response to disease, as long as there is sufficient oxygen in the body. Many people have reported success with dilute doses of hydrogen peroxide taken orally, but until properly controlled studies are carried out, this must be considered risky. The reason is that the long-term effects on the intestinal tract are unknown. However, the treatment is clearly highly effective when given intravenously by a doctor. The reason for this appears to be that enzymes in the blood very quickly convert the hydrogen peroxide into safe oxygen and water. The gastro-intestinal tract may not contain adequate levels of these enzymes, and therefore most of the hydrogen peroxide would not be converted. The possible side-effects of this are unacceptable. As a therapy there is documented evidence of its use as far back as the 1800s.

In New Zealand, a company called Oxides International Limited has developed a formulation of mineral salts (Genesis 1000) with a high pH rating that also oxygenates the blood. The ingredients are sodium chlorite, sodium carbonate, sodium sulphate and deionised water. Research shows that the ingredients break down in the stomach and release oxygen. The freed chlorite increases the blood oxygen levels by improving the efficiency of enzymes used in the respiratory chain.

It is interesting to note that the traditional cleansing diet used as a cancer therapy largely contains the very ingredients which increase cellular oxygen levels. That is, raw fruit and vegetables, juices, wheatgrass, beetroot and barley juice, sprouted seeds and pulses, vitamin C and beta carotene. This diet also supplies high levels of potassium to maintain the electrical balance of cell walls.

In terms of prevention, we have to ask ourselves why our cells may have become low in oxygen. One of the answers may be a poor diet low in raw fruits and vegetables, and high in paralysing cooked and processed food. However, the cancer may also be due to over-eating, lack of exercise, stress, poor liver or intestinal function, and in fact anything which increases body toxicity. Contributory factors are external air pollution, drugs, microbial toxins and the loss of rain forests.

Amino acids

A fascinating study was reported last year by a Dr G G Meadows, where amino acids were manipulated to raise immunity and destroy tumours. A protein formula was given to patients, which contained very low levels of the amino acids tyrosine and phenylalanine. They were restricted to 2.4mg and 2.5mg per kilogram of body weight respectively. Three weeks on a casein formula, plus fruit and vegetables, resulted in increases of killer T-cells by 93% and T-helpers by 45%. Platelet aggregation was reduced and the helper/suppressor ratio hardly altered.

In layman's terms, this means greatly enhanced cancer destruction and prevention, through considerably improved immune function. These amino acids are highest in meat – which is a very good reason for becoming a vegan. Where killer T-cells are high and sticky platelets are low, there is a greatly reduced chance of cancer spreading, reduced tumour growth and even regression.

Shark cartilage

This substance has been the subject of many clinical studies in recent years because of its apparent ability to shrink tumour size. Scien-

tists first discovered that sharks do not get cancer, and then realised that this is probably because of their cartilage skeletons where no blood vessels are needed for nourishment. Subsequent research indicated that shark cartilage contains proteins which actually inhibit the growth of new blood vessels. Cancerous growths require an increased network of blood vessels to supply nutrients for growth, and anything inhibiting these networks will logically also shrink the tumour. Because the blood vessels that are developed by tumours grow too quickly, they are fragile and need constant replacement. Shark cartilage prevents the regrowth. A Dr J Prudden in USA first used cartilage as a wound-healer, and then in a study of 31 cancer patients with impressive results. Only 6% failed to improve, and all the rest experienced total or partial tumour regression. In another study of terminally ill patients with only 6 months to live, the cartilage decreased the tumours by 33-100% in seven of the eight subjects.

It is important to use whole cartilage and not the isolated proteins because the cartilage also contains immune-regulating and anti-inflammatory mucopolysaccharides. Shark cartilage has its best effect on the solid type of tumour which is constantly developing its own capillary network. It is not so useful in treating leukaemia, lymphoma or Hodgkin's disease. Growing children and anyone who is pregnant or has a cardiovascular disorder should not take cartilage without professional advice. For more detailed information, the reader should buy *Sharks Don't Get Cancer*, by Dr I W Lane and Linda Comac.

Free radicals

These are described in Part Two, but a brief note is important here because free radical damage to the cell's mitochondria (energy producing area) is what initiates cancer. The mitochondria is like a cell within a cell, and it has its own DNA. Carcinogenic substances zero in on this DNA in order to create a cell with cancerous characteristics. This cell then divides and multiplies very rapidly by cleverly using the energy-producing mechanism.

Free radicals are caused by processed oil and margarine, rancid fats, burnt food and a lack of nutrients like vitamins A, C, E and selenium. They are also a natural end-product of energy production in every cell in the body, which we easily mop up when we're young.

Free radicals can be immobilised as we get older by antioxidants – vitamins A, C, E and the mineral selenium, and scavenging enzymes like SOD found in raw juices from wheatgrass and barley greens. Other natural food chemicals known as carotenoids and flavonoids have a broad-range effect, and are ten times more effective than vitamins as antioxidants. Carotenoids are in carrots, apricots, melons, mango, yams, pumpkins, greens and sweet potatoes. Flavonoids are found in pollens, propolis, beetroot, berry fruits and many herbs, such as milk thistle, catechu, vine, hawthorn berries and ginkgo. Quercetin is a powerful flavonoid in supplement form.

A five year Chinese study completed in 1993 showed conclusively that antioxidants greatly reduce the incidence of cancer. 30,000 people were divided into four groups, each given different supplements. In those taking beta carotene, vitamin E and selenium the death rate from stomach and oesophageal cancer reduced by 21% and all cancer by 13%. Had the diets also been improved, the results would have been even more impressive.

Sticky platelets

Platelets are blood cells with several functions related to arresting bleeding. Three quarters of cancer patients are said to have platelets which clump together when they ought not, and when this occurs various chemicals are released which medical researchers believe increases the spread of cancer. The process is stimulated by stress, animal fat, sugar, white flour, smoking, disease and a lack of seeds and oily fish in the diet – all of which are also involved in coronary artery disease. Omega-3 fatty acids in flaxseeds and oily fish prevent the problem.

Aspirin is used by orthodox medicine to prevent sticky platelets but it is surely better to address the fatty acid imbalance or take one of the following supplements, all of which prevent platelet aggregation – garlic, EPA 3g daily, bromelain 500mg daily or vitamin C 3g daily. Vitamin E, 1000iu daily, prevents the release of chemicals from the platelets when they become fragmented as a result of sticking together.

The diet is of prime importance in preventing sticky platelets, so remember to use oils correctly, avoid white flour and sugar and learn to cope with stress adequately. This alone may obviate the need for supplements to do the job. As you can see, the same dietary factors surface over and over again in every aspect of cancer protection.

Stress

The role of stress in cancer has been widely publicised. Internalising problems is a major factor in cancer, as it weakens the immune system, quite aside from causing sticky platelets. People who are worried or unhappy grow cancer cells faster. Young cancer victims often have unhappy marriages, others may have concerns about children or may be crying out for emotional support of some kind. Being depressed, anxious, despairing, angry, bitter, resentful or lonely for any length of time is stressful and will weaken the immune system, and therefore the ability to destroy the cancer cells that we form on a daily basis.

Stresses in our lives have all been measured but even simple things like feeling guilty or hurt, irritably sitting in traffic jams, or having to adapt to change, all cause stress accumulation. When life gets too hectic and our coping ability fails, illness results and cancer cells grow faster.

The body has a mechanism for dealing with stress called the 'Fight or Flight Syndrome'. Children obey the instinct and strike out with their fists or voices, but adults over-ride the impulse and allow stress to accumulate internally.

Certain personalities are more likely to get cancer than others. Examples are: people who are prone to feelings of helplessness, the saintly who feel it is wrong to express emotions, defensive types and those always trying to create a good impression. Heavy smokers who don't get cancer are usually very gregarious people who discharge negative emotions readily. Perhaps that is why Winston Churchill survived into his 90s on high levels of alcohol, tobacco and rich food.

Usually a series of events leads to the final outcome of cancer. It may start with a restrictive or unhappy childhood and be followed by a run of adult miseries such as a broken marriage, trouble with children or financial insecurity. Being unable to cope leads to immune deficiency and cancer.

Eradicating stresses on a routine basis is of prime importance. Anger must be vented harmlessly so that it does not become resentment. Jealousies should be resolved and injustices forgiven and forgotten. It is also important to be responsible for your own life and not blame others for any problems. Feeling sorry for oneself is part of being helpless.

It has been firmly established that we can grow or shrink a tumour with our thoughts. The Simontons, in their book, taught patients how to destroy cancer with visualisa-tions involving war between the immune system and the cancer. This works for some but many need more gentle visualisations. You can use visions of a healing coloured light coursing through the body, a healing water-fall, the sun's rays or anything else which appeals to you in particular. Once into a relaxed meditative state, use whatever method comes naturally and feels right to you. In this way you will joyfully anticipate your daily self-healing sessions. Everyone should read Bernie Siegel's wonderful books on this subject, partly because he is an authoritative figure (a surgeon), and partly because he is so positive about the sheer simplicity of self-healing.

Having read chapter III:3 on Stress, you will understand that the release of stress hormones damages cells because the message to all parts of the body is that distress exists. Then the cells malfunction and can become cancerous. However, when we are happy, cells release chemicals like interleukin, which increase immune function and lead to the destruction of cancer cells. Therefore rather than take the toxic drug form of interleukin, you can make oodles of your own just by being happy. The greater the level of joy in your life, the higher the release of inter-leukin. Tumours too, are known to release unhappy stress hormones like cortisole, and this in turn *causes* depression. Sad cells do not function properly and are then more likely to become cancerous. Conversely, it has been noted that when a cancer patient makes a mental shift into a positive outlook about his or her condition the depression lifts, which means the cells are no longer secreting sad chemicals – instead they are healing.

There are thousands of cases documented in medical literature where large malignant growths have just disappeared with time, when the patient was told that her illness was not malignant. The enormous relief and joy resulting from the news would release large amounts of interleukin. There is a lot to be said for not telling a patient that they have cancer, if bad news would prevent an optimistic outlook.

Techniques for stress management

• Counselling and talking things over with a friend.
• Relaxation techniques, such as autogenics, yoga, healing visualisation and meditation, for half an hour every day, is an essential part of cancer treatment. Three times weekly is enough for prevention.
• Moderate exercise increases the natural killer cells, which inhibit the spread of cancer via the bloodstream.
• Bach flower remedies, to rebalance emotions which are out of control.
• Laughter is of great value, so watch an amusing film, read a funny book and seek out people who are fun as often as possible. Laughter equates with happiness, the most positive emotion. Even smiling increases immune function so practise this when alone as well as with people. If you walk down the street with a smile on your face, your white cell count will increase.
• Take time every day for yourself, and walk, sit in the sun, listen to music, do something creative, or enjoy the company of friends.
• Love is probably the greatest healer, so reach out to others – give and receive. Most of all, begin by learning to love your inner self. He or she is your best friend, loves you dearly and will lead you, when you're ready, to a meaningful communication with your God in meditation periods. This will always happen in a way which is comfortable for you. Touch is also very healing, be it massage or giving and receiving hugs.
• Above all, never worry about getting cancer, as the mind is very powerful and can grow or destroy cancer cells with chemical messages from the brain.

At a seminar in Australia, Dr A Sali emphasised the fact that cancer patients fit the following profile:

• Always stressed in some way.
• Have an inadequate diet.
• Allergies are present.
• Low levels of hydrochloric acid and digestive enzymes.
• Bowel flora levels are inadequate.
• Immune function is deficient.
• Sticky platelets are a feature.

A good diet and emotional balancing techniques will correct all these features, so enjoy changing all the negative parts of your life into positive health-giving features.

TREATMENT

Diet

Enough conflicting dietary advice has been given to thoroughly confuse the average person. Should they go the macrobiotic route, follow the Gerson diet or something in between? It is important to understand your own body type when choosing a long-term eating pattern. A diet high in grains (macrobiotic) will suit one person very well and cause untold problems in another. Some are natural fish and vegetable eaters, while others are natural vegetarians.

However, when treating an existing cancer, the most important consideration is to first thoroughly cleanse all the tissues. The liver is the most important organ to work on as it has the job of detoxifying any harmful substances entering the body and then removing them to the gut. A toxic bowel will re-poison the system and overload the liver, so this is another area which requires close attention. Dr Gerson maintains that poor liver function is central to the development of cancer. Only juice fasting will effectively detoxify all systems. Frequent coffee enemas to detoxify the liver may also be essential for some in the early stages. Alternatively, several days of one tea-spoon of epsom salts in 1 litre of water may be taken. If fasting produces unpleasant symp-toms, it means that the body is releasing large amounts of toxins which must be flushed out.

Juice fasting

Juices only, for weeks on end initially, if you have a qualified person to supervise. Freshly-pressed juices contain living enzymes which absorb directly from the gastro-intestinal tract. The body always breaks down waste, and faulty cells first, so there is no need to fear the loss of healthy tissue through weight loss. Many years ago a Dr Brand in South Africa decided to treat her cancer with water fasting. Although the growth was reduced it still remained and she became increasingly weak. Once she changed to fasting on grapes, all traces of the cancer were destroyed in a matter of weeks. Many other such case histo-ries have been documented by Dr Brand and others. Juices are of inestimable value in can-cer treatment for their living enzymes and oxygenating properties.

Juices also increase the body's potassium levels, which in turn increase the pH of tu-mours. Research has shown that when the pH of cancer cells reach 7.5, they become dor-mant.

$1\frac{1}{2}$lbs of juiced raw carrots with juiced raw beetroot is important in cancer regression. The beetroot flavonoids normalise cell oxida-tion, are powerful antioxidants and detoxify the liver. The carotenoids in carrots are powerful antioxidants, and negate the genes that programme a cancerous cell.

Wheatgrass juice, with its enzymes, chlo-rophyll and antioxidants, is a miracle food for all chronic disease. Buy a book on sprouting and grow your own wheatgrass. Spirulina powder could be added to juice for its potent blend of food form vitamins, minerals and proteins, which are actually alkaline forming. Spirulina contains more beta-carotene than carrots but it is important to use a brand grown in clean water.

Post-fasting diet

After the fasting period, the following diet is of proven great value because of its high 'live' content. However the juices should also be continued on a daily basis.

- *Total veganism* for at least three months. All foods should be organically produced. 75%-90% should be eaten raw.
- *75% of the diet* should be a mixture of fruit, vegetables and sprouted foods (nuts, seeds, pulses and grains). This level will al-kalise the tissues.
- Add organically-grown whole fruit and vegetables after the fast, and if possible eat 90% of it raw. Add other foods at the rate of one each day and listen to the body to see what suits it best.
- Apples, grapes, pears and bananas should be emphasised, but eat a wide variety of all fruit and vegetables, and remember to in-clude onions and garlic, as well as broccoli, cauliflower, cabbage and Brussels sprouts. Take Kyolic garlic capsules if not eating any in its raw state.
- *25% of the diet* is made up with solid foods to include small amounts of raw nuts, seeds and especially flaxseeds.
- Eat whole grains (especially millet, corn spelt, quinoa and rice), and dried peas, beans, lentils and buckwheat within this 25%.
- If following a vegan diet, consult the veget-able protein-combining chart to make com-plete protein every day.
- *Once off the vegan diet*, add the following if desired, but only as a part of the 25% solid foods: oily fish such as mackerel, trout,

salmon and sardines, three times weekly in small servings.

• Free-range eggs. They contain sulphur proteins important in restoring normal oxygen levels in cells.

• A little homemade cottage cheese or goat cheese.

• A live natural yoghurt or kefir.

• Natural grain-eaters can slowly alter the ratio of these with vegetables, into a macrobiotic pattern.

• *Water* should be filtered, or use distilled water and take kelp tablets for natural minerals. Drink herbal teas, water, freshly-pressed juices, miso, vegetable broth or Japanese green tea (can inhibit cancer).

• *Oils* – make dressings with flaxseed (linseed) oil that is genuinely cold-pressed. Failing this, soak flaxseeds overnight in water, and add the resulting jelly-like substance to a dressing made from extra virgin olive oil and lemon juice. Flavour with lots of raw garlic and herbs.

• To stir fry, only wipe the pan with some coconut oil, and then splash water in as you are cooking to stop food burning. Olive oil may be used in cooking, but keep the temperature low, or the molecular structure will be damaged.

• *Fats* in total should be restricted to 18% of your diet or less, and ensure that the omega-3 and -6 oils form the major proportion. To achieve this, you really need to remain a virtual vegan, with a little oily fish added, and an occasional egg or serving of cheese.

• *Brewer's yeast* contains all the essential amino acids, and is an excellent source of B vitamins and chromium.

• *Liver juice* is rich in nutrients, and forms an essential part of the Gerson diet. An organic source would be vital, as animals also store dangerous chemicals in the liver.

Avoid

• All processed and refined foods, and everything made from them (white flour and sugar make platelets sticky).

• Added salt and unfiltered tap-water. Cancer cells contain more sodium than normal cells, and this blocks the alkalising potassium in juices.

• Meat, unless it is organically grown. Other meat contains more pesticides and hormones than you would believe.

• Cereals that are not soaked, fermented or sprouted, as they leach minerals from the body. A loaf of bread has had the grain fermented and soaked.

• All margarines and processed oils.

• Alcohol, except a little organic wine occasionally.

• Coffee, tea, canned drinks, squashes and canned juices.

• Food to which you are allergic.

Supplements of value
Adult doses:

• *Vitamin C* – 6-20g daily, or to bowel-tolerance, as calcium ascorbate. Statistics show that this vitamin reduces the incidence of breast cancer in post-menopausal women by 24%.

• *Beta carotene* – 15-30mg daily, as well as carrot juice for a wider range of carotenes. Derivatives of these penetrate the DNA of cancer cells and suppress the genes which induce a cell to become malignant. Countless studies have conclusively indicated that high levels of carotenes in the blood protect against all types of tumour development.

• *Vitamin E* – 200-400iu daily, suppresses genetic cancer induction (as does beta carotene) and prevents sticky platelets. A low-serum vitamin E is a cancer prediction.

• *Selenium* – 200mcg daily.

• *Vitamin D* – 400iu daily.

- *Zinc* – 50mg daily + *molybdenum* 100-300mcg + *manganese* 5-10mg daily.
- *B-complex* – 50mg once daily.
- *Calcium* and *magnesium* – 500mg of each daily.
- *Pangamic acid* – 100mg twice daily, to oxygenate the body, or use *Genesis 1000*.
- *Hydrogen peroxide treatment*, for oxygenation.
- *Cysteine* 500mg, and *flaxseed oil* 1tbsp, 3 times daily before meals, is another oxygenation option.
- *Flavonoids* – 2g daily, as pollens, propolis, quercetin, silymarin, beetroot or berry fruit extracts.
- *Antioxidant enzymes* – these scavenge free radicals, and can be bought as a single supplement.
- *HCl acid, pancreatic digestive enzymes* and *bromelain* 1g, just before each meal.
- *EPA* – 2-6g daily, depending on availability of food sources.
- *Evening primrose oil* – 500mg once daily.
- *Arginine* – 3g daily for one month, stimulates the thymus to produce T-cells that destroy cancer cells – stress depresses this gland.
- *L acidophilus* – a lactobacillus supplement twice daily.
- *Potassium iodide* – 200-300mg, to block breast cancer cells and restore the electrical potential in cells. It balances the positive and negative charges in all cell walls.
- *Shark cartilage* – as a treatment for solid tumours - 1g for every 15lb of body-weight, three times daily, half an hour before food. Rapid absorption is important so that digestive enzymes do not denature the cartilage. Therefore the cartilage is taken with a little juice on an empty stomach.
- *Béres Drops Plus* – 15 drops three times daily. This product has been used in Europe for 22 years in cancer treatment. It restores the immune system's ability to fight back and

increases the body's pain-killers. It also reverses the millions of micro-organisms found in cancerous tissue. The disease is not caused by these, rather they develop as the direct result of total nutrient depletion in the cancer tissue. Many researchers believe that the micro-organisms paralyse the immune system's ability to destroy faulty cells.

I am not suggesting that every cancer patient should take all of these supplements. They should be taken according to individual requirements and choice.

It is always very helpful to see a naturopath, for a few visits initially, so that you can get expert help with your diet, do a proper body-cleanse and find out exactly which supplements you need.

Herbs

- *Silymarin* – 50mg three times daily if necessary, to improve liver function.
- *Suma* – a Brazilian herb with strong anti-cancer properties. Many cures have been reported using this herb. It regulates hormones and increases intracellular oxygenation, which normalises faulty cells. Suma also strengthens the immune system and regulates the acid/alkaline balance in the body. Dosage at 20g daily is safe, although reported cures have occurred using as little as 8g. This herb is contra-indicated during the first three months of pregnancy.
- *Pau d'arco* – another Brazilian herb with anti- tumour properties. It contains high levels of oxygen, which is released when brewed as a tea.
- *Iscador* – an extract of the herb mistletoe which initiates an immune response and is given by intra-muscular injection. It is specifically toxic to tumour cells and it has been shown to increase immune system functions.
- *Shitake mushroom* – is anti-viral, anti-cancer and a powerful immune stimulant, available in tablet form.

- *Mandrake*, *podophyllum*, *colchicum*, *vinca rosea*, *thuja*, *turmeric*, *sweet violet* and *berberis* herbs – all of these are capable of destroying cancer cells.
- *Echinacea* restores immune function.

Many herbalists successfully shrink some tumours that are resistant to modern drugs. They do this with nothing more than a simple herbal blend, along with dietary improvements.

John Hoxey's herbal recipes against cancer are internationally famous. Here is one which has the effect of returning cell DNA to normal, balancing the acids/base levels and cleansing the bowel, the lymph and the blood as well as stimulating circulation. Four parts *licorice root* and *red clover*, two parts *burdock root*, *stillinger root*, *golden seal root*, and *poke root*, one part *cascara*, *prickly ash bark* and *buckthorn bark*. Make the herbal mixture into an infusion and drink one cup three times daily. Potassium iodide is added to this recipe, and 300mcg daily is the recommended dose.

Herbs are nature's pharmacy, and you might like to choose some of these along with your dietary regime. The important thing is to *enjoy* your new approach to health.

Homeopathy

Constitutional treatment by a very experienced classical homeopath has produced some remarkable cures, and will at least improve the quality of life.

- *Euphorbia* – for the deep searing pain of cancer.
- *Arsenicum Alb* 30c – for fear of death. It is important to be positive.

Radiotherapy and chemotherapy protection

Chemotherapy and radiation cause nausea, hair loss, severe fatigue and a sensation of systemic poisoning.

Homeopathy – for nausea. *Sol* 30c – three doses two hourly after radiation, or *phosphorus* 200c – one dose after each exposure.

Herbs – Chinese research clearly indicates that the taking of particular herbs during radiotherapy or chemotherapy significantly improves survival rates. A good blend is as follows – *astragalus*, *ganoderma*, *eleuthero*, *ginseng*, *ligustrum*, *atractylodes*, *schizandra*, *codonopsis* and *licorice*. The dose is one tablespoon of the blended powdered herbs three times daily. Eleuthero ginseng would be of value alone, for those who cannot source the Chinese herbs. The Chinese blend prevents growth of metastases and protects dramatically against the destruction of white blood cells caused by such toxic invasive treatment.

Supplements – *vitamins C, E, B5* and *B6*. *Béres Drops Plus*. *Brewer's yeast* and *spirulina* powders, three tablespoons daily.

In my experience, patients taking the herbs, Béres Drops and a homeopathic remedy sail through treatment with no nausea or loss of energy, and minimal hair loss.

Cancer cells are disordered cells, and just as any production line can produce abnormal products, so can the human body. We all produce cancerous cells but an alert surveillance system mediated by immune function destroys them as they arise. However, if our immune system is weakened by a poor lifestyle, drugs and radiotherapy we may lose the ability to destroy rogue cells.

Science is spending billions looking for a cure which would be better spent in demonstrating the fact that prevention is in our own hands. In fact, *the number of people working in the cancer field is said to be far greater than those with the disease*. In spite of this, the death rate from cancer is still climbing at an alarming rate. In 1900 one person in thirty died of the disease, and by 1980 the rate was up to one in five. Now we have a situation where one person in three develops cancer. All the screening processes have done nothing to halt the upward spiral.

Furthermore, in most cancers, radiotherapy and chemotherapy produce only short-term benefits – in the long-term, statistics show that there is no difference in survival between those who undergo these treatments and those who don't. Even the highly respected British medical publication, *The Lancet*, published an editorial in April 1991 concluding that chemotherapy was at best a treatment of doubtful benefit. A real downside of this treatment is that it inhibits white blood cell production, and once some cancer cells are destroyed, the remaining ones often multiply more rapidly. Chemotherapy seeks to block the DNA of cancer cells, but some usually remain untouched, and as soon as the drugs are discontinued, those cells can start multiplying into new tumours – a diet high in carotenes might prevent this from happening.

Only a strong immune system can search and destroy every single cancerous cell in the body. A professor from the department of medicine at the University of California has published statistics indicating that patients who avoid surgery, drugs and radiation live at least three times longer than those who receive these treatments.

Correcting the diet, using supplements where applicable, coping with stress and emotions properly, and especially dealing with the pollution of air, water and food, would alone precipitate a dramatic drop in the incidence of cancer. This disease hardly existed a century ago. It is a condition of modern times caused by minds and bodies that have been sadly neglected for a variety of reasons.

No one should ever lose hope of a cure, and anyone whose resolve is failing should read Dr Ian Gawler's wonderful book about his own cure of a so-called terminal cancer. A very important part of the treatment is to take charge of your life as a whole. If your doctor is making your treatment decisions, then you still have a victim attitude. Only by charting your own course do you have the greatest chance of 100% recovery. Read widely, listen to all the advice and then sit down and draft out the direction of your own treatment plan.

Think positively and be of good cheer. Those happy chemicals will do you a power of good.

III: *39. AIDS*

An enormous amount of information has been published about AIDS, using all sorts of confusing categories. However, the blunt fact is that if an individual is HIV positive he will almost certainly develop AIDS unless he restores his health for a greater chance of very long-term survival. The virus is present inside his CD4 T lymphocytes, monocytes and macrophages, all of which are part of his immune system. The full-blown condition results once the T4 count is decimated. Whether or not this occurs depends on the mental and physical health of the individual and his ability to fight back. Certainly it is possible to be HIV positive with anti-bodies to the virus and remain symptom-free for many years. There is growing evidence that some people carry the virus and never develop AIDS, and there is also evidence that about 5-10% of people with AIDS are not even infected with the HIV virus. This suggests that the virus is not necessarily the *cause* of the disease, rather the result of it.

At the Pasteur Institute, Professors Duesberg and Montagniel believe that AIDS may be an auto-immune disease whereby the body is destroying its own immune system. They believe that the HIV virus is an opportunist and not the actual cause of AIDS. That is, the virus takes advantage of an already-weakened body and is then able to enter and multiply within human cells. If this is an auto-immune disease, then it is the most serious of all because in this case the immune system is destroying one of its own components (CD4 helper T-cells). In other auto-immune diseases, the immune system destroys tissue such as joints, but it does not self-destruct.

Another theory is that the immune system is not self-destructing but just annihilating the white cells in which the virus replicates (CD4 helper T-cells) and therefore we should be concentrating on increasing the CD8 T-cells which will eradicate the virus.

One certain fact is that those who develop AIDS or become HIV positive already have compromised immune systems. They have usually suffered from allergies, candida, herpes, hepatitis or glandular fever, and have taken antibiotics frequently. In addition, there may be a long history of poor diet, late nights, inadequate rest, sleep, exercise, recreation and long-term stress – all conditions which compromise the immune system.

When the diet is poor, or antibiotics and other drugs have been used indiscriminately, the gut environment becomes very unhealthy. Eventually a series of events leads to a toxic porous gut and resultant allergic reactions. The immune system, already weakened by a faulty lifestyle, is called upon to fight increasing levels of fungi, foreign protein and undesirable bacteria or parasites in the intestines, blood and tissues. Is it any wonder that an opportunist virus can then invade a body where the surveillance system is tired and overstretched in fighting self-inflicted ills?

Consider the fact that although there is a world-wide epidemic, the disease has not struck down well-nourished healthy communities in the way that it is decimating those (even whole populations) who have unhealthy lifestyles. It is the latter which weakens the immune system and makes us vulnerable, not only to attack from viruses but also to developing an auto-immune disease. As we destroy the earth, we also destroy our immune systems with the resulting polluted air, water and food, and become more and more weak as a species. AIDS is almost like a punishment for our incredibly selfish treatment of the world. At the very least we should look at it as a final warning to clean up our act before those who are still healthy also have their immune systems compromised – to the extent that the risk of AIDS is a real probability.

Treatment of the HIV-positive person is directed at detoxifying the gut and tissues, maintaining a strong immune system, strengthening cells against viral invasion and healing his or her life. A very comprehensive programme is required with the following necessities: a healthy diet, clean water and air, sunshine, exercise, stress-management, adequate sleep, relaxation, visualisation, creative hobbies, a healthy happy lifestyle, a positive outlook, moral and emotional support. Patients using visualisation techniques to increase their white cell count have had before-and-after blood counts done in hospitals, which showed a marked rise after the imaginal exercises. Supplements and herbs are essential for increasing immune function and reducing viral activity. Regular massage is physically and mentally healing and a lovely way of introducing anti-viral herbal oils.

Whatever the cause turns out to be, it is absolutely essential to strengthen the immune system and detoxify those at risk of AIDS. There is a danger of people believing that being HIV positive is not so serious if they are presently symptom-free, thereby not recognising the need to take immediate and comprehensive steps to heal their physical and emotional lives and restore health and immune competence.

The development of full-blown AIDS is often the result of continuing with a poor diet, the taking of drugs or living with a polluted internal environment, because these all reduce immune competence. Repeated infections may also trigger the onset, but *a life which is not healthy is the most potent trigger of all*. However, do not despair if you already have AIDS, because there are significant numbers of people in this situation who have remained well on a long-term basis because of their healthy lifestyles.

The power of the mind

It cannot be overemphasised that one of the most important factors in any serious illness is a positive state of mind. Because every cell in the body has receptors for brain messages, we all have the capability of exercising control over every part of our bodies. Many people do this as a part of a visualisation or meditation session, and it has been demonstrated over and over that positive messages can lead to a complete arrest of very serious disease when used as a part of holistic healing. Conversely, it has also been demonstrated that this process can be reversed quite dramatically by an authoritative figure like a doctor, indicating pessimism or doubt.

Dr Bernie Siegal, a brilliantly sensitive American surgeon, has used the message system between mind and body in an even more basic form. As his patients are going under anaesthetic he instructs them to redirect their blood-flow so that blood-loss during the operation will be minimal, and he says it works every time. Any problems occurring during the surgery, such as a falling blood pressure, is rectified by a whispered instruction into the patient's ear, and you've guessed it – it happens. It is now known that patients in the operating theatre absorb all that is said. Those who hear positive statements from the surgical team heal quicker. Dr Siegal has demonstrated that even patients in comas hear and respond to messages that state powerful reasons for returning to consciousness and living. On an even more basic level this exceptional man has shown that positive statements to junior doctors on ward rounds will cure terminal illnesses in some patients who hear the discussion. Equally, the doctor who removes hope or expresses doubt is often administering a death sentence. In the early days, Dr Siegal was surrounded by sceptical colleagues, but they soon because completely convinced after spending a little time in the operating theatre with him.

If one person can have such a powerful effect on the body of another, just think what you could do for yourself on a daily basis. That inner self residing in you is capable of healing your life. It is a spark of energy which belongs to a God/force that loves you. Trust it, believe in it, love it, rely on its wisdom and tell it what you would like it to do for you. Bernie Siegal's greatest gift was to show us that healing the mind and the body can be achieved in this very simple way. Just put yourself into a relaxed peaceful state every day and then talk to your inner self. At the same time, surround yourself with supportive people and see a counsellor or dream analyst if necessary, in order to find any mental blocks which may be preventing healing.

Studies of long-lived AIDS patients have turned up a consistent pattern of people who are fighters. They work hard at being healthy in mind and body. Although they accept their disease, they never view it as a death sentence. The disease has been a means of healing their lives so that every day has become a joy, a reason for living, loving and valuing their families, friends and the gifts of nature. The disease has given them a sense of purpose, a sense of self-worth, an appreciation of the inner being and the ability to nurture themselves when necessary. Leading on from this, these same people are then able to get involved in helping others, and find a balance between giving, receiving and taking care of themselves.

HIV effects on the immune system

The HIV virus actually replicates inside the CD4 helper T-lymphocytes. Eventually the cells are destroyed and reduced in total number. However it is not certain whether the virus is responsible for the destruction or whether the immune system is self-destructing. The virus is found inside the T4 cells of most AIDS sufferers, whether asymptomatic, in a middle area or with the full-blown condition. However, research indicates that this disease also involves macrophages, and these are not destroyed by the HIV virus like the T4-cells. Rather they act as HIV reservoirs, and remain as chronically-infected cells. This adds further evidence to the theory that AIDS may be an auto-immune disease. If the virus destroys T4-cells, surely it would also destroy macrophages.

The diet is of vital importance to the health of the immune system, and here again the consumption of junk food, sugar, white flour and fats adversely affect it. Sugar dramatically lowers phagocytic activity. White flour is converted to fats, and where total fat and cholesterol are raised, T- and B-cell production is disordered. This means that antibody response goes awry, and the destruction of the infecting organisms is also inhibited. Where blood sugar levels are high as a result of sugar and other simple carbohydrates in white bread and pasta, hydrochloric acid and digestive enzymes are reduced, and so vital protein absorption is inhibited. All cells, including those of the immune system, require protein.

AZT

If you are HIV-positive, think long and hard

and read widely before allowing anyone to give you this toxic drug. Professor Duesberg has noted that the drug actually *causes* the *symptoms* of AIDS in healthy people who just happen to be HIV positive. There is also irrefutable evidence that once the drug is discontinued, white cell counts spontaneously increase, which means that the drug may be destroying these cells in some way. AZT is said to protect cells against viral invasion in the early stages, but there are many other completely non-toxic methods of doing this.

Long-term AIDS survivors tend to be those who do not take AZT or other drug therapy. In fact there is evidence that many people who are well suddenly start to go downhill very rapidly if they take AZT. In a German study, where AIDS victims were given AZT for a year, they experienced a 65% drop in their white blood cell counts. This drug is reported to have been tested on animals 15 years ago as a leukaemia treatment, but never tested on humans because of the massive toxicity discovered during the studies.

People who take AZT eventually suffer bone marrow destruction, and then they need regular blood transfusions. Obviously the AZT is massively immune-suppressive and blood transfusions certainly exacerbate this – the result is a downward spiral consisting of one serious disease after another. If you then continue with the orthodox approach to AIDS, the diseases call for more and more toxic drugs, which in turn have increasingly horrendous side-effects like kidney destruction and blindness. Can any logical mind want to follow this pathway?

The allopathic medical approach to AIDS does nothing to build health – rather it simply waits for deterioration, and at each new low level, instigates what it sees as the appropriate drug therapy. This approach just hastens the downward trend, and the side-effects of the drugs used, cause their own destructive diseases.

Because it is probable that AIDS only develops in those with already compromised immune systems, orthodox medicine is once again guilty of only treating symptoms – but in this case the drugs used frequently hasten the end with their powerful toxicity. Worse still, AZT may actually be *causing* AIDS in those in the borderline risk area. The only way to approach disease is by restoring our normal self-healing ability.

Bastyr clinic research

A one-year clinical trial carried out at this respected naturopathic clinic in Seattle indicated very positive results. All the patients already had many AIDS-related symptoms, and were first instructed on how to eat correctly. Supplements were taken to strengthen the immune system and herbs were used for anti-viral activity at a cellular level. Hydrotherapy was employed to raise the core temperature of the body to 102°F for 40 minutes, twice weekly, for three weeks at a time. This was repeated four times during the year. Raising core temperature by means of total immersion in a controlled temperature bath has an anti-viral effect.

Additionally, some patients received acupuncture while others were treated homeopathically. All received psychological counselling to heal their lives. Individual problems were always treated, as they arose, with relevant vitamins, herbs or other nutritional support. The impressive result was that 100% survived and not one person's condition progressed to a more serious stage. Similar studies using placebo or AZT always indicate a high percentage of cases progressing to full-blown AIDS, and many deaths during the year long trial periods.

TREATMENT
Diet
Follow the naturopathic diet and lifestyle to the letter, which includes the instructions on exercise, stress-release, relaxation and recreation. One of the most important things to be aware of is listening to your body-signals. Never push yourself to the extent of feeling fatigued, as this will decrease your immune function. When you feel tired, drop what you are doing and rest for as long as your body requires. Remember that avoidance of junk, sugar, refined carbohydrate, margarine, processed oils and excessive saturated fat is of utmost importance to the immune system, as is dealing with anything causing stress.

The immune system components are made of cells in the same way as the rest of the body. This means that they have cell walls composed of various fatty acids, just as in all other cells. The structure of the wall determines the flow of anything in and out of the cell, including viruses. If it is too rigid because of a lack of unprocessed polyunsaturates, then viruses can readily enter. Equally damaging to cell wall fluidity is an excess of saturated fat, any margarine or chemically-processed oils, sugar and white flour – all the products that fill a major percentage of supermarket shelves. Studies in Africa with polyunsaturates have indicated that those taking evening primrose oil and EPA (from oily fish) suffered less fatigue, diarrhoea, skin-rashes, infections, fevers and weight-loss.

A high-fibre vegetarian diet, with a little oily fish if desired, is best. Emphasis should be placed on the use of sprouted foods (because of the greatly increased nutrient value), raw food and fermented foods like sourdough wholegrain bread, sauerkraut, yoghurt and rejuvelac, which is made from grains. Food-combining is vital where digestive processes are inadequate. A wide variety of food should be eaten for exposure to a maximum number of vitamins, minerals and enzymes. Organically-grown food is also important and the diet must be 75% alkaline-forming. If the tissues are acidic, HIV will flourish. Viruses, bacteria and fungi are inhibited by alkaline conditions.

Emphasise the carotenoid orange and yellow-coloured fruits and vegetables, and the flavonoid-containing foods like beetroot, berry fruits, cherries, grapes, blackcurrants and hawthorn berries.

A US study indicated a dramatic effect on immunity when the amino acids tyrosine and phenylalanine were severely curtailed in the diet for three weeks. Killer T-cells increased by 93%, cytotoxic cell activity increased by 80% and helper T-cells increased by 45%. The ratio of T-helpers to T-suppressors improved from 1.75:1.93 to 1.73:1. When the diet was stopped there was an immediate regression to former levels. However, the study is extremely interesting, and no doubt more research will be built upon it. A vegetarian diet reduces the intake of these two amino acids.

A recent French study has indicated that a 'Stone Age' diet dramatically improves the health of HIV subjects. This basically means 75% alkaline-forming food, mostly raw food, nothing processed, as well as avoidance of all dairy products and gluten grains.

Any malabsorption problems must be promptly sorted out with the use of enzymes or betaine HCl acid tablets, and diarrhoea must be treated with herbs and garlic, as well as allergen avoidance. Supplements are better taken in capsule form so that absorption is more likely. Free form amino acids in capsule form may be necessary in cases of weight-loss, poor digestion or diarrhoea. Where candida is present, the diet becomes very restrictive, as yeast foods, ferments, fruit juice, dairy products and farmed meat have to be avoided.

Supplement explanation

Vitamin C is antioxidant, anti-viral and supports immune function. The Noble Laureate, Linus Pauling, has published evidence that large doses of the vitamin has reduced P24 antigens in laboratory studies by 90%, which indicates a profound HIV-inhibitory effect. With large doses, it is important to prevent kidney stones with adequate levels of magnesium citrate, B6 and plenty of water. 10g daily is the lowest dose at which anti-viral activity is seen. Many AIDS patients take 50 to 60g daily. With high doses of vitamin C, calcium depletion and nervous symptoms may occur, therefore 0.5 to 1g of calcium citrate should be added for every 10g of vitamin C.

Flavonoids have anti-viral and immune-stimulating activity. They are found in nature combined with vitamin C, and enhance its function. Some good ones to take as supplements are quercetin, pignaginol and catechin. The latter also breaks down bowel toxins.

Beta carotene, vitamin E, selenium, zinc, manganese, iron and B vitamins are all discussed in chapter III:1 on the Immune System. In AIDS, beta carotene increases natural killer cells. 180mg daily has been shown to lead to 20% more CD4 helper T-cells.

Glutathione, a blend of three individual amino acids, is depleted by the HIV virus, as are other antioxidants. HIV-positive people who do not yet have symptoms have 30% less glutathione than normal in the bloodstream, and 60% less in the lungs, and this may account for the onward progression of the disease. This amino acid is important for the proper activity of T- and B-cells as an antioxidant against free radicals, and it plays a part in maintaining the integrity of all cell walls. Where cell walls function properly, nutrients pass in and out correctly and viral invasion cannot occur. A new report indicates that L-cysteine inhibits the HIV virus – this amino is a component of glutathione. Another study found that under test tube conditions, glutathione powerfully inhibits HIV. Arginine, which is also an amino acid, not only activates killer T-cells but increases their number. In a study using 30g daily for just three days, natural killer T-cells increased by 91%. This dosage would almost certainly be toxic for longer than a few days, but no doubt research will reveal the optimal safe dosage. Arginine is known to stimulate the thymus gland to be more active in processing T-cells.

Calcium EAP (ethanoleamine phosphate ester) is a natural precursor to the formation of lecithin. In the case of AIDS its real value is in its ability to restore cell membrane integrity to prevent viral replication. It does this by altering the electrical charge mechanism in the cell wall. Calcium EAP is explained in detail in chapter III:37 on Multiple Sclerosis.

Three very effective western anti-viral herbs are echinacea, licorice root and greater celadine. Garlic increases killer T-cells and contains the sulphur amino acid cysteine. Others are cinnamon, myrrh, thyme, eucalyptus, lavender, black pepper, juniper and geranium. All of these can be found as essential oils that can be absorbed during a daily massage or bath.

Some clinical studies indicate that bitter melon juice can increase the CD4 count dramatically within three months – by as much as 300%. It is also capable of reversing other HIV-related conditions, such as neuropathy, tuberculosis, arthritis and herpes. Bitter melon has long been used to treat psoriasis and diabetes, and has known anti-tumour properties. The active ingredient inhibits viral replication, and has an interferon-type effect by preventing one cell from infecting another.

The following are Chinese herbs which

have been found to inhibit HIV replication: arctium, epimedium, lonicera, woodwardia, viola, senecio, andrographis, coptis, prunella, lithospermum, alternanthera, licorice, astragalus and cassia seed. Dr Subhuti Dharmananda and his colleagues in Seattle have done valuable pioneer work in the use of Chinese herbs against HIV and other viruses. Several formulas are sold by the Institute for Traditional Medicine in Seattle, which are specific to various conditions associated with AIDS. Astragalus 10+ formula or Astra 8 are anti-viral immune enhancers. Shitake mushrooms and reishi mushrooms are powerfully anti-viral and supportive of the immune system. These are normally taken with the astragalus formula. Some of these were used in the Bastyr College clinical study.

Since AIDS reduces antioxidants, adding free radical scavenging enzymes is of value. Wheatgrass juice and barley greens are rich in antioxidant enzymes. Additionally the immune stimulating vitamins and minerals also have antioxidant activity.

Supplements

Adult doses:
- *Vitamin C* – to bowel-tolerance, 10g daily is the minimum, 30g would be better. Use calcium ascorbate as every one gram of ascorbic acid leaches 100g of calcium.
- *Flavonoids* – 500mg three times daily, of a mixed kind.
- *Beta carotene* – 45mg daily, plus carrot juice.
- A good multi-vitamin/mineral designed for AIDS can be bought from several manufacturers. Failing this the approximate doses individually are as follows, and the dosage is for a complete day's amount:
- *Vitamin E* – 400iu.
- *Vitamin D3* – 200-400iu.
- *Vitamin B-complex* – 25-50mg + 50mg extra of B1 and niacinamide (B3), and 500mg

extra of choline and pantothenic acid. B12 folic acid and biotin must be part of the B-complex, but in small amounts.
- *Selenium* – 200mcg.
- *Magnesium citrate* – 300-500mg.
- *Calcium citrate* – 300-500mg, only if not taking calcium EAP.
- *Zinc citrate* – 25-30mg.
- *Iron citrate* – 100mcg.
- *Manganese* – 10-20mg.
- *Molybdenum* – 100mcg.
- *Chromium polynicotinate* – 200mcg.
- *Potassium iodide* – 200-300mcg.

The following are taken separately:

- *Flaxseed (linseed) oil* – 1 tablespoon daily.
- *Cider vinegar* in water daily, before breakfast.
- *Evening primrose oil* – 1g daily.
- *Calcium EAP* – 600mg, three times daily.
- *Béres Drops Plus* – 3 times daily.
- *L acidophilus* supplement – twice daily.
- *Oxyplex* – 4-6 capsules daily, or some other mixed antioxidant enzyme product. Take them daily before food.
- The components of *glutathione*: L-cysteine, L-glycine and L-glutamic acid, at the rate of 1g each daily before food.
- Intravenous *hydrogen peroxide* treatment by a doctor is worth considering – see chapter III:38 on cancer.

The supplements are chosen primarily for their ability to restore immune function to normal. Some also have specific anti-viral activity and others restore the integrity of the cell wall.

Any candida must be vigorously treated, and the bowel wall healed. As other conditions arise they should be treated by appropriate natural means. Remember that drugs suppress the immune system – the very thing that needs all the help it can get.

Herbs of value
Adult doses:
Choose from the following, or better still, see a naturopath or medical herbalist for guidance in choosing the best blend for you.

- *Astragalus* 10+ – 1 tablespoon twice daily (11g daily).
- *Reishi mushroom* and *shitake mushroom* extract - 3 tablets twice daily.
- *Echinacea* and *golden seal* – 1g each, three times daily.
- *Pau d'arco* fluid extract – quarter to half teaspoon three times daily.
- *Greater celadine* – 1g with *blood root* 5mg, twice daily.
- *Licorice root* – 0.5-1g three times daily.
- *Bitter melon* as juice or as concentrate in capsule form.
- Anti-viral *essential oils* daily.
- *Garlic* cloves – 4 added to salads.

Homeopathy
Constitutional treatment was shown in the John Bastyr study to have a marked effect on increasing T4 cells, when given as a part of the holistic programme.

Don't forget that in order to be healed and live a full life-span, you must treat your body as a whole and heal it on a physical, mental and spiritual level.

III: *40. ALZHEIMER'S DISEASE*

This condition is rapidly increasing in incidence and is affecting people at a younger age than previously. There has been a tenfold increase in diagnosed cases in this century and it is believed that the situation will worsen dramatically. Currently it is the fourth highest cause of death in the Western world.

Although a definitive diagnosis is only possible on autopsy, conclusions can be drawn by exclusion. Once a diagnosis of dementia has been made, then various tests are necessary to determine the cause. Many elderly people are in this situation through nutritional deficiencies, toxic conditions or cardiovascular disorders. Much of this arises because they don't eat properly. Only 50% of cases of dementia are due to Alzheimer's. Other causes are pharmaceutical drugs, low thyroid function, low blood sugar, diabetes, alcoholism, Parkinson's disease or tumours. However, research indicates that patients with Alzheimer's also have a high incidence of thyroid disease.

In Alzheimer's, brain dysfunction tends to be diffuse and this is highlighted on an EEG examination of brain function. The typical Alzheimer's person has tangled brain cells with heavy metals like aluminium, lead and mercury trapped in the mesh. There is also heavy plaque formation containing these metals. Both disorders are most marked in the olfactory area of the brain and for this reason it is hypothesised that inhaled environmental toxins play a causative role. This may be so, but a 1991 study highlighted the case of an Alzheimer's patient who was found to have a severely-disordered olfactory region, whereby nothing could possibly have entered the brain through the protective bone structure. However, she still had the typical tangled nerve cells in that part of her brain. In spite of this isolated case one cannot ignore the relationship between the rapidly increasing incidence of Alzheimer's and the deterioration in the quality of the air we breathe.

The quality of our food and water is of equal importance. Modern processing adds aluminium to our food and governments add it to our water to remove any cloudiness. They also add fluoride because of the unproven hypothesis that it will prevent tooth decay. Unfortunately research has indicated a clear association between fluoride and Alzheimer's, in that the fluoride combines with aluminium in the bloodstream and prevents it from being excreted by the kidneys. Instead it is stored in the bones and the brain.

Many people believe that Alzheimer's will be the most dreaded disease of the next century and that may well be so unless we stop ingesting fluoride, mercury, aluminium and pesticides in our food and water.

Causes

Although it is known that aluminium and other heavy metals accumulate in the brain of an Alzheimer's victim, we do not know why or even *if* this is the only reason for the disease. Research indicates that Alzheimer's may involve a mixture of genetics, heavy metal absorption, circulatory problems and nutritional factors.

When circulation is poor, brain levels of nutrients are also depleted, and certain proteins such as cysteine and glutamic acid can become toxic. The latter is an excitatory protein which is badly affected by lack of oxygen to the brain. Poor circulation because of deficient heart function or hardened arteries is often present in the elderly and this reduces the oxygen supply. One study showed that those *without* Alzheimer's have high brain levels of zinc, and this mineral certainly blocks the toxic effects of excess glutamate, as does the amino acid taurine. Low zinc has been found in association with an accumulation of several other amino acids in the brain of dementia patients and is another frequently deficient nutrient in elderly people.

The amino acid called cysteine, which is widely available in the food chain, is made in the brain and present in the environment and becomes toxic if not metabolised correctly. Vitamins C, B6, B12 and folic acid are all required for the proper function of cysteine. Studies indicate that Alzheimer's patients have low B12 in their cerebro-spinal fluid (the fluid protecting the brain and spinal cord) and elevated levels of cysteine.

Improving liver function as well as blood circulation to the brain has been shown to reduce dementia symptoms markedly, and many studies also indicate that improving nutrient levels increases brain function. The elderly are notoriously deficient in many vitamins and minerals. A wide range of minerals are needed by the brain such as zinc, copper, manganese, molybdenum, selenium, iron, iodine, chromium, boron, calcium and magnesium, along with all the B vitamins in particular. These will all be present if a naturopathic diet is followed.

It is hypothesised that aluminium is found in abundance in the brain of Alzheimer's victims because these people lack the ability to remove this metal from the body – possibly because they lack the chelating protein transferrin, which normally removes aluminium to the kidneys. Aluminium is also known to ac-

cumulate wherever calcium and magnesium levels are low and this can occur in those drinking fluoridated water. The fluoride combines with other minerals and renders them unavailable for use. In addition, calcium is used up alkalising the blood in a high-protein diet and magnesium is lost in food-processing.

A deficiency of B vitamins may also be involved in Alzheimer's, as B12, B6 and folic acid have been found to inhibit the absorption of aluminium from water. One study in UK indicated that there was a 50% higher incidence of the disease in areas of high levels of aluminium in water. This metal is also thought to interfere with the uptake of iron by the body's iron transport protein. Perhaps low levels of iron in those with a family history of Alzheimer's should be followed up with tests for aluminium toxicity. When aluminium levels are too high in the brain, choline (a B vitamin) is negatively affected. Eventually a lack of this means that brain messages cannot be passed from one nerve cell to another or from nerve cells to organs. This results in poor function of everything. Alzheimer's victims also lack the enzyme needed to produce the actual chemical messenger (acetylcholine) that is made from choline.

Aluminium is found as the major ingredient in under-arm deodorants, is present in significant amounts as an additive in processed foods, baking powder, infant formulas, canned soft drinks, antacids, cosmetics, toothpaste, buffered aspirin, processed cheese, and in common salt as an anti-caking agent. Acids like citric or phosphoric greatly enhance the absorption of aluminium, so fruit juice in cans or fresh juice taken with a food source of aluminium will increase the body level. Cooking in aluminium pans, as well as using aluminium foil, increases the risk of toxic loads in food. Tomatoes, spinach and eggs absorb measurable levels from aluminium cookware, and the metal will also dissolve into tea, coffee, meat and turnips.

To avoid aluminium, use deodorants which specify that they do not contain this metal, use natural cosmetics, herbal toothpaste and paracetamol instead of aspirin. Use quality cheeses and sea-salt, and cook only in stainless steel, enamel or ceramic pans. Wax paper can be used in the oven in place of foil, sandwiches can be wrapped in plastic, turkeys can be wrapped in gauze soaked in oil for cooking, and food can be stored in glass or ceramic dishes. Buy bottled water or use a kitchen tap filter which specifies that it removes fluoride and aluminium. Most of all, prepare food from fresh natural ingredients and resist the quick-processed option.

Mercury, the other common metal found in the brain of Alzheimer's sufferers, is a major ingredient in amalgam fillings, and there is no doubt that mercury gas leaks from this source constantly. Since the teeth are close to the olfactory region of the brain this aspect is of significance. Canned tuna is the highest food source of mercury, but lobster, shrimp and large sea-water fish contain significant levels, as does wheat that has been treated with methyl mercury fungicides. Use fresh salmon or sardines instead of tuna, and buy organically-grown flour for making bread and baking. Insist on dental fillings that do not contain amalgam – more and more countries are banning its use in dentistry. Germany did so in 1993. Silica is the most powerful known antagonist to mercury. In fact, it assists the kidneys in removing this metal from the body. It also has a proven effect against aluminium. Researchers have noted that a diet deficient in silica corresponds to higher levels of aluminium in the brain. Silica is found in unprocessed grains and horsetail herb.

Organophosphates found in pesticides is another suspected cause of Alzheimer's. These chemicals are also used to make rubber, cellophane, cling film, and for the chemical extraction of oils from olives and palm. Cling film is safe if not heated, but if it is used to cover food being heated the steam condenses at the under surface and drips back into the food. These drops of water then contain dangerous chemicals. Cover food to be heated with ceramic or Pyrex lids. Wrapping fatty foods like cheese in cling film also leads to the chemicals migrating into the food.

Finally, it is thought that free radical attacks on the brain could be partially responsible for Alzheimer's. These more readily cause damage as we age, and the elderly are frequently deficient in the antioxidant nutrients needed to neutralise the effect of free radicals. A study in 1992 has discovered that brain tissue in Alzheimer's victims has twice as much of the antioxidants glutathione and vitamin E as in other elderly people. This is thought to be because the body is trying to compensate for greater-than-normal free radical activity.

Symptoms

Symptoms of Alzheimer's are considered to be a failure of recent memory and progressive mental deterioration, until the individual is incapable of carrying out normal daily-life functions. Particular features seem to be difficulty in learning new things, failure to recognise familiar faces and forgetting how to use familiar objects – such as not realising that a key is for unlocking a door or for starting the engine of a car, or that the oven has to be switched on in order to cook the food inside or that an ice cream cone is for eating. By this stage the disease is well advanced and cannot be reversed, although nutritional support has been shown to improve mental function.

Prior to obvious symptoms of memory-loss

there is often a general slowing down of body function, and many of the symptoms at this very early stage match the homeopathic remedy alumina. This is a particularly interesting area, as perhaps the whole disease could be aborted with homeopathic treatment.

Homeopathic alumina

This remedy, according to George Vithoulkas, a world-renowned homeopath, is characterised by delayed action, both mental and physical. The slow physical reactions are due to an initial delayed nervous system reaction.

On the mental level the person is slower to comprehend information and figure out what to do about it. He is confused, vague and ideas are hazy. He may have difficulty expressing himself, and finding the correct words takes longer than usual. Speech is slower for this reason.

On the emotional level there is a sense of being hurried, of not being able to do things quickly enough, of time passing too slowly and apprehension over not achieving goals. A pervasive fear of impending trouble may be present. Anxiety, anxious dreams and frequent waking at night may feature.

On the physical level, the slow function leads to weakness. Bowel function can be slow even though the urge to go is strong. Bladder function is disturbed if one has to get up in the night, or if the flow is slow to start. Digestion may be affected by reduced function of the walls of the gut, which means that food sticks in the gullet or passes through the intestines very slowly. These people are usually slow eaters. The genital area has very relaxed musculature and sex drive disappears. Legs become increasingly heavy and weak and go their own way because of a lack of nervous control over the muscles. Numbness of the soles of the feet may develop due to delayed nerve reflexes.

Not every person who suits the homeopathic remedy alumina is going to have all of these symptoms by any means, but one or two from each level may be present.

Mucous membranes can become dry because poor nerve function means poor circulation. For the same reason the skin may be dry and itchy, including around the anus – but no rash is present. Dry crusts on the skin and in the nose correlate with dry skin and mucous membranes. The eyes may itch and the areas particularly affected are the inner corners and lower lids. Dry eyes produce a burning sensation, agglutination at night and a perception of halos around lights. Poor eye-muscle function can cause cross eyes, double or dim vision and drooping of the eyelid.

Unusual pertinent features are a tendency to sneer at everything and be obstinate and contradictory. Alumina patients are almost always intolerant of alcohol and may have adverse symptoms with potatoes, spices and starch foods. These people long for fruit and vegetables and may even crave indigestible things like charcoal.

Just because a person may fit this remedy, it doesn't imply that he will get Alzheimer's – not at all. However, for those with a family history of the disease who notice a slowing down of mental and physical function in middle age, it may be that homeopathic alumina would prevent the disease or at the very least slow its progression, where a genetic predisposition exists. Look for itchy burning eyes and skin, bladder or bowel weakness, slow eaters who can't swallow food properly and an intolerance of alcohol.

Dosage of alumina would be 30c every twelve hours for three doses, and then repeat monthly if necessary. Sometimes symptoms stay away for longer and repeats are utilised less frequently.

Prevention and treatment

An excellent quality diet where food is organically-grown and all processed foods are avoided is the most important step, so follow the naturopathic diet.

- Increase calcium in the diet, from green vegetables, salmon and sardines. Just 1oz of sardines contains 125mg of calcium, and a moderate serving of red salmon contains 600mg. The quality of calcium from these sources is far superior to that found in dairy products.
- Increase magnesium by eating nuts, seeds, soya beans, brewer's yeast and wholegrains.
- Increase B vitamins, from brewer's yeast, wholegrains, vegetables, lamb's liver or kidneys, soya and nuts, sunflower seeds and bananas.
- Increase zinc, from lamb's liver, fish and shellfish, cheese and seeds. Although zinc is present in vegetables and cereals, it is not so well absorbed.
- Increase beta carotene from carrots, green vegetables, apricots, melons and peaches.
- Eat adequate amounts of complete protein daily.
- For the elderly who can't eat the fruit and vegetable content of the naturopathic diet, juice a large percentage of the raw portion and take cooked vegetables as soup.
- Improve liver function with dandelion coffee, lemon, beetroot and green vegetable juices.
- Improve circulation to the brain by following the recommendations in chapter III:31 on Atherosclerosis, to clear cholesterol plaque from blood vessel walls.
- Clean the air in the house with an air purifier.
- Exercise regularly at an aerobic rate.
- Practise stress-release techniques.
- Avoid sources of fluoride, aluminium, mercury and lead in your daily life. Read labels on everything carefully.
- Hair mineral analysis would determine the presence of heavy metals in the body. If present, follow a natural chelation programme using vitamins, minerals and amino acids.

Supplements of value

- *Phosphatidyl choline* – 25g daily is the dose for existing Alzheimer's. Take this in the form of a 90% preparation, to reduce the likelihood of side-effects – nausea, abdominal bloating and pain, and diarrhoea. This is the best substance for increasing serum choline levels.
- *Antioxidants* – beta carotene 15mg, vitamin C 3g, vitamin E 400iu, selenium 200mcg, all daily.
- *Coenzyme Q10* – 50mg daily, oxygenates the brain and improves memory. Take with B6, B3 and iron.
- *Zinc* – 50mg daily on an empty stomach, as citrate or picolinate, with manganese 5-10mg.
- *Silica* – 100mg daily, reduces aluminium absorption from water.
- *Vitamin B12* – 1000mcg of a high-assimilation type.
- *Folic acid* – 1-5mg daily.
- *B-complex* – 25-50mg daily, and extra *vitamin B6* (100mg twice daily in total).
- *Calcium* and *magnesium* – 1g each daily, as amino acid chelate or as EAP, as this is a precursor of phosphatidyl choline (an ingredient of lecithin).
- *Evening primrose oil* – 500mg times three daily.
- *Brewer's yeast* – 1 tablespoon daily, for chromium and B vitamins.

Each person should be assessed individually for nutritional deficiencies. It may be that other nutrients such as molybdenum, iron, iodine, boron or vitamin D3 are needed in some cases. If the diet is greatly improved, then many of these supplements can be reduced.

Herbs

- *Ginkgo biloba* – 40mg of the extract three times daily, improves brain circulation and is antioxidant to the brain.
- *Hawthorn berries* – 0.5-1g three times daily, improves cardio-vascular function and circulation.
- *Silymarin* – 50mg three times daily is protective of the liver. This is an extract of milk thistle herb.
- *Dandelion coffee* – improves liver function.

Appendices

Appendix one

CELLOIDS®

The celloid minerals are a system of therapy centred on balancing the twelve base minerals, of which the human body is largely composed. These same minerals are the indestructible part of all living things, and as such are of great importance to health.

Symptoms of illness are matched to specific cation/anion combinations of minerals, rather than to just potassium, iron, sodium, calcium or magnesium. Every combination has a completely different effect. For instance, potassium phosphate (PP) is a nerve nutrient, whereas potassium chloride (PC) has its effect on all conditions where congestion occurs in tissue. Iron phosphate (IP) has an anti-inflammatory effect, and so in combination with potassium chloride (PCIP) it is excellent for treating such diverse conditions as colds and arthritis.

The system was originally developed by a Dr William Schüssler in the 1870s, but in homeopathic form. His remedies are still in widespread use as 'tissue salts'. In the earlier part of this century, Maurice Blackmore of Australia decided that a pharmacological dose of minerals rather than a homeopathic system was the only way to return cell chemistry to normal over the long-term. In this manner, he reasoned that even chronic illness could be reversed.

Blackmore went on to develop a system of changing the crude minerals from the earth's crust to the form which is found in living plants (colloidal) so that the human body could assimilate them quickly and com-

pletely. In this way, larger doses can be given without any risks, just as large amounts of minerals in food cause no harm. Only children under 2 years old take less than the adult dose. All life occurs in colloidal form, and therefore any nutrients supplied in this manner will be readily used by the human body.

Blackmores have two ranges of products: over-the-counter and those for practitioner-prescribing only. The products in this book are practitioner ones, but you can find close equivalents in over-the-counter products from health food shops in Australia, New Zealand, Hong Kong, Singapore, Malaysia, and the United Kingdom. The practitioner products are also available from naturopaths and chiropractors in all the countries mentioned. Anyone in other countries can obtain information from Blackmores at 23 Roseberry Street, Balgowlah, NSW 2093, Australia. Alternatively these minerals can be bought worldwide in homeopathic 6x potency as 'tissue salts', which are very effective in acute conditions. Take these tablets at the same rate as suggested for the Celloids® versions. Because they are homeopathic, there is no need to reduce the dose for children under two years of age. Tissue salts cannot be used to reverse chronic illness: only the celloids, with their physiological doses of minerals, will achieve that goal.

Celioid® minerals are listed in the supplement section by practitioner title, and there follows a list of the full names for those who want to find equivalents over the counter. The tissue salt equivalents are alongside.

PC	potassium chloride	kali mur
PS	potassium sulphate	kali sulph
PP	potassium phosphate	kali phos
CS	calcium sulphate	calcarea sulph
CP	calcium phosphate	calcarea phos
CF	calcium fluoride	calcarea fluor
SP	sodium phosphate	natrum phos
SS	sodium sulphate	natrum sulph
MP	magnesium phosphate	magnesium phos
IP	iron phosphate	ferrum phos
S79	silica	silicea

Maurice Blackmore did not develop the twelfth salt (Natrum Mur) which is sodium chloride (common salt). All of these minerals come in various combinations, to reduce the numbers of tablets needed.

Appendix two

HERBAL PREPARATIONS

Tea

This is the easiest way of taking herbal medicine, but it is important to prepare it correctly.

The quantities are always one ounce of herbs to one pint of boiling water. Leave the herbs to infuse in a teapot with a lid for fifteen minutes before straining and drinking the required amount. Normally 1 pint of tea is one day's dosage, and is divided into three parts for use before every meal.

If the herb is in leaf form, an ounce will be a lot in terms of volume, and if it is in root form, one ounce will be a small amount. For making tea, herbs should be chopped small (root or bark) or crumbled (leaf). Using a fine powder results in a tea with sludge which must be strained through a coffee filter after the fifteen minute infusion. When using fresh herbs for tea, crush the stalks and leaf veins with a mortar and pestle before pouring over the hot water. Herbal tea can be kept in the fridge for three days if being used as compresses or an eye-wash.

Decoctions

These are usually made from roots, bark, tough leaves or seeds, which need longer heating to extract their chemical constituents.

The quantities are two ounces of herbs to one pint of boiling water, in an enamel or stainless steel saucepan. The herbs must be well-chopped or crushed, and they are simmered gently for fifteen minutes. The liquid will reduce by half, and the resulting drink will have a stronger flavour than a tea. It may be necessary to put some herbs through a coffee grinder in order to break them down enough, as a mortar and pestle has little effect on some roots.

Powdered herbs

Some herbs can be bought from herbal shops already powdered, but others come only in chopped form. Use a coffee grinder to reduce these to powder. Dried herbs can be kept in good condition for a year in a cool place (in the fridge in the tropics), and roots and bark last even longer if stored correctly. It is better to powder small amounts at a time, in order to preserve the plant's essential oils.

Essential oils

These are quite easy to make if you are prepared to spend a little time, but only fresh herbs can be used. Crush these to a pulp and put one ounce into a jar with one tablespoon of cider vinegar and one pint of olive, almond or avocado oils that are cold-pressed. Put the jar in an airing cupboard, or it can be put outside in hot sun during the day. However, it must be protected from light by being covered by a layer of sand, which will also increase the heat of the jar.

Shake the jar vigorously once daily for ten days. If the oil is not strong enough after this time, discard the herbs, add a fresh lot to the same oil and repeat the process.

Store your essential oil in a cool place and in amber glass bottles.

Tinctures

These are made by soaking one ounce of herbs in five ounces of 70% alcohol. It is best to use vodka – never use surgical spirit or any cheap alcohol. For those who can't tolerate even half a teaspoon of alcohol three times daily, the tinctures can be made from cider vinegar. Again the herbs need to be chopped very finely or ground, if they are root or bark, and it is also best to powder leaves when one ounce in whole form is very bulky.

Tinctures keep indefinitely, and the alcohol will extract some ingredients that are not readily released in water. Put the herbs into a screw-top jar with the vodka and shake vigorously once daily for two weeks. Strain the liquid through a gauze bag. Squeeze it tightly to extract as much as possible and store the tincture in dark bottles.

Skin creams

These are very simply made with herbal tincture and aqueous cream. A 1:10 solution is made with one tablespoon of tincture thoroughly mixed into ten tablespoons of aqueous cream. Store it in a wide-necked jar in the fridge.

A good standby cream is calendula, using marigold flowers for the tincture. Calendula will heal up any cuts or wounds, nappy rash or chafing sores.

Poultices

Mix a powdered herb with just enough water to make a thick paste, or use a double decoction and whisk in enough slippery elm powder to make the paste. Put a plate over a pan of boiling water, lay a piece of doubled gauze on the plate, put the paste in the centre and fold the edges of the gauze over it. Place the poultice directly onto the skin with a warm cloth on top to keep the heat in. Be careful that the poultice is not so hot that it burns the skin. To maintain the heat, the overlying towel can be reheated from time to time.

Herbal syrups

Make a double-strength decoction, strain it, and add one quarter of its volume of honey. This is useful for children who can't take tinctures or powders.

Gargles

Half a cup of water, plus half a cup of glycerine, and 10mls of tincture. Blend these together, gargle, and swallow a little at the end. Alternately, herbal teas can be used as a gargle.

Children's herbal dosage

To determine the correct dosage for a child in terms of a fraction of the adult dose, divide the child's age by his or her age plus twelve as follows: 4 divided by $(4+12) = 0.25$. 10 divided by $(10+12) = 0.45$. Therefore the four-year old takes one quarter, and the ten-year old one half of the adult dose. Another method is to dose on the basis of one fifth of the adult dose for every 10kg of body weight.

Appendix three

DETERMINING VITAMIN & MINERAL DEFICIENCIES

The best way of doing this is by a symptom analysis, because all deficiencies produce symptoms. However, it is best to seek the help of a naturopath or nutritionist here, a. symptoms do overlap widely. For instance, tingling of the toes and fingers, shortness of breath and becoming easily fatigued could look like a vitamin B1 deficiency – however, if the person concerned also flushed easily on exertion, was prone to infections, healed slowly and had bleeding haemorrhoids, his deficiency would actually be iron phosphate and not vitamin B1.

Hair analysis, blood tests, sweat tests, taste tests and enzyme tests are all valuable in determining deficiencies. However the problem is that each test is specific to a narrow range of nutrients. For instance a blood serum test for calcium will not indicate tissue levels of calcium, and in fact high serum calcium is often caused by the mineral being leeched from bones, or because there is an insufficiency of another ingredient for its deposition in bone. For this reason accurate laboratory analysis of nutrients requires a great many tests to be done. For instance, hair analysis is accurate for heavy metals like mercury and aluminium, and reasonably so for chromium and selenium, but no other minerals. Serum zinc tests are inaccurate, but white blood cell levels and the sweat test are reliable. The only accurate magnesium test is done by testing red blood cell levels, and B6 tests are only reliable from a fasting blood sample. So you

can see that accurate laboratory analysis is time-consuming and costly. Symptom analysis will pinpoint problems in most cases.

If you have one of the conditions examined in part 3 of this book then take the supplements recommended, but if you are relatively well, then just buy a quality multi-vitamin/mineral tablet for daily use.

I do think that every home should have a book on vitamins and minerals, so that you have a reference for the many symptoms produced by deficiency of a single nutrient. There are hundreds of such books on the market, so browse a little and buy one which is presented in a manner that is most appealing to you.

Supplements

The balanced diet in terms of vitamins and minerals is now a myth. As you can see from the earlier chapters, even natural food is deficient in a wide range of nutrients. If you follow the naturopathic diet, and almost all the food eaten is organically-produced, then supplements will not be required as a routine – only as therapy when necessary. However the reality for most of us is that we at least need good multi-vitamin/mineral supplements every day.

Choosing your multi

This is the tricky part, as some are much better than others. Ask your local health food shop for advice if in doubt. Always buy from health food stores, as 'multis' made by drug companies tend to use synthetic vitamins where natural ones are better, and they also use allergenic binders and fillers all too frequently.

Any multi-mineral should contain a wide range, to at least include calcium, magnesium, zinc, manganese, selenium, chromium and iron. Any copper should be balanced by much higher levels of zinc. There is a divergence of opinion amongst the experts concerning the best carriers. For instance, some gluconates have been found to absorb well, and others not at all. Iron bound to fumarate is toxic and ferrous sulphate poisoning can be fatal to children. Selenium is best absorbed as seleno-methionine and zinc as picolinate or citrate. Calcium absorbs well as amino acid chelate, with citrate, lysinate or aspartate, but some other carriers are also adequate. Chromium is best absorbed as polynicotinate, and some minerals can be bound to orotates while others should not be taken in this form. This subject would fill a book on its own, and you will never find an ideal product in relation to *every* ingredient in the tablet. Your safest bet is to buy according to advice from your naturopath, nutritionist or health food store.

Any multi-vitamin should contain vitamin A or beta carotene, vitamin B1 (thiamine), vitamin B2 (riboflavin), vitamin B3 (niacinamide, nicotinic acid, niacin), vitamin B5 (pantothenic acid, calcium pantothenate), vitamin B6 (pyridoxine), vitamin B12, folic acid, PABA, biotin, choline, inositol, vitamin C, vitamin D, and vitamin E as d-alpha tocopheryl. The synthetic form is written as dl-alpha tocopheryl. A reliable company will put adequate levels in every tablet and state the dosage for adults and children. The best way of judging the quality of a product is by how you feel after taking it for a few weeks. A product with easily-assimilated ingredients will improve your sense of well-being and energy levels. It is not necessary for all ingredients to be natural, as some are effective in synthetic form. Linus Pauling stated that ascorbic acid was as effective as natural vitamin C, and synthetic Bs do a good job as long as natural ones are present in the diet as brewer's yeast or wholegrains and green vegetables. However vitamin A is best as beta carotene for high doses, vitamin E should be natural, and if possible vitamin D is preferable as D3 (cholecalciferol). Vitamin B6 is often needed in its active form of pyridoxine-5-phosphate.

Labels

These must list all the ingredients, with the carriers (in the case of minerals), and their amounts in terms of micrograms (mcg), milligrams (mg), grams (g) or international units (iu). All fillers, binders, excipients and colours must be declared. Natural things like guar gum, gum acacia, alginic acid, cellulose, silica and dicalcium phosphate are completely acceptable. Good products will state that they are free of lactose, wheat, corn, soy, salt, sugar and yeast, as well as preservative, artificial colours and sweeteners. Hypo-allergenic products usually come in capsule form, because in this way a manufacturer can use very few excipients.

Appendix four

PROSTAGLANDINS

See chapter II:6.
PGE2 is responsible for inflammatory reactions, water and sodium retention in the tissues, constriction of blood vessels, high blood pressure and tumours. It also depresses the immune system although vitamin E in the diet helps counteract this by inhibiting PGE2 synthesis in the body. This prostaglandin is largely made from the arachidonic acid in animal protein.

PGE3 is a powerful anti-inflammatory tissue hormone which has its greatest beneficial effect on the cardio-vascular system, saturated fats, cholesterol, triglycerides, the nervous and the immune systems. It reduces arachidonic acid release from animal protein, and in this way controls all those inflammatory chemicals causing blood clots, hypertension and atherosclerosis. The inflammatory PGE2 is muzzled by PGE3, which also means control over illnesses like eczema, asthma and arthritis. Triglycerides are dramatically lowered and cholesterol is controlled. The white blood cells of the immune system are all increased in number and activity, and auto-immune reactions prevented. This is the reason for EPA's remarkable effect on tumour regression. It also stores sunshine in the body which explains why races living in the far north do not suffer winter depression. Their cold-water fish contain very high levels of EPA, which is a highly polyunsaturated fat. Prostaglandin E3 is made from the omega-3 fats found in oily fish and flaxseeds in particular.

PGE1 is the best known prostaglandin, and an enormous amount of research has been published about it because of its connection with evening primrose oil. It controls the immune system and so is of benefit in infections, auto-immune diseases like rheumatoid arthritis, lupus, psoriasis and allergic reactions. The effect on the cardio-vascular system prevents clots, hypertension and atherosclerosis as well as lowering cholesterol. The hormones are also beneficially affected by PGE1, and this is why evening primrose oil is given for menstrual disturbances, weight control and even to make insulin work better.

The nervous system cannot function without PGE1, as it ensures that nerve messages are passed from one nerve to another and from nerves to muscles and other cells. PGE3 is thought to be of equal importance here. All messengers, both nervous and hormonal, are controlled by PGE1, as is the rate of cell-division and metabolism. PGE1 also has a controlling effect on the inflammatory PGE2.

Pathways of oils to prostaglandins

Once an EFA has been digested and absorbed into the blood and then carried to the cells, it has to undergo many chemical changes before becoming a prostaglandin. Unfortunately it is seldom a smooth path and the biggest stumbling block occurs at the first chemical change. If the necessary vitamins and minerals are not present, nothing can happen, but even if you've solved that problem, the reaction can still be blocked by stress, drugs, moderate or high levels of alcohol, excessive mono-unsaturated and saturated fat or cholesterol, white flour or sugar, aging and sickness, but most of all by chemically-processed oils, margarines and shortenings – in future I shall bring these three together as 'processed oils'. Even commercially-roasted nuts and seeds contain damaged oils. So, these things are not only of no use to us but they block the activity of the essential natural oils. Follow the 'fatty acid pathways' chart now, on page 53 in Part II Chapter 6.

Omega-6 pathway – linoleic acid is converted in the presence of protein, A, B and C vitamins, zinc and magnesium to GLA which is the substance found in evening primrose oil, borage and blackberry seeds. The next stop (DHGLA) leads directly to the formation of the prostaglandin E1 series (PGE1), which is anti-inflammatory. It is possible for us to make some into arachidonic acid but man largely lacks the enzyme to do this and prefers to make the very important PGE1. Have a look at the chart for a visual memory of this pathway. It's really quite simple. Only the names are strange. Now you can see why so many people benefit from taking evening primrose oil. Either they are not getting the precursor oils in the diet or their conversion is being blocked by a poor lifestyle and diet.

Omega-3 pathway – alpha linolenic acid is converted to EPA which occurs naturally in the oily fish previously mentioned. The final step is to DHA and prostaglandins of the E3 series (PGE3). This is also an anti-inflammatory PG. For those who are not converting the seed oils to EPA, we give a supplement of it or recommend oily fish in the diet.

Arachidonic acid pathway – this must be discussed here although it is no longer consid-

ered an EFA simply because the body can make some from omega-6 oils. However our major source of this fatty acid is animal protein and most people ingest an excessive amount. Look at the chart and you'll see that arachidonic acid makes two groups of chemicals and almost all of them are of a potent inflammatory nature; prostaglandin E2 being one. They cause blood vessel damage, blood clots, high blood pressure, the initiation and spread of cancer and the inflammatory reactions seen in asthma, eczema, psoriasis and chronic upper respiratory tract infections like chronic otitis media.

BIBLIOGRAPHY

Cancer

Oxides International Ltd, 117 Khyber Pass Road, PO Box 74347, Auckland, New Zealand.

Begin M E, 'Fatty acids, lipid peroxidation and diseases', *Proc Nutr Soc* 49, 261-267 (1990).

Bennett F C & Ingram D M, 'Diet and female sex hormone concentrations: an intervention study for the type of fat consumed', *Am J Clin Nutr*, 52, 808-812 (1990).

Bristol J B, 'Sugar, fat and the risk of colorectal cancer', *Brit Med J*, 291: 1457, 1885.

Burns C P & Spector A A, 'Effects of lipids on cancer therapy', *Nutr Rev*, June 1990; 1.

Cameron E & Pauling L, *Cancer and Vitamin C*, The Linus Pauling Institute of Science and Medicine, 1979.

Chen F, Cole P, Mi Z, Xing L, 'Dietary elements and oesophageal cancer morality in Shanxi, China', *Epidemiology* 3, 1992.

Colditz G A *et al*, *Am J Clin Nutr* 41:32-6, 1985.

Daly J M, Reynolds J, Sigal R K *et al*, 'Effect of dietary protein and amino acids on immune function', *Crit Care Med* 1990; 18 (2):S86-S93.

DeCosse J J, Miller H H, Lesser M L, 'Effect of wheat fibre and vitamins C & E on rectal polyps in patients with familial adenomatous polyposis', *J Natl Cancer Inst* 1989; 81: 1290-7.

Dharmananda, Subhuti, *Chinese Herbal Therapies for Immune Disorders*, Inst for Trad Med and Prev Health Care.

Doll R, 'Symposium on diet and cancer', *Proc Brit Nutr Soc* 49, 119-131 (1990).

Gerson Max, *A Cancer Therapy*, Gerson Institute, California.

Goldin B R *et al*, 'Estrogen exretion patterns and plasma levels in vegetarian and omnivorous women', *New Eng J Med* 307: 1542-47, 1982.

Graham S *et al*, 'Dietary factors in the epidemiology of cancer of the larynx', *Am J Epidemiol* 113 (6): 675-80, 1981.

Grotz Walter, *A Report*, Box 126, Delano, MN 55328, USA.

Ho J H, 'Nasopharyngeal carcinoma', *Advanced Cancer Research*, 15, 1972.

Ho J H, 'Salted fish in Southern China', *Lancet* 2, 1978.

Huang D F, *et al*, 'Analysis for volatile nitrosamines in salted preserved foodstuffs traditionally consumed by Southern Chinese', *IARC Science Publ* 20, 1978.

Hughes R E, 'Hypothesis: a new look at dietary fibre', *Human Nutr: Clin Nutr* 40C: 81-86, 1986.

International Clinical Nutrition Review, Vols 8-13.

Journal for Alternative and Complementary Medicine, UK, 1988-1993.

Kelly W D, *One answer to cancer*, Kelly Research Foundation, 1971.

Knekt P, Albanes K, Seppanen R *et al*, 'Dietary fat and risk of breast cancer', *Am J Clin Nutr* 52, 903-908 (1990).

Kolonel L N *et al*, 'Association of diet and place of birth with stomach cancer incidence in Hawaii, in Japanese and Caucasians', *Am J Clin Nutr* 34(11):2478-85, 1981.

Kune G A, 'Eating fish protects against some cancers: epidemiological and experimental evidence for a hypothesis', *J Nutr Med* 1990; 48(6): 223-40.

Kusaaka Y, Kondou H, Morimota K, 'Healthy lifestyles are associated with higher natural killer cell activity', *Prev Med* 21, 602, 1992.

Lee H P, Gourley L, Duffy S W *et al*, 'Dietary effects on breast-cancer risk in Singapore', *Lancet* 337, 1197-1200 (1991).

Lee M J, 'Relationship between stool pH and butyrate levels', *Nutr Cancer*, 16(2) 75-76 (1991).

Longcope C, 'Relationships of oestrogen to breast cancer, of diet to breast cancer and of diet to oestradiol metabolism', *J Nat Cancer Inst* 82 (11), 96-97 (1990).

Lovestone S, Fahy T, 'Psychological factors in breast cancer' *Br Med J* 302, 1219-1220 (1991).

McCabe E, *Oxygen therapies*, Energy Publ, Morrisville NY, 1988.

Negri E, La Vecchia C, D'Avanzo B, Franceschi S, 'Calcium, dairy products, and colorectal cancer', *Nutr Cancer* 13, 255-262 (1990).

Rosenberg L *et al*, 'Breast cancer and alcoholic beverage consumption', *Lancet* 1:267, 1982.

Sali A, *International nutrition seminar 1986*, sponsored by Bioglan Laboratories.

Salonen J *et al*, 'Risk of cancer in relation to serum concentrations of selenium and vitamin A and E: matched case- control analysis of prospective data', *Brit Med J* 290:417, 1985.

Sauer L A, Dauchy R T, 'The effect of omega-6 and omega-3 fatty acids on H-thymidine incorporation in hepatoma 7288CTC perfused in situ', *Brit J Cancer* 66, (1992).

Seeger P G, Wolz S, *Successful biological control of cancer*, Neuwwieder Verlagsgesellschaft, Neuwwied, Germany 1990.

Seeger P G, *Krebs - Problem ohne Ausweg?*, Verlag f Medizin, Heidelberg, Germany, 2nd edn 1988.

Shklar G, Schwartz J, Trickler D, Reid S, 'Regression of experimental cancer by oral administration of combined alpha-tocopherol and beta-carotene', *Nutr Cancer* 12, 321-325 (1989).

Simonton Carl MD, Matthews-Simonton Stephanie, Creighton James L, *Getting well again*.

Skrabanek P, 'False premises and false promises of breast cancer screening', *Lancet* August 10, 1985.

Tuyns A, 'Alcohol and cancer', *Proc Nutr Soc* 49, 145-151 (1990).

Wagner D A *et al*, *Cancer Res* 45:6519-22, 1985.

Wald N J *et al*, 'Plasma retinol, beta carotene and vitamin E levels in relation to the future risk of breast cancer', *Brit J Cancer* 49:321-4, 1984.

Warburg Otto, 'On the origin of cancer cells', *Science* 123 (1956).

Watson R *et al*, 'Cancer prevention by retinoids: role of immunological modification', *Nutr Res* 5:663-75, 1985.

Willett W C, MacMahon B, 'Diet and cancer: an overview', *New Engl J Med* 310(11): 697-703, 1984.

Willett W C *et al*, 'Prediagnostic serum selenium and the risk of cancer', *Lancet* 2:130-3, 1983.

Wolfe Derek, 'A report', *Int Journal of Alternative and Complementary Medicine*, Feb 1993.

Wright Jonathan V MD, 'The oestrogen quotient', *Int Clin Nutr Rev* July, 1991.

Wynder E L, Cohen L A, 'A rationale for dietary intervention in the treatment of post-menopausal breast cancer patients', *Nutr Cancer* 3 (4) 195-199, 1982.

Yu Mimi C *et al*, *NPC in Malaysia and Hong Kong*, National Cancer Institute, Monog 69.

Yu Mimi C, 'Nasopharyngeal Carcinoma in Chinese - salted fish or inhaled smoke?' *Prev Med* 10, 1981.

'Antioxidant vitamins and B-carotene in disease prevention', *Am J Clin Nutr*, (supple to vol 53), Jan 1001.

'Serum vitamin and provitamin A levels and the risk of cancer', *Nutr Rev* 42 (6):214-5, 1984.

Cardio-vascular disease

A textbook of natural medicine, J Bastyr College Publication.

Ammon H P T and Handel M, 'Crataegus, toxicology and pharmacology', *Planta Medica* 43:101-120, 318-22, 1981.

Anderson J W, Spencer D C C, *et al*, 'Oat-bran cereal lowers serum total and LDL cholesterol in hypercholesterolaemic men', *Am J Clin Nutr* 52, 495-499 (1990).

Anonymous, 'Coffee drinking and acute myocardial infarction', *Lancet* 2:1278-9, 1972.

'Antioxidant vitamins and B-carotene in disease prevention' *Am J Clin Nutr* (suppl to vol 53), Jan 1001.

Bordia A K, Josh H K, Sanadhya Y K, 'Effect of garlic oil on fibrinolytic activity in patient with CVD', *Atherosclerosis* 28:155-9. 1977.

Check W, 'Switch to soy protein for boring but healthful diet', *J A M A* 247:3045-6 1982.

Drexel H *et al*, 'Lowering plasma cholesterol with beta sitosterol and diet', *Lancet* 1:157, 1981.

Dyckner T, Wester O, 'Effect of magnesium on blood pressure', *Br Med J* 286: 1847-9, 1983.

Eichner E R, 'Alcohol versus exercise for coronary protection', *Am J Med*, 79 (2):231-40, 1985.

Ernst E *et al*, 'Garlic and blood lipids', *Brit Med J* 291:139, 1985.

Ferrannini E *et al*, 'Insulin resistance in essential hypertension', *N Engl J Med* 317, 350 (1987).

Flaten H, Hostmark A T, Keirulf P *et al*, 'Fish oil concentrate: effects on variables related to cardiovascular disease', *Am J Clin Nutr* 52, 300-306 (1990).

Fraser G E *et al*, The effect of various vegetable supplements on serum cholesterol', *Am J Clin Nutr* 34:1271-7, 1981.

Goodliffe Colin, *How to avoid heart disease*, Blandford Press, 1987.

Hanaki Y, Sugiyama S, Ozawa T, 'Ratio of low density lipoprotein cholesterol to ubiquinone as a coronary risk factor', *N Engl J Med* 1991; 325: 814-5.

Hargreaves A D, Logan R L, Thomson M *et al*, 'Total cholesterol, low density lipoprotein cholesterol, and high density lipoprotein cholesterol and coronary heart disease in Scotland', *Br Med J* 303, 678-681 (1991).

Hartung G H, Foreyt J P, Mitchell R E *et al*, 'Relation of diet to high density lippoprotein cholesterol in middle aged marathon runners, joggers and inactive men', *N Engl J Med* 302: 357-61, 1980.

Henry H J, McCarron D A, Morris C D, Parrott-Garcia M, 'Increasing calcium intake lowers blood pressure', *J Am Diet Assoc* 85:182-5, 1985.

Hodges R, Rebello T, 'Carbohydrates and blood pressure', *Ann Int Med* 98: 838-41, 1983.

Hughes A, Tonks R S, 'Platelets, magnesium and myocardial infarction', *Lancet* 1:1044-6, 1965.

International Clinical Nutrition Review, Vols 8-13.

Jenkins D J A *et al*, 'Effect of pectin, guar gum, and wheat fiber on serum-cholesterol', *Lancet* May 17 1975, pp1116-7.

Journal of American College of Nutrition, Vol 10, p66.

Kamikawa T, Kobayashi A, Yamashita T *et al*, 'Effects of coenzyme Q10 on exercise tolerance in chronic stable angina pectoris', *Am J Cardiol* 56:247, 1985.

Kark J *et al*, 'Coffee, tea and plasma cholesterol: the Jerusalem lipid research clinic prevalence study', *Brit Med J* 291(6497):699-704, 1985.

Katan M B, Mensink R P, 'Isomeric Fatty Acids and Serum Lipoproteins', *Nutr Rev* 50 (4), (1992).

Kirby R W *et al*, 'Oat-bran intake selectively lowers serum low-density lipoprotein cholesterol concentrations of hypercholesterolemic men', *Am J Clin Nutr* 34(5):824-9, 1981.

Krumdieck C, Butterworth C E, 'Ascorbate cholesterol lecithin interactions: Factors of potential importance in the pathogenesis of atherosclerosis', *Am J Clin Nutr* 27:866-76, 1974.

Landsberg L, 'Insulin and hypertension', *N Engl J Med* 317 (6), 378 (1987).

Lewis B *et al*, 'Towards an improved lipid-lowering diet: Additive effects of changes in nutrient intake', *Lancet* December 12 1981.

Little P, Girling G, Hasler A *et al*, 'The effect of a combination low sodium, low fat, high fibre diet on serum lipids in treated hypertensive patients', *Eur J Clin Nutr* 44, (1990).

Maebashi M *et al*, 'Lipid-lowering effect of carnitine in patients with Type IV hyper-lipoproteinemia', *Lancet* Oct 14 1978, p805-7.

Makheja A N, 'Onions, garlic and platelet aggregation', *Lancet* April 7, 1979.

Malinow M R *et al*, 'Alfalfa', *Am J Clin Nutr*, 1810-12, 1979.

Mattson F H *et al*, 'Optimizing the effect of plant sterols on cholesterol absorption in man', *Am J Clin Nutr* 35:697-700, 1982.

McCully K S, 'Atherosclerosis, serum cholesterol and the homocysteine theory: a study of 194 consecutive autopsies', *Am J Med Sci* 1990; 299(4):217-21.

Murphy S P, Subar A F, Block G, 'Vitamin E intakes and sources in the United States', *M J Clin Nutr* 52, 361-367 (1990).

Nestel P, 'Cholesterol and fish oil', *Am J Clin Nutr* 43:752-57, 1986.

'New ideas on CHD pathology', *Int Clin Nutr Rev* July 1992, p183.

Oh S Y, Ryue J, Hsieh C H, Bell D E, 'Eggs enriched in w-3 fatty acids and alterations in lipid concentrations in plasma and lipoproteins and in blood pressure', *Am J Clin Nutr* 54, 689-695 (1991).

Opie L H, 'Role of carnitine in fatty acid metabolism of normal and ischemic myocardium', *Am Heart J* 97: 373-8, 1979.

Oriando G, & Rusconi C, 'Oral L-carnitine in the treatment of chronic cardiac ischaemia in elderly patients', *Clin Trials J* 23:338-44, 1986.

Patki P S, Singh J, Gokhale S V, Bulakh P M, Shrotri D S, Patwardhan B, 'Efficiency of potassium and magnesium in essential hypertension: a double blind, placebo controlled cross over study', *Br Med J* 301, 521-523 (1990).

Potter J D, Topping D L, Oakenful D, 'Soya, saponins, and plasma cholesterol', *Lancet* 1:223-4, 1979.

Pritikin N, McGrady P, *Pritikin Program for Diet and Exercise*.

Ramirez J, Flowers N C, 'Leukocyte ascorbic acid and its relationship to coronary artery disease in man', *Am J Clin Nutr* 33:2070-87, 1980.

Renaud S, Nordoy A, 'Small is beautiful: alpha linolenic acid and eiscosapentaenoic acid in man', *Lancet* 1:1169, 1983.

Riales R R, Albrink M J, 'Effect of chromium chloride supplementation on glucose tolerance and serum lipids including high-density lipoprotein of adult men', *Am J Clin Nutr* 34:2670-8, 1981.

Riemersma R A, Wood D A, Macintyre C C A *et al*, 'Risk of angina pectoris and plasma concentrations of vitamins A C E and carotene', *Lancet* 337, 1-5 (1991).

Rouse I L, Belin L J, Mahoney D P *et al*, 'Vegetarian diet and blood pressure in a population', *Lancet* ii:742-3, 1983.

Sali A, *International nutrition seminar*, Sydney. 1986.

Salonen J T *et al*, 'Association between cardiovascular death and myocardial infarction and serum selenium in a matched-pair longitudinal study', *Lancet* 2: 175-9, 1982.

Saynor R, 'Effects of omega-3 fatty acids on serum lipids', *Lancet* 2:696-7, 1984.

Saynor R, 'Effects of omega-3 fatty acids on serum lipids', *Lancet* ii:696, 1984.

Schuitemaker G, 'Oxy-cholesterol in food', *Int Clin Nutr Rev*, 9, p5, 1989.

Seelig M S & Heggtveit H A, 'Magnesium interrelationship in ischemic heart disease: A review', *AM J Clin Nutr*, 27:59-79, 1974.

Seelig M S, Heggtveit H A, 'Magnesium interrelationship in ischaemic heart disease: a review', *Am J Clin Nutr* 27:59-79, 1974.

Simons L A, Hickie J B, Balasubramaniam S, 'On the dietary effects of dietary n-3 fatty acids (Maxepa) on plasma lipids and lipoproteins in patients with hyperlipidemia', *Atherosclerosis* 54:75-88, 1985.

Simopoulos A P, Salem Jr N, 'Egg yolk as a source of long- chain polyunsaturated fatty acids in infact feeding', *Am J Clin Nutr* 55, 411-444 (1992).

Simpson H *et al*, 'Low dietary intake of linoleic acids predisposes to myocardial infarction', *Brit Med J*, 285:684, 1982.

Singh R B, Sircar A R, Mehta P J, Laxmi B, Garg V, 'Nutrition intervention in acute myocardial infarction', *J Nutr Med* 1, 179-186 (1990).

Singh R B, Rastogi S S, Verma R *et al*, 'Randomised controlled trial of cardioprotective diet in patients with recent acute myocardial infarction: results of one year follow up', *Brit Med J*, 304, (1992).

Skrabal F, Aubock J, Hortnagl H, 'Low sodium/high potassium diet for prevention of hypertension: Probable mechanisms of action', *Lancet* ii:895-900, 1981.

Smith G D, Shipley M J, Marmot M G, Rose G, 'Plasma cholesterol concentration and mortality. The Whitehall study', *J A M A* 267 (1), 70-76 (1992).

Suh I, Shaten J, Cutler J A *et al*, 'Alcohol use and mortality from coronary heart disease: the role of high density lipoprotein cholesterol', *Ann Intern Med* 116, 881-887 (1992).

Taussig S & Nieper H, 'Bromelain: its use in prevention and treatment of cardiovascular disease, present status', *J Int Assoc Prev Med* 6:139-51, 1979.

Truswell A S, 'Reducing the risk of coronary heart disease', *Brit Med J* Vol 291, July 6, 1985.

Tsai A C, Mazeedi H A, Mameesh M S, 'Dietary beta-carotene reduces serum lipid concentrations in spontaneously hypertensive rats fed a vitamin A fortified & cholesterol-enriched diet', *J Nutr* 122, 1768, 1992.

Turlapaty P D M V & Altura B M, 'Magnesium deficiency produces spasms of coronary arterties: relationship to etiology of sudden death ischemic heart disease', *Science* 208:199-200, 1980.

Violi F, Practico D, Ghiselli A *et al*, 'Inhibition of cycloxygenase independent platelet aggregation by low vitamin E concentration', *Atherosclerosis* 82, 247-252 (1990).

Vorster H H, Spinnler Benade A J, Barnard H C *et al*, 'Egg intake does not change plasma lipoprotein and coagulation profiles', *Am J Clin Nutr* 55, 400-410 (1992).

Walker A R P, Walker B F, Glatthaar I I, 'Sugar - a love-hate situation', *Int Clin Nutr Rev*, Jan 1991, p10 & editorial.

Willis A L, 'Dihomo-gamma-linolenic acid as the endogenous protective agent for myocardial infarction', *Lancet* ii:697, 1984.

Wood D A, Butler S, Riemersma R A *et al*, 'Adipose tissue and platelet fatty acids and coronary heart disease in Scottish men', *Lancet* 2:117-21, 1984.

Woodcock B E, Smith E, Lambert W H *et al*, 'Beneficial effect of fish oil on blood viscosity in peripheral vascular disease', *Br Med J* 288: 592-4, 1984.

Woodcock B E *et al*, 'Beneficial effects of fish oil on blood viscosity in peripheral vascular disease' *Brit Med J* 288:592- 4, 1984.

Yacowitz H, 'A study on calcium cholesterol and tryglycerides', *Brit Med J* May 1965.

Yudkin J *et al*, 'Effects of high dietary sugar', *Br Med J* 281:1396, 1980.

Zemel P C, Zemel M B, Urberg M, Douglas F L, Geiser R, Sowers J R, *Am J Clin Nutr* 51, 665 (1990).

AIDS

Archer D L & Glinsman W H, 'Intestinal infection and malnutrition initiate acquired immune deficiency syndrome (AIDS)', *Nutr Res* 5:9-19, 1985.

Beutler E, 'Nutritional and metabolic aspects of glutathione', *Annu Rev Nutr* 1989; 9: 287-302.

Cathcart R F, 'Vitamin C in the treatment of acquired immune deficiency syndrome (AIDS)', *Med Hypoth* 14:423-3, 1984.

Chaitow L & Martin S, *A world without AIDS*, Thorsons 1988.

Curran J, 'The epidemiology and prevention of the acquired immunodeficiency syndrome', *Ann Int Med* 103: 657-62, 1985.

Dharmananda S, *At the Institute for Traditional Medicine - technical information*, 2442 S E, Sherman, Portland, OR, USA.

Dharmananda Subhuti, *Chinese Herbal Therapies for Immune Disorders*, Inst for Trad Med and Prev Health Care.

Dharmananda S, *Your Nature, Your Health*, Inst for Trad and Prev Health Care.

D'Adamo P, 'Chelidonium and sanguinaria alkaloids as anti-HIV therapy', *J Naturopathic Med*, 31-34 1992.

Editorial, 'The secret low-amino diet', *Med Tribune* 31 (3):18, 1990.

Glasgow B J, Anders K, Layfield L J *et al*, 'Clinical and pathological findings of the liver in the acquired immune deficiency syndrome (AIDS)', *AM J Clin Pathol* 83: 1985.

Grody W W, Fligiel S, Naeim F, 'Thymus involution in the acquired immunodeficiency sydrome', *Am J Clin Pathol* 84:85-95, 1985.

Grotz, Walter, *Information on hydrogen peroxide research*, from: Box 126 Delano, MN 55328, USA.

Hong Dr Yen Hsu, *How to treat yourself with Chinese herbs*, Oriental Healing Arts Institute, 88205 Sepulveda Blvd, Suite 205, Los Angeles, CA (1980).

Jain V K & Chandra R K, 'Does nutritional deficiency predispose to acquired immune deficiency syndrome?' *Nutr Res* 4:537-43, 1984.

Lancet, January 27, 1990, pp234-6.

Lauritsen John, *Poison by prescription: the AZT story*, ISBN 0-943742-06-4.

Nash M, 'Low amino diet immune boost', *Med Tribune* 1990; 31(3) 1,12.

Neiper Hans, *Townsend Letters for Doctors*, Nov 1990.

Park K G M *et al*, 'Stimulation of lymphocyte natural cytotoxicity by L-arginine', *Lancet* 1991; 337:645-6.

Peters B S *et al*, 'Ineffectiveness of AL721 in HIV disease', *Lancet* March 3, 1990; p545-6.

Philips A N *et al*, 'Serial CD4 lymphocyte counts and

development of AIDS', *Lancet* 1991; 337:1992.

Revici E, 'Research and theoretical background for treatment of AIDS', *Townsend Letter for Doctors*, No 45, 1987.

Salahuddin S Z, Markham P D, Redfield R R *et al*, 'HTLV III symptom-free seronegative persons', *Lancet* ii: 1418-20, 1984.

Seegal, Bernie Dr, *Peace, love and healing*, Rider, 1990.

Turner R J, 'AIDS - a report on the John Bastyr study', *J A C M* February 1991.

Asthma

Bray G W, 'The hypochlorhydria of asthma in childhood', *Quart J Med* 24:181-97, 1931.

Brunner E H, Delabroise A M, Haddad Z H, 'Effect of parenteral magnesium on pulmonary function, plasma cAMP, and histamine in bronchial asthma', *J Asthma* 22:3-11, 1985.

Collip P J, Goldzier III S, Weiss N *et al*, 'Pyridoxine treatment of childhood asthma', *Ann Allergy* 35: 93-7, 1975.

Foreman J C, 'Mast cells and the actions of flavonoids', *J Allergy Clin Immunol* 73: 769-74, 1984.

Freedman B J, 'A diet free from additives in the management of allergic disease', *Clin Allergy* 7:417-21, 1977.

Haury V G, 'Blood serum magnesium in bronchial asthma and its treatment by the administration of magnesium sulphate', *J Lab Clin Med* 26:340-4, 1940.

Hosker H *et al*, 'Adult caeliac disease presenting with symptoms of worsening asthma', *Lancet* November 15, 1986, pp1157-58.

Lindahl O *et al*, 'Vegan diet regimen with reduced medication in the treatment of bronchial asthma', *J Asthma* 22:45-55, 1985.

Oehling A, 'Importance of food allergy in childhood asthma', *Allergol Immunopathol Suppl* IX: 71-3, 1981.

Ogle K A, Bullock J D, 'Children with allergic rhinitis and/or bronchial asthma treated with eliminination diet', *Ann Allergy* 39:8-11, 1977.

Rolls G *et al*, 'Reduction of histamine-induced bronchoconstriciton by magnesium in asthmatic subjects', *Allergy* 42, 186-8, 1987.

Rowe A H, Young E J, 'Bronchial asthma due to food allergy alone in ninety five patients', *J A M A* 169: 1158-62, 1959.

Tan Y, Collins-Williams C, 'Aspirin-induced asthma in children', *Ann Allergy* 48:1-5, 1982.

Wester P O, 'Magnesium', *Am J Clin Nutr* 45 (5 suppl): 1305-12, 1987.

Wright Jonathan V, 'Treatment of childhood asthma with parenteral vitamin B12 gastric reacidification, and attention to food allergy, magnesium and pyridoxine: three case reports with background and an integrated hypothesis', *J Nutr Med* 1990; 1:277-82.

Contrasting Chinese & Japanese Diets

Baber F M, 'The current situation in Hong Kong', *Hong Kong Practitioner* 1981.

Field & Baber, *Growing up in Hong Kong*, 1973.

Ho J H, 'Salted fish and NPC in Southern Chinese', *Lancet* 2, 1978.

Koo Linda L C, *The nourishment of life*, Commercial Press, 1982.

Yu Mimi C *et al*, 'NPC in Malaysia and Hong Kong', *Nat Cancer InstMonogr* 69, 1985.

Yu Mimi C *et al*, 'Nasopharyngeal carcinoma in Chinese - salted fish or inhaled smoke?', *Prev Med* 10, 1981.

Eczema

Eppic J, 'Seborrhea capitis in infants: a clinical experience in allergy therapy', *Ann Allergy* 29:323-4, 1971.

Horrobin D F & Stewart C, 'Evening primrose oil & atopic eczema', *Lancet* 336, 1990.

Lee T, Hoover R, Williams J *et al*, 'Effect of dietary enrichment with eicosapentaenoic and docosahexanoic acids on invitro neutrophil and monocyte leukotriene generation and neutrophil generation', *N E J M* 312:1217-24, 1985.

Manku M, Horrobin D, Morse N *et al*, 'Reduced levels of prostaglandin precursors in the blood of atopic patients: Defective delta-6-desaturase function as a biochemical basis foratopy', *Prostaglandins Leukotrienes and Medicine* 9:615-28, 1982.

Nisenson A, 'Treatment of seborrheic dermatitis with biotin and vitamin B complex', *J Ped* 51:537-49, 1957.

Renaud S and Nordoy A, 'Small is beautiful: alpha-linolenic acid and eicosapentaenoic acid in man', *Lancet* i:1169, 1983.

Soter N & Baden H, *Pathophysiology of dermatologic disease*, McGraw-Hill, NY, 1984.

Strosser A V, Nelson L S, 'Synthetic vitamin A in the treatment of eczema in children', *Ann Allergy* 10:703-4, 1952.

Wright S, Burton J L, 'Oral evening primrose seed-oil improves atopic eczema', *Lancet*, November 20, 1982, pp1120- 22.

Candida

Technical information:

Biocare Ltd, UK.

Nutribiotic, California.

Blackmores Ltd, Australia.

Wakunaga Co Ltd, Japan.

Balsdon M, Pead L, Taylor G, Maskell R, 'Corynebacterium vaginale and vaginitis', *Clin Ob Gyn* 24:439-60, 1981.

British Herbal Pharmocopoeia.

Crook William G MD, *The yeast connection*, Random House Inc, 1983.

Miles M R, Olsen L, Rogers A *et al*, 'Recurrent vaginal candidiasis - importance of an intestinal reservoir', *J A M A* 238:1836-7, 1977.

Rochlitz Steven, *Allergies and Candida*.

Spiegal C A *et al*, 'Anaerobic bacteria in non-specific vaginitis', *N Eng J Med* 303 (ii), 1980.

Truss O, *The missing diagnosis*, PO Box 26508, Birmingham, AL, USA, 1983.

Weiss Rudolf Fritz MD, *Herbal medicine*, Beaconsfield Publ, 1988.

Fats versus oils

Ahola I, Jauhiainsen M, Aro A, 'The hyper cholesterolaemic factor in boiled coffee is retained by a paper filter', *J Intern Med* 230, 293 (1991).

Anderson J W, Gilinsky N H, Deakins D A *et al*, 'Lipid responses of hypercholestrolaemic men to oat-bran and wheat-bran intake', *Am J Clin Nutr* 54, 678-683 (1991).

Beisson G J, *Lipids in human nutrition*, Durgess, 1981.

Bland J S, *Year Book of Nutritional Medicine*, Keats, 1985.

Bland J S, *Your health under seige*, Stephen Green Press, 1981.

Blankenhorn D H *et al*, 'The influence of diet on the appearance of new lesions of human coronary arteries', *J A M A* 1990;263 (12) 1646-52.

Bonaa A K *et al*, 'Effect of eicosapentaenoic and docosahexaenoic acids on blood pressure in hypertension', *N Eng J Med* 1990; 322:795-801.

Budwig J, *op cit*.

Derr J, Kris-Etherton P M, Pearson T A, Seligson F H, 'The role of fatty acid saturation on plasma lipids, lipoproteins, apolipoproteins: the plasma total and low-density lipoprotein cholesterol response of individual fatty acids', *Metabolism* 42, 130-134 (1993).

'Different effects of dietary saturated fatty acids on cholesterol metabolism in nonhuman primates', *Nutr Rev* 49 (9), 277- 278

(1991).

Diet & Nutrition: a holistic approach, Himilayan Intnl Inst, 1978.

Editorial, 'Trans-fatty acids and serum cholesterol levels', *Nutr Rev* 49 (2), 57-60 (1991).

Erasmus Udo, *Fats & Oils*, Alive Books, 1986.

Hill E G et al, 'Intensification of essential fatty acid deficiency in the rat by dietary trans-fatty acids', *J Nutr* 109:1759-67, 1979.

Hornstra G, Kristensen S D, 'Effect of (n-3) fatty acids on plasma lipoprotein metabolism', *Eur J Clin Nutr* 45, (suppl 2) (1991).

Horrobin D F, *Efamol Research Institute - technical information*, Eden Press, 1982.

Horrobin D F, *Clinical uses of essential fatty acids*.

Kris-Etherton P M et al, 'The effect of diet on plasma lipids, lipoproteins and coronary heart disease', *J Am Diet Assoc* 1988; 88:1373-1400.

Lindahl B, Johansson I, Huhtassari F et al, 'Coffee drinking and blood cholesterol-effects of brewing-method, food- intake and life-style', *J Intern Med* 230, 299-305 (1991).

Martin W, 'Margarine (not butter) the culprit?', letter to the Editor, *Lancet* 2:407, 1983.

Mattson F H, 'A changing role for dietary monounsaturated fatty acids', *J Am Diet Assoc* 1989, 89:387-91.

McDonald B E et al, 'Comparison of the effect of canola oil and sunflower oil on plasma lipids and lipoproteins and on in vivo thromboxane A2 and prostacyclin production in healthy young men', *M J Clin Nutr* 54, 599-605 (1991).

Mead J F, Fulco A J, *The unsaturated and polyunsaturated fatty acids in health and disease*, Charles C Thomas, 1976.

Mensink R P et al, 'Effects of monounsaturated fatty acids v complex carbohydrates on serum lipoproteins and apoproteins in healthy men and women', *Metabol* 1989; 38(2):172- 8.

Middaugh J P, 'Cardiovascular deaths among Alaskan natives, 1980-86', *Am J Public Health* 1990; 80(3):282-5.

Miller C C et al, 'Dietary supplementation with oils rich in (n- 3) and (n-6) fatty acids influences in vivo levels of epidermal lipoxygenase products in guinea pigs', *J Nutr* 1990;120:36-44.

Pritikin N, *The Pritikin programme for diet and exercise*, Bantam 1979.

Simons P, *Lecithin, the cholesterol controller*, Thorsons, 1983.

Simopoulos A P, Salem Jr N, 'Egg yolk as a source of long chain polyunsaturated fatty acids in infant feeding', *Am J Clin Nutr* 55, 411 (1992).

Simopoulos A P, 'Omega 3 fatty acids in health and disease and in growth and development', *Am J Clin Nutr* 54, 438- 463 (1991).

Sinclair H M, *Essential fatty acids*, Butterworths, 1958.

Superko H R, Bortz W, Williams P T et al, 'Caffeinated and decaffeinated coffee effects on plasma lipoprotein cholesterol, apolipoproteins, and lipase activity: a controlled, radomised trial', *Am J Clin Nutr* 1989, 50:1382-8.

Szostak W B, 'Homocysteine and cardiovascular disease', *Eur J Clin Nutr* 45 (suppl 2) 110-112 (1991).

Varela G, Rulzz-Roxo B, 'Some effects of deep frying of dietary fat intake', *Nutrition Review* 50 (9) 1992.

Vorster H H, Spinnler Benade A J, Barnard H C et al, 'Egg intake does not change plasma lipoprotein and coagulation profiles', *Am J Clin Nutr* 55, 400-410 (1992).

Williams R J, *Nutrition against disease*, Bantam, 1973.

'Fish oils and diabetic microvascular disease', *Lancet* March 3, 1990.

'Palm Oil', *Int Clin Nutr Rev* April 91, p115.

Metabolic types

Healthexcel, Box 495, Winthrop, WA 98862, USA.

Bieler H, *Diet is your best medicine*, Bantam, 1978.

Bland Jeffrey, *Your personal health programme*, Thorson, 1984.

D'Adamo Peter ND, 'Gut Ecosystem Dynamics 111', *Townsend Letter for Doctors*, Aug/Sept, 1990.

Kelley W D, *One answer to Cancer*, Kelley Research Foundation, 1971.

Mourant A E, *Blood Types and Diseases*.

Williams Roger J, *Biochemical individuality*, Bantam, 1973.

Bowel toxaemia

A Textbook of Natural Medicine, John Bastyr College Pubs.

Ackerson A, Resnick C, 'Effects of L-glutamine, NAG, GLA and Gamma Oryzanoll on intestinal permeability', *Townsend Letter for Doctors*, Jan 1993.

Airola Paavo, *Health secrets from Europe*, Arco, 1972.

Airola Paavo, *How to get well*, Health Plus, 1974.

Aiuti F, Paganelli R, 'Food allergy and gastrointestinal diseases', *Ann Allergy* 51:220-1, 1983.

Ballard J, Shiner M, 'Evidence of cytotoxicity in ulcerative colitis from immunofluorescent staining of the rectal mucosa', *Lancet* i:1014-7, 1974.

Bentley S J, Pearson D J, Rix K J B, 'Food hypersensitivity in irritable bowel syndrome', *Lancet* ii:295-7, 1983.

Bircher-Benner M, *The prevention of disease by correct feeding*, 1934.

Bircher-Benner M, *Raw food in health and disease*, 1947.

Bjarnason I, Ward K, Peters T J, 'The leaky gut of alcoholism: possible route of entry for toxic compounds', *Lancet* i:28, 1984.

Buchler M, Malfertheiner B, Griener B et al, 'The influence of large bowel on pancreatic enzyme secretion and content', *Digestion* 30:88-9, 1984.

Chart H et al, 'Linoleic acid inhibition of adhesion of enteropathogenic Escherichia coli to HEp-w cells', *Lancet* 1991, 338:126-7.

Crisati D, 'Glucosamine : Basement membrane builder', *J Alt & Compl Med*, Mar 1993.

Cummings J H, 'Fermentation in the human large intestine: evidence and implications for health', *Lancet* i:1206-8, 1983.

Editorial, 'Antigen absorption by the gut', *Lancet* ii:715-7, 1978.

Friend B A, Shahani K M, 'Nutritional and therapeutic aspects of lactobacilli', *J App Nutr* 36: 125-36, 1984.

Goldin B R, Gorbach S L, 'The effect of milk and lactobacillus feeding in human intestinal bacterial enzyme activity', *Am J Clin Nutr* 39:756-61, 1984.

Goodman M J, Kent P W, Truelove S C, 'Glucosamine synthetase activity in colonic mucosa in ulcerative colitis and Crohn's disease', *G U T* 1975, vol 16.

Grant D & Joice J, *Food combining for health*, Thorsons, 1984.

IARC Intestinal Microecology Group, 'Dietary fibre, transit time, fecal bacteria, steroids and colon cancer in two Scandinavian populations', *Lancet* ii:207-10, 1977.

Jones V A, McLaughlan P, Shorthouse M et al, 'Food intolerance: A major factor in the pathogenesis of irritable bowel syndrome', *Lancet* ii:1115-7, 1982.

Lederman E K, *Good health through natural therapy*, Pan, 1978.

Monro J, Brostoff J, Carini C, Zilkha K, 'Food allergy in migraine', *Lancet* ii:1-4, 1980.

Parke A L & Hughes G R V, 'Rheumatoid arthritis and food: a case study', *Br Med J* 282:2027-9, 1981.

Saarinen D R, Backman A, Kajosaari M, Siimes M A, 'Prolonged breast-feeding as prophylaxis for atopic diseases', *Lancet* ii:163-6, 1979.

Savage D C, 'Factors involved in colonization of the gut epithelial surface', *Am J Clin Nutr* 31:S131-8, 1978.

Shahani K M, Ayebo A D, 'Role of dietary lactobacillin in gastrointestinal microecolgy', *Am J Clin Nutr* 33:2448, 1980.

Stephansson K, Dieperink M E, Richman D P *et al*, 'Sharing of antigenic determinants between the nicotinic acetylcholine receptor and proteins in Escherichia coli, Proteus vulgaris and Klebsiella pneumoniae', *N Eng J Med* 312:221- 5, 1985.

Tryphonas H & Trites R, 'Food allergy in children with hyperactivity, learning disabilities and/or minimal brain dysfunction', *Ann Allergy* 42:22-27, 1979.

Turner R N, *Naturopathic Medicine*, Thorsons, 1984.

Béchamp v Pasteur

Adam J, *The Genuine Works of Hippocrates*, Williams & Williams, 1939.

Béres J, from notes sent to me by Dr J Béres, 1146 Budapest, Chazar Andras, U G, Hungary.

Hume E D, *Bechamp or Pasteur*, Lee Foundn for Nutr Research, 1923.

Ouseley John, *The Blood & its Third Anatomical Element*, 1912.

Weikang Ltd, 100 Elderpark St, Glasgow, Scotland, for information re:- Gaston Naessens.

Otitis media

Buist Robert, 'Editorial on breast feeding and the prevention of otitus media', *Int Clin Nut Rev* 41, 1983.

Diamant M, Diamant B, 'Abuse and timing of use of antibiotics in acute otitis media', *Arch Otol* 100:226-32, 1974.

Hagerman R J, Falkenstein A R, 'An association between recurrent otitis media in infancy and later hyperactivity', *Clin Ped*, May 1987.

McMahan J T, Calenoff E, Croft D J *et al*, 'Chronic otitis media with effusion and allergy: Modified RAST analysis of 119 cases', *Otol Head Neck Surg* 89:427-31, 1981.

Mendelsohn Robert S, MD, *How to raise a healthy child in spite of your doctor*, Ballantine, 1987.

Mygind N, Meistrup-Larsen K I, Thomson J *et al*, 'Penicillin in acute otitis media: A double-blind placebo-controlled trial', *Clin Otol* 6:5-13, 1981.

Saarinen U M, 'Prolonged breast feeding as prophylaxis for recurrent otitis media', *Acts Ped Scand* 71:567-71, 1982.

Van Buchen F L, Dunk J H, Van Hof M A, 'Therapy of acute otitis media: Myringotomy, antibiotics, or neither?', *Lancet* 2:883-7, 1981.

Naturopathy
Homeopathy
Vitalists v Mechanists

A Textbook of Natural Medicine, John Bastyr College Publications.

Benjamin H, *Everybody's guide to nature cure*, Thorsons 1981.

Blackie Margary G, *The Patient Not the Cure*.

Brennen T *et al*, 'Incidence of adverse effects & negligence in hospitalised patients', *N E J M* 324, 1991.

British Homeopathic Journal.

Campanella M, *The History and Philisophy of Naturopathy*, written for Health Schools Intl, used in part by kind permission of the director, Dr Peter Derig, PO Box 876, Runaway Bay, QLD 4216, Australia.

Cheraskin E & Rengsdorf W, *Predictive Medicine*, Pacific Press, 1973.

Finkel H, *Health via Nature*, Soc for Publ Health Education, 1925.

Haehl Richard, *Samuel Hahnemann - His Life and Work*, 1922.

Kent James Tyler, *Lectures on Homeopathic Philosophy*, 1979.

Lindlahr H, *Philosophy of Natural Therapeutics*, C W Daniel, 1975.

Robert Dr H A, *The principles and art of cure by homeopathy*, 1976.

Schubert R, *Mechanism & Vitalism*, Soldern Univ of Notre Dame

Press, 1962.

Vithoulkas G, *Homeopathy, Medicine of the New Man*, Thorsons, 1985.

Vithoulkas G, *The science of homeopathy*, Grove Press, 1979.

Williams R, *A physicians handbook on orthomolecular medicine*, Keats, 1977.

Wood Dr Clive, *Say yes to life*, Dent, 1990.

Wright Elizabeth, *Brief Study Course in Homeopathy*, 1977.

Immune system

Beisel W R, 'Single nutrients and immunity', *Am J Clin Nutr* 35 (suppl) 1982.

Beisel W R, 'Single nutrients and immunity', *Am J Clin Nutr* 35:417-68 (suppl) 1982.

Besdonsky & Sorkin, 'What do the immune system and the brain know about each other?', *Immunology Today* 4/1/1983.

British Herbal Pharmapoedia, 1985.

Chang H M, But P P, *Pharmacology and Applications of Chinese Materia Medica*, Vol 2, World Scientific Publishing, 1987.

de Vries Jan, *Viruses, Allergies and the Immune System*, Mainstrom Publ, 1988.

Dharmananda Subhuti PhD, *Chinese Herbal Therapies for Immune Disorders*, Inst for Trad Medicine & Prev Health Care, CA.

Erdmann Robert & Jones Meirion, *The amino revolution*, Century, 1987.

Grieve M, *A Modern Herbal* Penguin, 1980.

Park K G M *et al*, 'Stimulation of leukocyte natural cytotoxicity by L-arginine', *Lancet* 337, 1991.

Weidermann, Smith, Bon Gray *et al*, *Exercise and the Immune System*, Today's Life Science, July 1992.

Wood Dr Clive, *Say Yes to Life*, Dent, 1990.

Free radicals

Bioglan Laboratories, Sydney, Australia - technical information.

Health Schools International, Australia -technical information.

Sali A, *Seminar*, sponsored by Bioglan, International Nutrition, 1986.

Sluggish liver

A Textbook for Natural Medicine, John Bastyr Publications.

Airola Paavo, *How to Get Well*, Health Plus Publishers.

Arria A M, Tarter R E, Warty V *et al*, 'Vitamin E deficiency and psychomotor dysfunction in adults with primary biliary cirrhosis', *Am J Clin Nutr* 52, 383-390 (1990).

British Herbal Pharmocopaeia, 1983.

Cowan R, 'Soya bean lecithin may prevent cirrhosis', *Sci News*, 1991.

Duff G L *et al*, *Am J Med* 11:92, 1951.

Gerson Max, *A Cancer Therapy*, Gerson Inst, 5th Edn, 1990.

Pixley F *et al*, 'Effect of vegetarianism on development of gall stones in women', *Brit Med J* 291:11-12, 1985.

Planta Medica 50, 1984, and 49, 1983.

Reuben D, *The save your life diet*, Ballantine, 1981.

Sachan D S, Rhew T H, Ruark R A, 'Ameliorating effects of carnitine and its precursor on alcohol induced fatty liver', *A J C N* 39:738, 1984.

Science News, Dec 1990.

Homeopathy

Boericke W, *Materia Medica with Repertory*, Boericke and Tafel, Philadelphia, 1927.

Cheraskin E, Ringsdorf W M, Clark J W, *Diet and Disease*, Keats Health Science, Connecticut, 1977.

Clark J H, *Clinical Repertory*, Homeopathic Publ Co, London, 1904.

Clark J H, *Dictionary of Materia Medica*, 3 vols, Homeopathic

Publ Co, London, 1925.

Clark J H, *The Prescriber*, Homeopathic Publ Co, London, 1952 (8th edn).

Gerson M, *A Cancer Therapy*, The Gerson Inst, CA, 1990.

Jensen B, *Tissue cleansing through bowel management*, Bernard Jensen, CA, 1980.

Kent J T, *Materia Medica*, 2nd edition, Sinha Roy, Calcutta, 1970.

Lessell C B, *Homeopathy for Physicians*, Thorsons, 1983.

Pfeiffer C, *Mental and Elemental Nutrients*, Keats Publ Co, Connecticut, 1975.

Pratt N, *Homeopathic Prescribing*, Beaconsfield Publ, 1980.

Roberts A H, *The Principles and Art of Cure by Homeopathy*, Homeopathic Publ Co, London, 1936.

Smith Trevor, *Homeopathic Medicine*, Thorsons, 1982.

Tyler, Margaret L, *Homeopathic Drug Pictures*, Health Science Press, 1952.

Wheeler C E, *The Principles and Practice of Homeopathy*, Heinemann, 1940.

Ziff S, *The toxic time bomb*, Thorsons, 1984.

Vegetarianism
Juices
Wholefoods
Naturopathic lifestyle

Airola Paavo O, *How to keep slim with juice fasting*, Health Publishers, 1971.

Ballentyne Rudolph, *Diet & nutrition: A holistic approach*, Himalayan International Institute 1978.

Beiler Henry G, *Food is your best medicine*, Random House, 1965.

Bieler Henry, *Diet is your best medicine*, Bantam, 1978.

Bircher R, *Way to positive health*, Bircher-Benner Verlag, Erlenbach, Zurich, 1967.

Bircher-Benner M, *Eating your way to health*, Penguin, 1973.

Bland Jeffrey, *Medical application of clinical nutrition*, Keats, 1984.

Brown H, *Protein nutrition*, Charles C Thomas Publ, 1974.

Buist Robert, 'Editorial - A reappraisal of water fluoridation', *Int Clin Nut Review*, Apr 1990.

Cheraskin E, Ringsdorf W M, Clark J W, *Diet & disease*, Rodale Press, 1968.

Clarke James, *The prevention of incurable disease*, 1981.

Effects of heating on foodstuffs, Applied Science Publishers, London, 1979.

Hall R H, *Food for nought: The decline in nutrition*, Random House, 1974.

Kenton Leslie & Suzannah, *Raw energy*, Century Hutchison, 1984.

Lappe Frances Moore, *Diet for a small planet*, Ballantine, 1971.

McCarrison Robert, *Nutrition & health*, McCarrison Society, London, 1982.

Null M, *The new vegetarian*, William Morrow & Co, 1978.

Pahlow Mannfried, *Living medicine*, Thorsons, 1980.

Pfeiffer E, *Formative forces in crystallization*, Rudolf Steiner Publications, 1936.

Pfeiffer Carl C, *Mental and elemental nutrients*, Keats Publishing, 1975.

Pfeiffer C & Banks J, *Total nutrition*, Simon & Schuster, 1980.

Prasad A S, *Trace elements in human health & disease*, Academic Press, 1977.

Priestley R J, *Nutrition Almanac*, McGraw Hill, 1979.

Pritikin Nathan & McGrady Patrick M Jr, *The Pritikin programme for diet and exercise*, Bantam, 1980.

Shelton Herbert M, *Fasting can save your life*, Natural Hygiene Press, 1964.

Strehlow Dr Wighard, *Spelt - the wonder food*, Purity Foods Inc, 2871 W Jolly Rd, Okemos, MI 48854, USA.

The yearbook of agriculture, US Govnmt Printing Office.

Thompkins P & Bird C, *The secret life of plants*, Allen Lane, London, 1974.

Walker N W, *Raw vegetable juices*, Harcourt Brace Jovanovich, 1978.

Wigmore Ann, *Recipes for longer life*, Rising Sun Publ, 1978.

Wigmore Ann, *The wheatgrass book*, Avery.

Yudkin John, *Pure white and deadly, the problem of sugar*, Davis Poynter, 1972.

Stress

Alberti K G, Nattrass M, *Lancet*, 2:25-9, 1977.

Bach Edward, *The twelve healers*, CW Daniel, 1933.

Blackmores *Prescribers Reference for Botanicals*, 1986.

British Herbal Pharmocopoeia.

Chopra Deepak, *Perfect health*, Harney Books, 1990.

Dubos R, *Man adapting*, Yale Univ Press, 1966.

Fink D H, *Release from nervous tension*, Unwin, 1945.

Gardner G W et al, 'Physical work capacity and metabolic stress in subjects with iron deficiency anemia', *Am J Clin Nutr*, 30(6):910-17, 1977.

Gawain Shakti, *Creative visualization*, Bantam, 1979.

Kermani Kai, *Autogenic training*, Souvenir Press.

Pfeiffer Carl C, *Mental and elemental nutrients*, Keats Publishing, 1975.

Rainey JM et al, *Psychopharmac bull.*, 20(1):45-9, 1984.

Ryman Danielle, *The aromatherapy handbook*, Century, 1984.

Scheffer Mechtfield, *Bach flower therapy*, Thorsons, 1986.

Selys H, *The stress of life*, McGraw Hill, 1956.

Shaw DL et al, 'Management of fatigue: A physiologic approach', *Am J Med Sci*, 243:758, 1962.

Shone Ronald, *Creative visualization*, Thorsons, 1984.

Siegal Bernie, *Love, medicine and miracles*.

Siegel Bernie, *Peace, love and healing*, Rider, 1990.

Simpson, L, 'Myalgic Encephelomyelitis', *J R S Medicine*, Oct 1991.

Weiss R F, *Herbal Medicine*, Beaconsfield Publishers, 1988.

Werbach M R MD, *Nutritional influences on illness*, Third Line Press, 1987.

Wheeler F J, *The Bach remedies repertory*, CW Daniel, 1952.

White Ian, *Australian Bush Flower Essences*, Bantam.

Wood Clive Dr, *Say Yes to life*, Dent, 1990.

Wright H B, *Executive ease & disease*, Gower Press, 1975.

Allergy & rotation diets

Amella M et al, 'Inhibition of mast cell histamine release by flavanoids and human basophil histamine release', *Int Arch Allergy Applied Immuno*, 77:155-7, 1985.

Arshad S H, Matthews S, Gant C, Hide D W, 'Effect of allergen avoidance on development of allergic disorders in infancy', *Lancet* 339, 1493-97, 1992.

Clemetson C A, 'Histamine and ascorbic acid in human blood', *J Nutr* 110(4):662-68, 1980.

Coca Arthur F, *Familial nonreaginic food allergy*, CC Thomas, Springfield MA, 1942.

De Vries, Jan, *Viruses allergies and the immune system*, Mainstream Publ, 1988.

Eagle Robert, *Eating & allergy*, Thorsons, 1986.

Feingold B, *Why your child is hyperactive*, Random House, 1974.

Kuvaeva I et al, 'The microecology of the gastrointestinal tract and the immunological status under food allergy', *Nahrung*, 28(6-7):689-93, 1984.

Lapp Doris J, *Allergies and the hyperactive child*, Sovereign Books.

Lewith G T & Kenyon J, *Clinical ecology*, Thorsons.
Mackarness Richard, *Chemical vitamins*, Pan Books, 1976.
Mackarness Richard, *Not all in the mind*, Pan Books, 1976.
Mandell Dr Marshall & Scanlon Lynne Waller, *5 day allergy relief system*, Pocket Books, 1984.
Pastorello E *et al*, 'Evaluation of allergic etiology in perennial rhinitis', *Ann Allergy*, 55:854-56, 1985.
Paterson, Barbara, *The allergy connection*, Thorsons.
Pearce F *et al*, 'Mucosal mast cells, III: Effect of quercetin and other flavanoids on antigen induced histamine secretion from rat intestinal mast cells', *J Allergy Clin Immunol*, 73:769-74, 1984.
Randolph T G, *Human ecology and the susceptibility to the chemical environment*, Thomas, Springfield IL, USA, 1962.
Rinkel H J, 'Food allergy', *J Kansas Med Soc*, 37:177, 1936.
Rinkel R J, 'Food Allergy, IV: The function and clinical application of the rotary diversified diet', *J Pediat*, 32:266, 1948.
Rowe A H & Young E J, 'Bronchial asthma due to food allergy alone in 95 patients', *J A M A*, 169:1158, 1959.
Simmonds, Wendy, *Four day rotation diet - on which mine is based*.
Theron G, Randolph M D & Moss Ralph W, *Allergies - Your hidden enemy*, Thorsons, 1980.

Multiple sclerosis

Technical information from Biocare Limited, UK.
Agranoff B A, Goldberg D, 'Diet and geographical distribution of multiple sclerosis', *Lancet*, 2: 1061-66, 1974.
Barnes M P, Bates D, Cartlidge N E F *et al*, 'Hyperbaric oxygen and multiple sclerosis: short term results of placebo controlled, double blind trial', *Lancet*, i:297-300, 1985.
Bates D *et al*, 'Polyunsaturated fatty acids in the treatment of acute remitting multiple sclerosis', *Brit Med J*, 2:1390-1, 1978.
Bates D, Fawcett P R W, Shaw D A, Weightman D, 'Polyunsaturated fatty acids in treatment of acute remitting multiple sclerosis', *Br Med J* ii:1390-1, 1978.
Holman R T, Johnson S B, Hatch T F, 'A case of human linolenic acid deficiency involving neurological abnormalities', *Am J Clin Nutr*, 65:617-23, 1982.
Int Journal of Alternative & Complementary Medicine, UK, Jan 92.
Mai J, Sorensen P S, Hansen J C, 'High dose antioxidant supplementation to MS patients', *Bul Trace Elem Res*, 1990; 24:109-17.
Mertin H, Meade C J, 'Relevance of fatty acids in M S', *Brit Med Bull*, 33:67-71, 1977.
Millar J H D *et al*, 'Double-blind trial of linoleate supplementation of the diet in multiple sclerosis', *Brit Med J*, 2:765-8, 1973.
Millar J H D, Zilkha K J, Langman M J S *et al*, 'Double blind trial of linolate supplementation of the diet in multiple sclerosis', *Br Med J*, i:765-8, 1973.
Nieper, Hans A, 'Impairment of Digestive Potential in M S and Osteoporosis Patients', *Townsend Letter for Doctors*, Feb/Mar 1991.
Renaud S, Norday A, 'Small is beautiful: alphalinolenic acid and eicosapentaenoic acid in man', *Lancet*, i:1169, 1983.
Swank, R L & Pullen M H, *The multiple sclerosis diet book*, Doubleday 1977.
Wright H P, Thompson R H S, Zilkha K J, 'Platelet adhesiveness in multiple sclerosis', *Lancet*, ii:1109-10, 1965.
'Treatment of M S', *Townsend letter for Doctors*, Nov 90.

Arthritis

A textbook on natural medicine, John Bastyr College Pubs.
Adams Ruth & Murray Frank, *Arthritis*, Larchmont Books, 1983.
Airola, Paavo O, *There is a cure for arthritis*, Parker Publishing, 1968.
Airola, Paavo O, *How to keep slim with juice fasting*, Health Publ, 1971.
Amella M, Bronner C, Briancon F *et al*, 'Inhibition of mast cells histamine release by flavanoids and bioflavanoids', *Planta Medica*, 51:16-20, 1985.
Barton-Wright E C, Elliott W A, 'The pantothenic acid metabolism of rheumatoid arthritis', *Lancet*, 2:862-3, 1963.
Bellew B A & Bellew J G, *The desert Yucca*, Spacity Graphics, CA.
Bingham R *et al*, 'Yucca plant saponin in the management of arthritis', *J Applied Nutr*, 27:45-50, 1975.
Bjarnason L *et al*, 'Intestinal permeability and inflammation in R.A: effects of non-steroidal anti-inflammatory drugs', *Lancet*, 2, 1984.
Bjarnason L, So A, Levi A J *et al*, 'Intestinal permeability and inflammation in rheumatoid arthritis: Effects of non-steroidal anti-inflammatory drugs', *Lancet*, ii:1171-4, 1984.
Campbell G W, *A doctor's proven new home cure for arthritis*, Thorsons, 1983.
Croft, John, *Natural relief from arthritis*, Thorsons 1979.
Darlington L G, Ramsey N W, Mansfield J R, 'Placebo-controlled, blind study of dietary manipulation therapy in rheumatoid arthritis', *Lancet*, i:236-8, 1986.
Dong C H & Banks J, *New hope for the arthritic*, Ballantine, NY.
Editorial, 'Green-lipped mussel extract in arthritis', *Lancet*, 1:85, 1981.
Hansen T M *et al*, 'Treatment of rheumatoid arthritis with prostaglandin E1 precursors cislinoleic acid and gamma-linolenic acid', *Scand J Rheum*, 12:85, 1983.
Highton T C, McArthur A W, 'Pilot study in the effect of New Zealand Green Mussel on rheumatoid arthritis', *NZ Med J*, March 12, 1975, p261.
Jarvis D C, *Arthritis and folk medicine*, Fawcett Publ, 1960.
Kjeldsen-Kragh J, Haugen M, Borchgrevink C F *et al*, 'Controlled trial of fasting and one-year vegetarian diet in rheumatoid arthritis', *Lancet*, 338, 899-902, 1991.
Kremer J, Michaelek A V, Lininger L *et al*, 'Effects of manipulation of dietary fatty acids on clinical manifestation of rheumatoid arthritis', *Lancet*, i:184-7, 1985.
Kuhnau J, 'The flavanoids: A class of semi-essential food components: Their role in human nutrition', *World Rev Nutr Diet*, 24:117-91, 1976.
Kurki P, Heliovaara M, Palosou T, Aho K, 'Food intolerance and rheumatoid arthritis', Letter, *Lancet*, 2, 1419-20, 1988.
Lee T H, Arm J P, 'Prospects for modifying the allergic response by fish oil diets', *Clin Allergy*, 16:89-100, 1986.
O'Farrelly C, Marten D, Melcher D *et al*, 'Association between villous atrophy in rheumatoid arthritis and a rheumatoid factor and gliadin-specific IgG', *Lancet*, 2, 819-822, 1988.
Panush R S, 'Delayed reactions to foods. Food allergy and rheumatic disease', *Ann Allergy*, 56:500-3, 1986.
Parke A L, Hughes G R V, 'Rheumatoid arthritis and food - a case study', *Brit Med J*, 282:2027-9, 1981.
Pfeiffer C, *Mental and elemental nutrients*, Keats Publ.
Seignalet J, *Diet, fasting and R A*, Letter in *Lancet* 339, 1982.
Stein H B *et al*, 'Ascorbic acid-induced uricosuria: A consequence of megavitamin therapy', *Ann Int Med*, 84(4):385-8, 1976.
Thompkins P & Bird C, *The secret life of plants*, Allen Lane, London 1974.
Wolfe M M, Soll A H, 'The physiology of gastric acid secretion', *N E J M*, 319 (26), 1988.
'Letter to the Editor about Boron', *Int Clin Nurt Rev*, Apr 91.

Macrobiotics
Food-combining
Acid - alkaline

Aihara Herman, *Acid & alkaline*, George Ohsawa Macrobiotic Foundation, 1971.

Bircher Ruth, *Your way to health*, Faber & Faber 1961.

Cannon G & Einzig H, *Dieting makes you fat*, Century, 1983.

Colbin Annemarie, *The book of whole meals*, Ballantine 1983.

East-West Journal - A US monthly magazine about macrobiotics.

Grant Doris & Joice Jean, *Food-combining for health*, Thorsons 1984.

Hay, William Howard, *A new health era*, Harrap.

Jensen, Bernard, *Chlorophyll magic from living plant life*, Jensen Pubs, 1973.

Kushi Michio, *The macrobiotic way*, Avery 1985.

Mervyn L, *Minerals & your health*, Allen & Unwin 1980.

Ohsawa George, *Zen macrobiotics*, Ohsawa Foundation 1965.

Paul A A & Southgate A T, *The composition of foods*, HMSO 1978.

Pfeiffer Carl J, *Mental & elemental nutrients*, Keats Publ Inc, 1975.

Shelton Herbert M PhD, *Food-combining made easy*, Dr Shelton's Health School, 1951.

Trowell Hugh, *Dietary fibre, refined carbohydrate foods and disease*, Academic Press, 1984.

Diabetes & Hypoglycaemia

A textbook for natural medicine, John Bastyr College Publications.

Akhtar M S, Athar M, Yaqub M, 'Effect of momordica charantia on blood glucose level of normal and alloxan diabetic rabibits', *Planta Medica*, 42:205-12, 1981.

Allen F M, 'Blueberry leaf extract: Physiologic and clinical properties in relation to carbohydrate metabolism', *J A M A*, 89:1577-81, 1927.

Anderson J W, Herman R H, 'Effects of carbohydrate restriction on glucose tolerance of normal men and reactive hypoglycemic patients', *Am J Clin Nutr*, 28:748, 1975.

Anderson J W, Ward K, 'High-carbohydrate, high-fiber diets for insulin-treated men with diabetes mellitus', *Am J Clin Nutr*, 32:2312-21, 1979.

Bhatt H R, Linnel J C, Matt D M, 'Can faulty vitamin B12 (cobalamin) metabolism produce diabetic retinopathy?', *Lancet*, 2:572, 1983.

Chakravarthy B K, Gupa S, Grambhir S S, Gode K D, 'Pancreatic beta-cell regeneration in rats by epicatechin', *Lancet*, 2:759-60, 1981.

Chakravarthy B K, Gupa S, Gode K D, 'Antidiabetic effect of (-)-epicatechin', *Lancet*, 2:272, 1982.

Cogan D G *et al*, 'Aldose reductase and complications of diabetes', *Ann Int Med*, 101:82-91, 1984.

Freund H *et al*, 'Chromium deficiency during total parenteral nutrition', *J A M A*, 241(5):496-8, 1979.

Hollenbeck C B, Lecklem J E, Riddle M C, Conner W E, 'The composition and nutritional adequacy of subject-selected high carbohydrate, low fat diets in insulin dependent diabetes mellitus', *Am J Clin Nutr*, 38:41-51, 1983.

Jamal G A *et al*, 'Gamma-linolenic acid in diabetic neuropathy', *Lancet* 1:1098, 1986.

Khan A *et al*, 'Insulin potentiating factor and chromium content of selected foods and spices', *Biol Trace Elem Res*, 1990; 24:183-8.

Liu V J and Abernathy R P, 'Chromium and insulin in young subjects with normal glucose tolerance', *Am J Clin Nutr*, 25(4):661-7, 1982.

Manson J E *et al*, 'Physical activity and incidence of non-insulin dependent diabetes mellitus in women', *Lancet*, 1991, 338:774-8.

Mertz W, 'Effects and metabolism of glucose tolerance factor', *Nutr Rev*, 33(5):129-35, 1975.

Offenbacher E, Stunyer F, 'Beneficial effect of chromium-rich yeast on glucose tolerance and blood lipids in elderly patients', *Diabetes*, 29:919-25, 1980.

Riales R R, Albrink M J, 'Effect of chromium chloride supplementation on glucose tolerance and serum lipids including high-density lipoprotein of adult men', *Am J Clin Nutr*, 34:2670-8, 1981.

Rivellese A *et al*, 'Effect of dietary fibre on glucose control and serum lipoproteins in diabetic patients', *Lancet*, 2:447, 1980.

Simpson H C R *et al*, 'A high-carbohydrate leguminous fibre diet improves all aspects of diabetic control', *Lancet*, 1:1-5, 1981.

Simpson H C R, Simpson R W, Lousley S *et al*, 'A high carbohydrate leguminous fiber diet improves all aspects of diabetic control', *Lancet*, 1:1-5, 1981.

Trowell H C, 'Dietary-fiber hypothesis of the etiology of diabetes mellitus', *Diabetes*, 24 (8): 762-65, 1975.

Uusitupa M, Kumpulainein J, Voutilainen E *et al*, 'Effect of inorganic chromium supplementation on glucose tolerance, insulin response, and serum lipids in noninsulin dependent diabetic', *Am J Clin Nutr*, 38:404-10, 1983.

Vinson J *et al*, 'In vitro and in vivo reduction of erythrocyte sorbitol by ascorbic acid', *Diabetes*, 1989; 38:1036-41.

Zonszein J, 'Magnesium and diabetes', *Pract diabetol*, March/Apr 1991; 10:1-4.

'High-carbohydrate, high-fiber diets for insulin-treated men with diabetes mellitus', *Am J Clin Nutr*, 32:2312-21, 1979.

Alzheimers

Adams J D, Klaidman L K, Odunze I N *et al*, 'Alzheimer's and Parkinson's disease. Brain levels of glutathione, glutathione disulphide and vitamin E', *Mol Chem Neuropathol*, 14, 213-26, 1991.

Arriagada P V *et al*, 'Neurofibrillary tangles and olfactory dysgenesis', *Lancet*, 1991, 337:559.

Birchal J D, Chappell J S, 'Aluminium, chemical physiology, and Alzheimer's disease', *Lancet*, 2, 1008-1010, 1988.

Burnet F M, 'A possible role of zinc in the pathology of dementia', *Lancet*, 1:186-8, 1981.

Burns A, Holland T, 'Vitamin E deficiency', Letter to the Editor, *Lancet*, April 5, 1986, pp805-6.

Colin-Jones D, Langman M J S, Lawson D H, Vessey M P, 'Alzheimer's disease in antacid users', *Lancet*, 1, 1453, 1989.

Cowburn J D, Blair J A, 'Aluminium chelator (transferrin) reverses biochemical deficiency in Alzheimer brain preparations', Letter, *Lancet*, 1, 99 (1989).

Deakin J F W, 'Alzheimer's disease: Recent advances and future prospects', *Brit Med J*, 287:1323-4, 1980.

Ebrahim S, 'Aluminium and Alzheimer's disease', *Lancet*, 1, 267, 1989.

Editorial, 'Aluminium and Alzheimer's disease', *Lancet*, 1, 82, 1989.

Levy R, Little A, Chuaqui P, Reith M, 'Early results from double blind, placebo controlled high dose phosphatydcholine in Alzheimer's disease', *Lancet*, 1:474-6, 1982.

Little A *et al*, 'A double-blind placebo controlled trial of high dose lecithin in Alzheimer's disease', *J Neurol Neurosurg & Psychiat*, 48:736-42, 1985.

Martyn C N, Barker D J P, Osmond C *et al*, 'Geographical relation between Alzheimer's disease and aluminium in drinking water', *Lancet*, 1, 59-62, 1989.

McLachlan D R C *et al*, 'Intramuscular desferrioxamine in patients with Alzheimer's disease', *Lancet*, 1991, 337:1304- 8.

Nordstrom J W, 'Trace mineral nutrition in the elderly', *Am J Clin Nutr*, 36:788-95, 1982.

Rhijn A G, Prior C A, Corrigan F M, 'Dietary supplementation with zinc sulphate, sodium selenite and fatty acids in early dementia of Alzheimers type', *J Nutr Med*, 1, 259-66, 1990.

Rosenberg G, Davies K L, 'The use of cholinergic precursors in neuropsychiatric diseases', *Am J Clin Nutr*, 36:709-20, 1982.

Smith J S and Kiloh L G, 'The investigation of dementia: Results in 200 consecutive admissions', *Lancet*, 1:824-7, 1981.

Weintraub S *et al*, 'Lecithin in the treatment of Alzheimer's disease', *Arch Neurol*, 40:527, 1983.

Wiener Michael, 'Aluminium and dietary factors in Alzheimer's disease', *J Aust Coll Nutr Environ Med*, Dec 16-18, 1990.

Zaman Z, Roche S, Fielden P *et al*, 'Plasma concentrations of vitamins A and E and carotenoids in Alzheimer's disease', *Age and Aging*, 21, 91-4, 1992.

U R T infections

Baird I, Hughes R, Wilson H *et al*, 'The effects of ascorbic acid and flavanoids on the occurence of symptoms normally associated with the common cold', *Am J Clin Nutr*, 32:1686-90, 1979.

Beisel W R, 'Single nutrients and immunity', *Am J Clin Nutr*, 35:417-68 (suppl) 1982.

Beisel W, Edelman R, Nauss K, Suskind R, 'Single nutrients effects of immunologic functions', *J A M A*, 245:53-8, 1981.

Bernestein J, Alpert S, Nauss K, Suskind R, 'Depression of lymphocyte transformation following oral glucose ingestion', *Am J Clin Nutr*, 30:613, 1977.

Brook I, 'Treatment of streptococcal pharyngotonsillitis', *J A M A*, 247:2496, 1982.

Buist Robert, 'Editorial on breast feeding and the prevention of otitus media', *Int Clin Nutr Rev*, 41, 1983.

Chandra R K, 'Excessive intake of zinc impairs immune response', *J A M A*, 252 (11):1443-6, 1984.

Couleham J L *et al*, 'Vitamin C and acute illness in Navajo school children', *New Engl J Med*, 295 (18): 973-77, 1976.

Diamant M, Diamant B, 'Abuse of timing of use of antibiotics in active otitis media', *Arch Otol*, 100:226-32, 1974.

Duchateau J *et al*, 'Influence of oral zince supplementation on the lymphocyte response to mitogens of normal subjects', *Am J Clin Nutr*, 34:88-93, 1981.

Eby G A, Davis D R, Halcomb W W, 'Antimicrobial agents and chemotherapy', *Lancet*, 25:20-4, January 1984.

Goodman Sandra, *Vitamin C, the master nutrient*, Keats, 1988.

Hagerman R J, Falkenstein A R, 'An association between recurrent otitis media in infancy and later hyperactivity', *Clinical Ped*, May 1987.

How to raise a healthy child in spite of your doctor, Contemporary Books, 1980.

Leevy C, Cardi L, Frank O, *et al*, 'Incidence and significance of hypovitaminemia in a randomly selected municple hospital population', *Am J Clin Nutr*, 17:259-71, 1965.

Mendelsohn Roberts MD, *Confessions of a medical heretic*, Warner Books, 1980.

Pauling Linus, *Vitamin C, the common cold and the flu*, W H Freeman & Co, 1976.

Prasad J, 'Effect of vitamin E supplementation of leukocyte function', *Am J Clin Nutr*, 33:606-8, 1980.

Ringsdorf W, Cheraskin E, Ramsay R, 'Sucrose, neutrophil phagocytosis and resistance to disease', *Dent Surv*, 52:46-8, 1976.

Saarinen U M, 'Prolonged breast feeding as prophylaxis for recurrent otitis media', *Acta Ped Scand*, 71:567-71, 1982.

Sanchez A, Reeser J, Lau H *et al*, 'Role of sugars in human neutrophilic phagocytosis', *Am J Clin Nutr*, 26:1180-4, 1973.

Schmidt M A, *Childhood ear infections*, North Atlanta Books 1990.

Swartz M N, 'Stress and the common cold', *N E J M*, 253, 1991.

Van Buchen F L, Dunk J H, Van Hof M A, 'Therapy of acute otitis media: Myringotomy, antibiotics, or neither?', *Lancet*, 2:883-7, 1981.

Waskerwitz S, Berkelhammer J, Mann G V, 'Food intake and resistance to disease', *Lancet*, 1:1238-9, 1980.

'Effect of zinc on thymus of recently malnourised children', *Lancet*, November 19, 1977, p1057-9.

INDEX